Family-centered community nursing

A SOCIOCULTURAL FRAMEWORK

Family-centered community nursing

A SOCIOCULTURAL FRAMEWORK

Edited by

ADINA M. REINHARDT, Ph.D.

Associate, Rocky Mountain Gerontology Center, University of Utah;
Health Care Coordinator, Division of Health Care Financing and Standards,
Utah State Department of Health,
Salt Lake City, Utah

MILDRED D. QUINN, R.N., M.S.

Professor Emeritus and Dean Emeritus,
College of Nursing, University of Utah,
Salt Lake City, Utah

VOLUME TWO

Illustrated

The C. V. Mosby Company

ST. LOUIS · TORONTO · LONDON   1980

VOLUME TWO

Printed in the United States of America

The C. V. Mosby Company
11830 Westline Industrial Drive, St. Louis, Missouri 63141

Library of Congress Cataloging in Publication Data

Reinhardt, Adina M   comp.
  Family-centered community nursing.

  Includes bibliographies and index.
    1. Community health nursing.   2.   Family—Health and
hygiene.   3.   Community health nursing—United States.
4.   Family—Health and hygiene—United States.   I.   Quinn,
Mildred D.   joint comp.   II.   Title.   [DNLM:
1.   Family.   2.   Public health nursing.   WY108 R369f 1973]
RT98.R44   362.1′0425   73-8681
ISBN 0-8016-4121-7

TS/M/M   9   8   7   6   5   4   3   2   1   01/A/230

Contributors

LEN HUGHES ANDRUS, M.D.
Professor and Co-Director, Family Nurse
Practitioner and Physician Assistant Program,
Department of Family Practice,
University of California at Davis,
Sacramento, California

BOND L. BIBLE, Ph.D.
Rural Health Consultant; formerly director of
AMA Department of Rural Health,
State College, Pennsylvania

KEVIN P. BUNNELL, Ed.D.
Director, Continuing Medical Education,
Colorado Medical Society,
Denver, Colorado

THERESA T. CHEN-LOUIE, D.N.Sc.
Associate Professor,
Department of Nursing,
San Francisco State University,
San Francisco, California

MICHAEL C. CHULADA, M.Ed.
Executive Director
Planned Parenthood Association of Utah,
Salt Lake City, Utah

SHARON L. CROSS, R.N., M.S.
Supervisor, Minneapolis Health Department
Combined Nursing Services; Lecturer,
Graduate Program in Public Health Nursing,
School of Public Health, University of Minnesota,
Minneapolis, Minnesota

ANNE CURRAN, M.S.W., M.C.J.
Research Assistant, The Children's Center,
Salt Lake City, Utah

SHARON V. DAVIDSON, R.N., M.Ed.
President, Continuing Professional Education
and Nursing Review Programs, Inc.,
Colorado Springs, Colorado

**JO ELEANOR ELLIOTT, R.N., A.M., F.A.A.N.,
Sc.D. (Hon), Ll.D. (Hon)**
Executive Director of
Nursing Programs, Western Interstate
Commission for Higher Education,
Boulder, Colorado

RAYMOND FELDMAN, M.D.
Formerly Director, Division of Mental Health
and Related Areas, Western Interstate
Commission for Higher Education,
Boulder, Colorado

DOROTHY J. HICKS, M.D.
Associate Professor, Department of Obstetrics
and Gynecology, School of Medicine,
University of Miami;
Director, Rape Treatment Center,
Jackson Memorial Hospital,
Miami, Florida

**MARGARET L. HORNYACK, R.N., M.S.,
C.O.H.N.**
Doctoral candidate in Public Health,
University of Texas Health Sciences Center,
School of Public Health,
Houston, Texas

ANNE E. JORDHEIM, R.N., Ed.D.
Chairperson, Community Health,
St. Joseph's College,
Brooklyn, New York

ROBERT H. KROEPSCH, Ed.D.
Formerly Executive Director, Western
Interstate Commission for Higher Education,
Boulder, Colorado

**MARGARET A. KESSENICH MEAGHER, R.N.,
M.S.,C.**
Clinical Specialist, Psychiatric Nursing,
Denver, Colorado

FERD H. MITCHELL, Jr., Ph.D.
Academic Administrator, Department of
Family Practice, School of Medicine,
University of California at Davis,
Sacramento Medical Center,
Sacramento, California

DENISE M. MORI, B.S.
Social Worker and Crisis Counselor,
Rape Treatment Center,
Jackson Memorial Hospital,
Miami, Florida

PAULA PALMER, M.A.
Formerly Staff Assistant, Western Interstate
Commission for Higher Education,
Boulder, Colorado

†CHARLOTTE R. PLATT, R.N.
Director of Nursing (retired),
Emergency Department,
Jackson Memorial Hospital,
Miami, Florida

MIRIAM S. ROSENBERG, R.N., M.A.
Instructor, Department of Nursing,
Herbert H. Lehman College
of The City University of New York,
Bronx, New York

ELLEN M. SCHEEL, R.N., B.S., P.H.N.
Community Health Nurse (retired),
Wausau Visiting Nurse Association,
Wausau, Wisconsin

DIANE SYNHORST, R.N., M.A.
Pediatric Nurse Practitioner,
formerly with Family Health Program,
Salt Lake City, Utah

JAN TENNEY, R.N., M.S.
Pediatric Nurse Practitioner, Child Nurse
Consultant, Utah Department of Health,
Salt Lake City, Utah

JOY K. UFEMA, R.N., A.A.
Nurse Thanatologist
Independent Consultant in Death and Dying;
Instructor, Harrisburg Community College;
Executive Director, Hospice,
Lancaster County, Pennsylvania

DONALD M. WATKIN, M.D., M.P.H., F.A.C.P.
Associate Research Professor,
Department of Medicine,
The George Washington University
School of Medicine,
Washington, D.C.

SUSAN J. WOLD, R.N., M.P.H.
University of Minnesota School of Nursing,
Minneapolis, Minnesota

LORA F. WORTMAN, M.S.W.
Director, Victim-Witness Counseling Unit,
Salt Lake County Attorney's Office,
Salt Lake City, Utah

---

†Deceased.

Today . . . is yesterday's tomorrow
It is now, it is here
The world . . . once mysterious and unknown
Is within all man's sphere . . .

Mildred D. Quinn

Foreword

A significant change in the tenor of the times is that people have come to regard health, education, and a degree of comfort in living, not as privileges but as rights to be expected and experienced. This kind of expectation requires corresponding change in the nature, scope, and outcomes of community health nursing, which is the concern of this book.

It is indeed fortunate that observers, students, and educators in the field of family-centered community nursing now have at their command a reference that gives demonstration of the changing nature of family nursing in the community setting and also emphasizes that the satisfaction of health care needs requires that community nursing enrich its tradition by adherence to certain new tenets.

These are tenets of a democratic, activist nature. They call for nurses to be able to size up and work against barriers to the health protection of individuals, families, and entire communities. They require recognition that true patient advocacy demands appreciation of patients' cultural roots and the nature of their socioeconomic experience and that it serves the patient advocate well to learn how the patient perceives himself.

The tone of this work on community nursing assumes that if nurses are to be teachers and patient advocates, they must set themselves to understand the totality of factors affecting health status; only through such understanding can nursing as a profession develop the suitable perspective for helping people prevent, correct, and/or live with debility; become more adept at self-management; deal with their personal stresses; comprehend and take care of their daily requirements for nourishing food, exercise, and medication; and—in fact—help design and proceed to follow a feasible and personally suitable health care regimen. This is a work which further emphasizes the nurse's responsibility for independence in crisis therapy, for facilitating timely patient entry into the health care system, and for coordinating all manner of health and health-related services that are basic to the realization of individual health potential.

Dealing carefully with unresolved issues in nursing, with progress in interdisciplinary collaboration, and with the components of family-centered nursing in an era of sociomedical change, the contributors to and editors of *Family-Centered Community Nursing* have produced a work that provides appropriate consideration of the current health care scene and will support the development of a more comprehensive, less fragmented system of health care on behalf of families in communities the country over. The tone, message, and content of this work, as well as its appearance at the dawning of our nation's third century when all of nursing is taking itself to account, combine to make it one of the more significant contributions to the nursing literature.

Jessie M. Scott

Assistant Surgeon General (ret.),
United States Public Health Service;
Director, Division of Nursing

Preface

There is little doubt that the community health nurse of the present and future will function as a family nurse practitioner providing primary health care services that must be continuous, comprehensive, coordinated, and dedicated to providing health care and promoting wellness for families, groups, and individuals in whatever setting they may be found. Today, there is a large and growing demand for community health services provided by such family nurse practitioners. Continuing fragmentation of the health care delivery system and proliferation of medical and allied health specialties have removed health care providers farther and farther from the needs of patients and families. It seems increasingly evident that the community health nurse is the essential element of the health care system at the family and community level.

From its beginnings, community health nursing has been concerned with the delivery of primary health care services to individuals, families, and groups. Today, community health nurses are assuming tasks formerly performed by the general practitioner, such as physical assessment of infants, children, and adults, health counseling, and education. These health care activities are performed by the community nurse in well-baby clinics, family practice settings, public health screening clinics, nursing homes, industrial environments, urban and rural community health care centers, schools, and the homes of chronically ill elderly and terminally ill patients.

The community health nurse must be able to make informed referrals to community resources and must have a general working knowledge of Medicare, Medicaid, and private programs that provide needed medical assistance to those persons eligible for the benefits of these programs.

In the past several years, significant social and economic changes have emerged that affect community health nursing. Among these changes, the following are most significant. First, the cost of health care to the consumer is escalating more rapidly than the consumer price index and impinging on the financial resources of individuals, families, and third-party payers. Second, the average health care consumer is becoming more cognizant of risk factors affecting health through a variety of informational media including campaigns undertaken by the federal government to educate the public about risks associated with smoking, obesity, hypertension, carcinogens, alcohol, and chemical substance (drug) abuse. Third, during the past several years, self-initiated health care consumer groups have begun to flourish. These groups emphasize the sharing of treatment strategies for specific diseases as well as the self-education and assumption of personal responsibility for "living with disabilities" and for health maintenance.

A fourth consideration is the dramatic

increase in the relative proportion of elderly persons and minorities in our population, which can be termed a demographic revolution. Health care strategies for working with these groups are now apparent in the community health nursing literature. The fifth recent trend is the increasingly effective political activism relating to health care and other social issues on the part of ethnic groups, homosexuals, feminist groups, the economically deprived, antiabortion and proabortion organizations, the elderly, and numerous other groups.

We believe that health care costs will continue to escalate, making it imperative that the community health nurse become a competent health care consumer advocate, viewing those consumers as interested in and capable of preserving their own good health and extending the healthy middle years of life. These consumers need support and guidance in risk avoidance and disability management and in adopting life-styles that promote and maintain health.

A community health nurse can and should function as a catalyst on the community level for increasing community consciousness of the need for family planning counseling, adoption of effective local and statewide health plans, meeting the physiological and psychosocial needs of victims of sexual assault, and developing innovative methods of providing support and home health care services to the chronically ill ambulatory elderly in order that they may continue to live independently in their own homes and avoid nursing home placement.

Community health nursing is expanding to include health and emotional counseling to the terminally ill to allow them to experience their remaining time in positive living and to become able to accept death with dignity in familiar environments.

The practice of community health nursing needs nurses who are assertive change agents with clients, families, and groups in the community—nurses who stimulate new behavior patterns of self-care, individual participation, and responsibility for health maintenance and promotion and who are able to evaluate the effectiveness of their practice. Community health nurses need to function even more effectively as teachers, consumer advocates, initiators, and motivators of client self-care behavior patterns. It is important to understand the distinction between patient education and self-care education. Patient education implies that teaching and learning are carried out between a health care giver and a dependent sick person. In contrast, self-care education assumes wellness (rather than illness) and responsible participation on the part of the consumer and is oriented to health maintenance.

The purpose of this book is to bring together material that concerns the changes taking place in community health nursing, for example, new roles for practice; new life-styles of clients and families; emerging problems in families such as increasing divorce rates, increasing child abuse, problems of adolescents, and problems of victims of sexual assault; needs of the chronically ill elderly for home health care; and supportive care for the dying.

All of the chapters are original and have been contributed by community health nurses and other health care professionals knowledgeable in the areas of practice addressed. We hope the book will be of value to undergraduate and graduate nursing students and practitioners in nursing and allied health disciplines.

Family-Centered Community Nursing is divided into four parts: Family-Centered Community Nursing in the 1980s, Family Life-styles Today, Health Services for Today's Population, and Perspectives on the Future of Community Health. These titles reflect the broad range of issues that should be the concern of today's community health nurse. Each part seeks to provide the reader with new knowledge and techniques that are applicable to today's practice. A look to the immediate future and the issues addressed by the contributors should stimulate the reader to move beyond current practice.

We believe that the goal of community health nursing should be an improved quality of health and an extended meaningful life expectancy for all social, economic, and cultural groups. Community health nurses who assertively challenge barriers to improve

health care for individuals, families, and communities and who promote change actively are essential to today's turbulent and evolving social system.

Contributors to this book have devoted many hours to seeking out the new, questioning the old, and presenting an accumulation of essential knowledge in meaningful language for all health care professionals. For sharing this knowledge with us, we are most grateful.

Adina M. Reinhardt
Mildred D. Quinn

Introduction

We strongly believe that the health care professional of today and the future must become increasingly competent and confident in the knowledge and skill base needed to understand all aspects of the provision of quality and personalized health care to members of all social and cultural groups.

We believe that the essential characteristics of quality care in any setting, which all happen to begin with the letter "C," are Competence, Caring, Confidence, Comprehensiveness, and Continuity. These characteristics we have used to develop a conceptual framework for this volume, along with a distinct emphasis on all psychosociocultural factors affecting the client's acceptance of nursing care delivery.

The first two characteristics—competence and caring—are essential and intertwined, "two sides of one coin," so to speak. Competence can be defined as the nurse's mastery of the basic skills required to carry out a comprehensive physical assessment of the patient. Among other things, this would include knowledge of heart and bowel sounds, taking of blood pressures, monitoring and counseling the patient regarding drug dosages and drug reactions, and teaching family members the techniques for caring for a bedfast patient. Competence, then, is reflected in the expertise the community health nurse has acquired in providing the physical care that the patient requires.

The notion of caring encompasses the nurse's sense of dedication and respect for human values; by this we mean that the nurse must approach each patient with respect for his basic humanness, regardless of social class or ethnic group membership. If the client or family senses any feeling of superiority or "putdown" suppressed by the nurse, this will probably destroy any helping relationship. Caring implies that the nurse have great sensitivity and empathy for the physical and emotional needs and suffering of clients.

The third characteristic—confidence—will stem from the nurse's strong belief in herself.* In addition, confidence grows in relation to mastery of both the technological skills just mentioned as well as knowledge, application, and a deep appreciation of the significant effect that psychosociocultural factors have on the client and family's acceptance and utilization of the nursing care and

---

*EDITORS' NOTE: Throughout this book, the use of the term *she* by the editors and contributors indicates no bias on our part, but rather is used for simplicity, to avoid awkwardness, and in recognition of the fact that the majority of nurses are women. The editors and contributors are aware of and respect the growing number of men in nursing.

counseling provided. This volume will strongly emphasize and provide numerous illustrations of the importance of these psychosociocultural aspects of nursing care delivery in the community. Likewise, confidence is experience-based; it increases through numerous successful encounters with clients in the community.

The last two "Cs" are continuity and comprehensiveness. We strongly believe that these characteristics are essential ingredients in quality nursing care delivery today. For example, as the proportion of elderly in the population increases, as more and more people with serious chronic disabilities are kept alive, as the poor and cultural ethnic minorities are given full access to "mainstream" health care, and the rich gain greater access to more health-threatening drugs and diversions, so the proportion of chronic to acute illness rises, the incidence of psychosomatic illness rises, and combined medical and socioeconomic problems increase. In all these situations, health care that is continuous and comprehensive is required. For a large percentage of the American public, care that is continuous and comprehensive is more a high-sounding phrase than a practiced reality. For example, a survey of newborn infants in two New York City health districts, one a slum and the other a middle-income area, disclosed there was no continuity of care for at least 40% of the babies of the white middle class, 75% of the babies of the minority middle class, and 90% of the babies of the minority lower class.[1] It appears that Milio[2] would agree that continuity and comprehensiveness are essential to quality care. Milio has recently criticized the "typical pattern of ambulatory care (that takes) a *segmented* approach rather than an *integrated* approach."[2] He states that "The more that service programs require individuals to arrange separate visits, with the personal logistical costs they entail, the less likely any service program has of a

sustained relationship with individuals, much less a familiarity with the interrelationships of their immediate world to the particular health problem which the facility focuses on."[2]

To deliver continuous and comprehensive care, the community nurse practitioner must become a skilled and aggressive patient advocate displaying a broad, comprehensive knowledge of the social, cultural, and health and welfare agencies providing services within a community. The community nurse will need skills in collaborating with an increasingly larger variety of professionals for the client's care, to develop relative independence of judgment in managing and synchronizing the various aspects of comprehensive care. According to Mauksch, the community nurse practitioner "is a new breed of nurse, is more assertive in her demands for a voice in decisions that affect her practice."[3] This nurse will be the primary decision-maker and manager, as well as the coordinator of client care, delivering care interdependently with other health professionals.

A host of new community practice settings await this new breed of community nurse practitioner. New roles for practice in any number of challenging new health care delivery settings are evolving daily, for example, primary care facilities, neighborhood health centers, community mental health centers, extended care facilities, independent group nurse practice clinics, and health clinics in apartment facilities for the elderly. In all these settings, the nurse will, in addition to health care delivery, have a growing responsibility for consumer health education and health counseling. The community nurse practitioner of the present and future needs to be independent, assertive, innovative, and creative, in addition to being a skilled provider of nursing care that is characterized by the five "Cs": Competence, Caring, Confidence, Comprehensiveness, and Continuity.

REFERENCES

1. Mindlen, R. L., and Densen, P. M.: Medical care of urban infants: continuity of care, America Journal of Public Health **59:**1294-1301, 1969.
2. Milio, N.: The care of health in communities: access for outcasts, New York, 1975, Macmillan Publishing Co., Inc.
3. Mauksch, I. G.: Nursing is coming of age . . . through the practitioner movement, pro, American Journal of Nursing **75:**1834-1843, 1975.

Contents

PART ONE

FAMILY-CENTERED COMMUNITY NURSING IN THE 1980s

1   Health manpower: education and training for the 1980s and beyond, 3

Jo Eleanor Elliott, Robert H. Kroepsch, Kevin P. Bunnell, Raymond Feldman, and Paula Palmer

2   The emerging role of the pediatric nurse practitioner, 17

Jan Tenney and Diane Synhorst

3   Maintenance, prevention, and promotion: changing public and private sector views of individuals' responsibility for personal health, 29

Donald M. Watkin

PART TWO

FAMILY LIFE-STYLES TODAY

4   Bicultural experiences, social interactions, and health care implications, 39

Theresa T. Chen-Louie

5   Alternate life-styles and the family, 60

Anne E. Jordheim

6   Separation, divorce, and subsequent coping problems of single-parent families, 70

Margaret A. Kessenich Meagher

7 Child abuse patterns in the family unit, 89
Sharon L. Cross

8 Fertility and family planning in the United States: progress,
programs, and challenges, 96
Michael C. Chulada

PART THREE

HEALTH SERVICES FOR TODAY'S POPULATION

9 Guidelines for creation and operation of community health care
systems in rural areas, 113
Bond L. Bible

10 The nurse and the adolescent in today's changing social
structure, 124
Miriam S. Rosenberg

11 Medical care for the rape victim, 135
Charlotte R. Platt, Dorothy J. Hicks, and Denise M. Mori

12 Diagnostic framework for victims of sexual assault, 145
Lora F. Wortman and Anne Curran

13 Home health care services for the family with an elderly parent, 156
Ellen M. Scheel

14 Occupational health nursing, 166
Margaret L. Hornyack

15 School nursing: problems and prospects, 178
Susan J. Wold

16 The dying patient, 194
Joy K. Ufema

PART FOUR

PERSPECTIVES ON THE FUTURE OF COMMUNITY HEALTH

17 Change processes in primary care, 211
Len Hughes Andrus and Ferd H. Mitchell, Jr.

18 Evaluating home health care, 221
Sharon V. Davidson

PART ONE

Family-centered community nursing in the 1980s

☐ Health care professionals today are looking at the present practice patterns and delivery of health care services on the community level and are projecting what these might well be in the immediate future. Many new nursing roles are emerging in positive response to the rapidly changing needs for health manpower development brought about by changing life-styles and changing social and cultural systems. These innovative community nursing roles and practice patterns reflect the growing needs of consumers for guidance and counseling in self-care and health maintenance and promotion.

In Chapter 1, Elliott et al. explore the training and educational programs that should be developed to meet changing health care needs. The authors describe and discuss new health systems responsive to these needs, the staffing of these innovative health care systems, and the necessary changes in educational patterns.

Tenney and Synhorst, two creative pediatric nurse practitioners, have contributed the second chapter, which focuses on the emerging role of the pediatric nurse practitioner. This material describes and discusses the development of this role and its scope of practice. The authors pose questions and discuss issues and problems inherent in the development of their unique practice patterns.

Chapter 3 perceptively emphasizes the cost-effectiveness of self-responsibility for personal health and defines health maintenance, prevention, and promotion as concepts. Watkins concludes that community health nurses play a vital role in educating consumers in self-care and health maintenance because of their closeness in working with and educating their clients to become actively involved in responsibility for their own health care. Readers can gain new insights and perspectives from an in-depth study of these chapters.

1

Health manpower

education and training for the 1980s and beyond

Jo Eleanor Elliott, Robert H. Kroepsch, Kevin P. Bunnell,
Raymond Feldman, and Paula Palmer

This chapter explores adapting education and training programs to meet new and rapidly changing needs for health manpower, with a view toward ultimately increasing accessibility to quality care for all Americans. It does not purport to speak to every issue of importance but to raise questions, offer one view of the future, and stimulate thought and discussion. The areas addressed are (1) the health system in the 1980s and beyond, (2) staffing the new health system, and (3) changing education for the new health system.

THE HEALTH SYSTEM IN THE 1980S AND BEYOND

Health education and training programs must continuously be reviewed and adapted to meet the new and rapidly changing needs for health manpower in this country. Changes in education must be directed toward a definite goal; that is, education must produce the personnel required to staff the health system in the 1980s and beyond. Therefore to speak of educational needs, we

Based on a paper prepared for the 1971 National Health Forum, San Francisco, California, March 14-16, 1971.

must first envision the health system of the future.

Following is an outline that speaks positively about the changes foreseen. The word "will," rather than "should" or "may," is used because of our confidence that the predictions will be realized eventually. Some of them—notably health maintenance and disease prevention—are already the subject of intensified concern. Some may not achieve immediate recognition, but significant trends are emerging that will launch a rapid process of change.

In the 1980s the health system in the United States will have the following characteristics:

Comprehensive health care will be accessible to an increasing majority of people.

1. Comprehensive health care means a full range of care and services including health maintenance, disease diagnosis, acute and intensive care, and restorative and extended care.

2. All aspects of human illness will be fully covered by the system including mental illness, alcoholism, and drug addiction.

3. All citizens will have equal access to all

3

elements of the health system. This means that groups of people that now have little access to the system will claim a far larger portion of health care resources than they do today.

4. Public information and health education programs will reach all of the people, which will increase their awareness of available services as well as willingness to participate in all phases of the health system.

5. Increasingly people will receive health care, especially at the maintenance and prevention levels, where they live, work, and go to school.

6. Consumers, because of their increased knowledge and concern, will require greater and more direct accountability from the health care providers.

Greatly increased attention will be given to health maintenance and disease prevention. This new emphasis will occur for several reasons:

1. Health maintenance has been grossly neglected by the present system of health care; an evolving system of health maintenance will fill this gap.

2. New scientific developments in preventive medicine will contribute to the trend of health maintenance.

3. The general public as well as persons responsible for the health system will recognize that prevention of illness is a less expensive undertaking than treatment of acute and chronic disease. Data will support this conclusion and cost containment pressure will expedite such recognition.

4. Environmental factors both in the living setting and in the work setting will be addressed, primarily as a result of public concern and ensuing pressures.

5. The holistic health movement's point of departure is that of promoting general well-being, using all modalities (for example, diet and exercise) to achieve and maintain a maximum state of health.

The health system will be built on national systems of health insurance. Insurance protection and health services will be provided for the poor and the aged and will be universally available to all others. Special coverage for long-term, disabling illness will be provided for every citizen.

The entire system will have a greater capacity for change than the present system. Responsiveness to the need for change will result from the following factors:

1. The ability to test quickly the implications of prospective management decisions through the use of econometric and mathematical models; computer predictions will reveal alternatives in minutes rather than in years.

2. The ability to determine accurately the unit costs of specific procedures; new management tools will enable identification of health care activities that are either less efficient or more costly than others. The demand for high-cost effectiveness will generate rapid, constructive change in areas of inefficiency.

3. The continued rapid development of scientific knowledge; frequent adjustments in the system will be required to take full advantage of these new developments.

4. The establishment of an efficient, well-utilized communications network; this network will employ the most modern technological devices for the rapid exchange of information among health personnel at all levels, thus greatly expanding each health worker's scope of vision.

5. The establishment of incentives to promote and encourage demonstration and evaluation of new ways and means—modified or radical—of providing health care.

6. The demands of consumers and taxpayers for both excellent and efficient health care services.

The roles and tasks of health professionals will be far less rigidly defined than they are today.

1. The use of health care teams will begin to obscure the sharp lines of demarcation between the tasks of the various professions. In different situations different members of the health care teams will assume responsibility for leadership and decision making.

2. New health occupations will emerge in response to new needs while others will change drastically to meet new demands, and outmoded occupations will disappear.

3. Licensure and certification requirements will be adjusted to support this new flexibility; qualifications for practice will be developed at a national level.

Continuing education for all members of the health system will be necessary to keep pace with rapid changes. Regular enrollment in programs of continuing education will be required of all health care personnel.

Management of the health system will respond to the increased consumer demand for optimum use of financial and human resources through scientific planning and management.

Consumers of health care will play an increasingly significant role in the planning, policy-making, and evaluation of the health system. Their voices will be heard through national and state consumer organizations, consumer advisory committees, councils, and similar organizations.

STAFFING THE NEW HEALTH SYSTEM
Health teams

The vision of a new health system assumes major changes in the categories of personnel responsible for delivering health care and services. Personnel highly trained in specialized fields will combine their talents in team structures that are organized to provide efficient and thorough health care. Team members will work together to identify specific tasks and goals, assign duties to the most qualified team members, coordinate the implementation of chosen activities, and evaluate the efforts of the team according to its established goals. Team structure will be flexible, evolving as needs change and as optimum relationships are recognized. The team approach will provide for efficient and coordinated use of health manpower, thereby improving health care for all citizens.

Membership in health care teams will rotate and/or overlap. Certain highly specialized health professionals will serve on several teams of one type or on several different kinds of teams. Team members will be encouraged to participate on each different type of team to gain an understandng of the entire scope of health care and services.

An increasing number of interested and able volunteer workers will assist in the delivery of health care, serving as essential members of every type of health care team. As their competencies improve they will assume some duties now performed by health professionals.

Management personnel of the health care system will work to ensure continuous communication among the different health care teams and coordination of their efforts. Health records will be passed rapidly from one team to another, as people progress through the ranges of care, individuals may assume responsibility for their own health records. Each team member will be knowledgeable about the entire health system and able to refer individuals to appropriate facilities and personnel outside his own area of competence and responsibility. Communication will also be facilitated among others involved in the health system—administrators, educators, researchers, and evaluators. The result of these efforts will be a unified, coordinated system of health care, designed to meet the health needs of every citizen at reasonable cost.

Several types of teams responsible for the direct delivery of health care will emerge: (1) *environmental teams* will identify unhealthy elements in the physical and social environment and work to correct them while *health maintenance/disease prevention teams* operate in a more limited community, supporting the work of the environmental teams and providing comprehensive screening for disease; (2) *acute and intensive care teams* will function within the walls of medical facilities, providing optimum care for seriously ill patients; and (3) *restorative and extended care teams* will render therapeutic physical and psychological services to patients recovering from various degrees of illness.

Environmental and health maintenance disease prevention teams

These teams will be responsible for health maintenance and disease prevention. First, environmental teams will study the physical and social environment of a large population, perhaps an area as large as a city or even a group of cities that constitute an environmental shed. To coordinate all relevant community resources, these teams will necessarily include ecologists, sanitarians, architects, social scientists, city planners, citizen representatives, and other as yet undefined specialists as well as health professionals. Their observations and recommendations will be carried to the public, governmental officials, and health agencies for action. The resulting laws and regulations, enforced, will help to prevent illness by providing a clean and stable living environment. Much attention will be given to the emerging role of environmental teams in an effort to define and direct their tasks.

Next, health maintenance/disease prevention teams will focus attention on one specific area within an environmental shed. Health maintenance team members will be associated with a specific local organization or facility serving a defined population. They will carry their services into the community, visiting families, schools industries, and community organizations. These teams will also combine the efforts of mental health specialists, social workers, veterinarians, midwives, ecologists, nutritionists, community liaison volunteers, and communications experts, in addition to those of physicians, nurses, and allied health workers. In many communities they will operate a special health maintenance facility for multiphasic screening and the diagnosis and treatment of symptomless diseases. They will facilitate entrance into the acute and intensive care systems for residents who are seriously ill.

Because the health maintenance system is dynamic rather than established, the roles and functions associated with environmental and health maintenance teams have not yet been clearly defined. Hence the workers who do those tasks will be able to function in a flexible, experimental fashion in identifying appropriate roles for team members. There will be considerable shifting of tasks among team members in the absence of fixed and rigid traditions. Team members will educate each other to perceive needs and identify problems outside the realm of their professional training. Complex procedures or techniques will be developed and tested by experts and then will be quickly taken over by other less specialized members of the team.

As a result of increased recruiting of ethnic minorities into the health professions, minority people will frequently serve their own communities as members of these teams, or they will serve as resources to the teams to ensure culturally sensitive care delivery. All care providers will have greater cultural awareness.

Health maintenance personnel will take on new responsibilites in industrial and commercial settings, elementary and secondary schools, colleges and universities, and neighborhood day care centers. These persons may or may not be members of health maintenance teams, but the teams will have regular contact with these workers, upgrading and coordinating their efforts and providing information to improve the services rendered.

Acute and intensive care teams

Compared to the neglected field of health maintenance, the acute care field is already well established in this country. However, several major changes will occur in the delivery of acute care:

1. The team approach to acute care will provide for more productive distribution of responsibilities and coordination of procedures.

2. The tasks of team members will shift as new technology conquers certain diseases and as new technological devices replace old procedures and techniques.

3. As the pressure increases to render care to the total population, there will be a tendency for highly trained professionals to assign relatively complex tasks to persons who are less highly trained; dental hygienists, for example, will perform some tasks now performed only by dentists.

4. Acute and intensive care will become increasingly centralized. The complexity and cost of new equipment for providing acute and intensive care will prohibit the distribution of such equipment to all hospitals. In cities, acute and intensive care facilities will be concentrated in large medical centers. Residents in large sparsely settled geographical areas, will be served by special services facilities. Rural residents with national or private health insurance coverage will demand excellent acute care, and improved transportation systems, including medical center heliports, will help develop a willingness to travel for such services.

Restorative and extended care teams

This category of health care will be second only to health maintenance in its emergent and developmental character. Increased at-

tention to restorative care will fill a second major gap in the present health system.

Persons working in this field will require an understanding of psychology and other behavioral sciences as well as specific skills of the profession. Personal skills in communication and human relations will be essential for those who render extended care to slowly recuperating patients since their problems are emotional as well as physical.

The focus of restorative and extended care team members will frequently be to strengthen the remaining and often latent abilities of their patients, to help rebuild strong personal identities and reestablish a sense of personal worth. The team members will bring a fresh approach and supply other kinds of "ego ideal" or conscience. They will have enthusiasm and patience; they will become involved with their patients, and their concern will often be contagious. Volunteers and family members with a high degree of personal commitment and some specialized training will be particularly helpful in restorative and extended care.

Restorative and extended care teams will function in acute care facilities, in new facilities especially designed for long-term treatment and rehabilitation, and in the home. Team members will meet the client when he no longer requires the services of intensive or acute care teams. Restorative personnel will help him to adjust to the new surroundings of an extended care facility, if necessary, treating him there as an in-patient, or offering care to him when he can live at home. Emphasis will be placed on returning the client as rapidly as possible to his home setting and/or independent living status.

Managers of the health system

New and traditional categories of management personnel will coordinate their efforts to serve and administer the health system. All persons who participate in the management of health services will have a working knowledge of the entire health system as well as a basic understanding of concepts of health and illness.

1. Health ombudsmen—consumer advocates. The function of these people will be to assist consumers to make full use of the health maintenance system, to facilitate their entrance into the acute or restorative systems, and to assist them in dealing with those systems. New participants in the health system may be overwhelmed and confused by its many components; for these people the ombudsman will provide counseling and a clear interpretation of the system. He will ensure that the consumer receives complete care, inform him of financial procedures and insurance provisions, and guide him to the appropriate health care facilities and personnel. He will refuse to be discouraged by bureaucracy or turned away by indifferent officials. Increasing activity by consumers themselves will be part of the consumer advocacy efforts. Organized groups of consumers will identify problem areas and may serve in the role of advocate. The role of ombudsman/consumer advocate might well be served by a highly trained health professional or a well-educated lay person.

2. Managers of health-related enterprises. Staff members who administer programs at the national, regional, state, and local levels often will not be members of traditional health professions. Yet they will be knowledgeable about health as they make administrative decisions about health education programs, health insurance, health and welfare planning, and so forth. New educational programs will make health generalists out of such administrators so that they can respond effectively and promptly to changing needs.

3. Health facility administrators. General managers will be needed for the new facilities for health maintenance and restorative care as well as for acute care centers. Special knowledge and skills will be required for the management of each type of health facility. Administrators will be knowledgeable about new techniques in health care delivery and will be responsible for encouraging the use of these techniques among their staffs. They will also facilitate coordination of the activities of the various health teams in keeping with the most current evaluations of optimal team structure and interactions.

4. Planning and management specialists. These people will design and operate the management information systems, which will be essential to the support of highly complex health structures. They will develop mechanisms to ensure interaction among all components of the health system; they will plan strategies for the resolution of conflict; and they will establish clear objectives for health care delivery, focusing all resources toward accomplishment of these objectives.

5. Health data specialists. This category of personnel will include both the data management and health professions. Health data specialists will conduct research on consumer characteristics, histories, and needs and will disseminate these data to appropriate persons in the health system.

Generators of change: researchers and evaluators

The health system will require personnel who will be responsible for generating change in a wide variety of areas. Provisions will be made for them to interface with managers on a regular basis.

1. Biological and environmental researchers. It will be essential to uncover new knowledge to improve the efficiency of all elements of the health care system to provide optimum care for all people.

2. Technical researchers. The invention and perfection of new medical equipment and technological devices will continue to improve the delivery of health care.

3. Clinical care researchers. Intensified research will continue to determine which approaches, activities, and techniques used in the direct care of patients result in optimum patient response and recovery.

4. Health care delivery researchers. A comprehensive system will be supported by a continuing program of research to improve the systems of delivery of health care according to consumer needs and responses. This will be accomplished through demonstration and evaluation of the different means of using various mixes of resources and changing personnel functions.

5. Management researchers. A continuing program of research will provide new techniques for efficient management and optimum cost effectiveness in health care.

6. Evaluation specialists. An efficient system of evaluation will require feedback from all operations, including both health care services and management of the system. The evaluation of both elements will provide continuing data to support changes in the direction of greater efficiency and effectiveness. Consumers will take an active part in the evaluation process.

Educators within the health system

The health system itself will embrace an educational component. Two categories of educators will serve within the health system:

1. Educators of health workers. The health care delivery system will assume increasing responsibility for staff training and development in close cooperation with educational institutions. Regular procedures for reexamination and recertification will be established as prerequisites for continuing practice.

2. Educators of consumers. When people are acutely ill it usually takes little education to convince them that they should seek medical help. It will require a far larger and more sophisticated educational program to con-

vince people who are well that they should take precise and aggressive continuing steps to maintain their health. A substantial cadre especially trained to perform this function will be required.

CHANGING EDUCATION FOR THE NEW HEALTH SYSTEM

The education and training of health workers at all levels will change dramatically and immediately in order to staff the health care delivery system of the 1980s. Educators, administrators, and practitioners will focus on the future and what it might be, rather than on the past and what it has been. The objectives of educational change will be founded on the needs of the health care delivery system in the 1980s and beyond. To produce the personnel who will coordinate and deliver health care in the future, innovation and experimentation, coupled with sound methods of evaluation, will permeate the entire educational system.

Changes in the people who educate

The education of health workers at all levels will continue to be under the direction of bona fide educators associated with educational institutions. Several sources of change in these educators will influence the educational system:

Persons who are not currently associated with health education will become faculty members in institutions of health education and training. They will include the following:

1. Experts in such fields of science as ecology and pollution control will train members of environmental and health maintenance/ disease prevention teams.

2. Social and behavioral scientists will orient health care workers to human perceptions, needs, and problems.

3. Experts in communication and its technology will illustrate the mechanisms of communication in a complex health system.

4. Management experts and systems analysts will educate all health workers in the utilization of scientific management techniques.

5. Educators will prepare students for new health careers as yet undefined.

6. Nontraditional health practitioners (for example, medicine men and curanderos) will broaden the spectrum and understanding of what "health care" is.

7. Health practitioners will share their knowledge of the field as well as their practical experience with students and professional educators.

8. Members of minority and ethnic groups will fully participate in the education of all health workers.

Consumers and volunteers will be trained as educators to teach the elements of health maintenance in their home communities. Such persons will be seen as a part of the educational system.

1. Selected residents of rural communities will serve as health maintenance educators in isolated areas.

2. Influential persons in ethnic communities, where distrust and language barriers prevail, will serve as educators for their people. Indigenous care givers will be identified and included.

3. Students will be trained to work part-time and during vacation periods as health educators for selected communities.

Faculty members will undergo changes in attitude, role perception, and educational priorities. Changes in the character of faculty members will revolve around the following themes—

1. People orientation. All faculty members will teach their students about health care for *people*, rather than only about care of patients. Webster defines a patient as "one who suffers or endures; a sick person, now commonly one under treatment or care, as by a physician, or surgeon, or in a hospital; or

the like." This concept is too limited for the 1980s. Although there will still be patients, the education of health care workers will be focused on the broader concept of the health care of people.

2. Development of leadership. Faculty members will be chosen for leadership roles on criteria other than seniority or formal credentials. Talent, creativity, interest in change, and orientation toward the future will be given far more consideration. The chairmen of departments and deans of schools who are resistant to change, who refuse to embrace changes, who represent the autocratic or authoritarian patterns of the past will not be reappointed.

3. Faculty development. Ways and means will be devised to make individual faculty members aware of the importance of keeping the content of what they teach relevant to the real world. Each faculty member will regularly have practical experience as a health worker outside the walls of the institution in which he teaches, preferably in a situation new and novel for him. This will be a requirement for continued employment. The faculty will use research findings as a source of updating and will participate in conducting research.

4. White faculty and ethnic minorities. To teach both ethnic students of color and white students who may serve minority groups, the faculty will be sensitive to the special problems, needs, and value systems of the non-white population and will use both students and community groups as resources to increase their knowledge and understanding of these populations. Efforts to educate the faculty and to promote racial understanding will be made in every educational setting. Faculty members will have practical experience working outside the institution in minority communities.

5. Cultural awareness. Faculty members will be knowledgeable about, and aware of, the cultural diversity of the students and of

the target groups of clients beyond racial awareness, for example, subculture groupings of Caucasians such as Irish, German, and the socioeconomically disadvantaged.

Changes in the categories of people who are educated

New categories of students in the health education institutions will include:

1. Ethnic and racial minorities. More opportunities to become leaders in the health professions will be provided to members of minority groups. This will result from concentrated efforts in recruitment and special provisions for financial aid. A system of admissions to ensure inclusion of ethnic students of color will be established in many institutions of health education.

2. Minorities by sex. Schools that prepare people for professions now dominated by women will actively recruit more men; schools that prepare people for professions now dominated by men will actively recruit more women.

3. People whose work is related to the health enterprise. Such people as community planners and administrators, welfare workers, social security administrators, providers of health insurance, managers of health facilities, and analysts of the health care system will require information about and understanding of the health care delivery system.

4. Health educators. Three levels of prospective health educators will be enrolled in training programs at institutions of health education:

   a. Prospective professors will require instruction in innovative teaching methods as well as in specialized fields of health knowledge.

   b. Practitioners who supervise students will require orientation toward the teaching-learning process and toward the educational preparation of their students.

   c. Consumers and volunteers who will teach health concepts in their communities will enroll in training programs at educational institutions.

5. Volunteers. Community people who want to serve on teams in health maintenance, acute care, and restorative care will enroll for training.

6. All health workers and continuing education. Every person who is part of the health care delivery system will be required to attend continuing education programs. Although continuing education has long been a function of the schools, the numbers of health workers and the variety of their services will expand markedly. Institutions will decentralize continuing education facilities to minimize the travel required of health workers. The focus of continuing education will be to expand the scope and depth of each health worker's knowledge of health fields both within and outside of his own specialty. The budgets of schools that teach health workers will reflect this new emphasis on continuing education. As continuing education becomes required for relicensure to practice, public monies will become available for assistance.

Changes in the content of education

Educational content and course requirements will be examined according to the objectives they seek to accomplish. For each health career, necessary competencies will be established. Course requirements will then be selected according to their contribution and relevance to the development of those competencies. This process of curricular development will permeate all programs of health education. Continual evaluation, revision, and expansion of educational content will assure each student a relevant, accurate, and up-to-date education.

Examples of new emphases in the content of education for health workers and related personnel will include:

1. Techniques of health maintenance and disease prevention. The education of every health worker will prepare him to take leadership to help resolve conditions and situations that work against the mental and physical health of the population. He will understand the problems of pollution of the environment, the lack of family planning, poor housing, and poor nutrition. He will also be attuned to the fact that money spent in these areas in the long run will reduce demands on the health care system. A significant portion of the practical experience of students in all health fields will occur in settings that are concerned with health maintenance and disease prevention.

2. Concepts of psychology. Every student being prepared to be a health worker will be exposed to the implications of the psychiatric and emotional factors related to physical illness. This is particularly true with regard to those consumers who are very young and very old. The teaching of these concepts will be expanded in all programs. This presupposes a basic grounding in the social and behavioral sciences.

3. Overview of the health system. To provide for the efficient communication and interactions of all health workers in the field, students will command a working understanding of all of the components of the health system. A course of this type will be required of every student in health services.

4. General concepts of health and illness. A series of courses will be developed to educate lay persons working in health-related fields, health management personnel, and persons with leadership roles in the community. Such a program will include concepts of health maintenance, an overview of the health system, current problems in health care delivery, and the problems of cost containment.

5. Techniques of scientific management and systems analysis. To promote the efficiency of the health system at all levels, an understanding of both management and evaluation concepts will be required of all health workers.

6. Relationships between health care and the law. Studies will be encouraged to explore the following:
   a. Legal provisions for pollution control and their responsiveness to health needs.
   b. Practitioner liability in the delivery of health care.
   c. Legal rights of the consumer in the health system.

7. New health careers programs.

Changes in the educational process

Changes in the content of education for health workers will be meaningless without simultaneous changes in teaching and learning methods. The following changes will occur:

1. Team teaching. Although experiments in team teaching exist nationwide, few of them reflect the true concept of teamwork. Teamwork in health education requires the following:
   a. An interdisciplinary approach to education. The resources and knowledge of all health and health-related fields will be integrated insofar as such integration is productive and meaningful. Psychology, for example, is a relevant component of physiology; its concepts should be incorporated into the study of physiology rather than isolated from it.
   b. Mutual respect among specialists in all health and health-related disciplines. Teamwork implies coordinated efforts among equals, each contributing his talents toward a common goal. The current "pecking order" attitude will be replaced by one that recognizes that specific situations will determine the appropriate source of leadership within the team structure. Respect for the tal-

ents and competencies of those in other professions will be reflected in the actions and attitudes of the faculty members.

c. Acceptance of the team concept in the delivery of health care as well as in education. The cooperative functioning of a teaching team demonstrates to students the advantages and dynamics of group work in health care delivery. Teaching teams will be responsible for the instruction of groups of students preparing for a wide variety of health careers. Future doctors, dentists, nurses, and paraprofessional personnel will study together, learning the values and contributions of each profession, in preparation for their work together in health care delivery teams. The education of health maintenance/disease prevention teams will bring together all the components of those teams in the classroom as well as in the community.

2. Maximum utilization of community resources. The educational plan wll be closely tied to the realities of the health system and the problems involved in that system. Practical experience will take students out into the community for observation and for participation in health care delivery services. Community leaders, planners, and practicing health workers will be brought regularly into the educational institutions to share their concerns with students and faculty. Knowledge of community resources—both human and physical—will be essential to all health workers.

3. Maximum utilization of all available technological teaching devices. Telecommunications systems and audiotape and videotape devices will transfer maximum amounts of information with minimum effort and cost. As these and other instructional devices are developed, their use will be immediately incorporated into the system of education.

4. Flexibility in the educational time span. Flexibility will be introduced into health educational programs to allow each student to progress at his own pace. High-ability students will be encouraged to complete degree requirements far ahead of the traditional schedule. Tutoring programs will assist slower students as they progress at their own speeds. Internship and residency programs for physicians and other health professionals will be revised and shortened.

5. The core concept of health education. All health workers will begin their preparation for health careers in a series of courses designed to offer basic knowledge of health concepts. Through such core studies, all health workers will share the same fundamental knowledge of the physical and social sciences, elements of health and its maintenance, and illness and its prevention. Relationships among students thus established in the classroom will support teamwork later in the field.

6. Diverging career patterns. Most health workers will choose one of two primary career patterns, which will emerge from the core studies. One track will emphasize practice that is essentially curative and restorative, as in institutional settings; the other will emphasize practice in community settings largely outside hospital walls, concentrating on health maintenance and disease prevention. Students will be encouraged to choose their career patterns according to their personal preferences and talents.

7. Utilization of all means of promoting and rewarding mobility and career development:

a. Credit by examination will be universally accepted by all educational institutions. Tested competencies will qualify the student for credit.

b. The concept of the external degree will be accepted both in theory and in practice. Examinations will be established to test required competencies for every academic degree related to health work. Highly motivated and mature students who pass such examinations will be awarded the appropriate degree, regardless of the time they have spent in educational institutions. Theoretically an unaffiliated student will be able to earn a degree without ever enrolling in a degree program at a school or university.

c. The opportunity to exercise options at various points on any health career continuum will be provided and encouraged. As a student's career interests shift, he will be able to move easily and rapidly into a new career program without course repetition or loss of credit.

Changes in where health workers are educated

To provide every student with a connecting link between his education and his role as a health worker, educational facilities will be increasingly decentralized and associated with the new facilities for health care delivery. Ambulatory clinics, outpatient facilities, extended care units, halfway houses, nursing homes, and neighborhood health centers will be used as educational laboratories in the preparation of all types of health care workers. A major part of each student's education will be provided in two new types of educational settings:

1. Neighborhood and small town health centers. Centers with facilities for the delivery of health maintenance care—together with limited facilities for emergency and restorative care—will include educational facilities for the formal instruction of students, continuing education of health workers, and health education of the surrounding population. Such centers will be located in every urban neighborhood and in small rural towns. Each facility will be a part of a network linked to larger centers from which specialists

will be available and to which referrals can be made.

2. Special services facilities. In sparsely populated areas, large special services facilities will be established to back up the surrounding network of small town centers, and to provide specialized, acute and extended care. These in turn, will be linked to a large medical center. The staff of each special services facility will have a significant component of highly qualified health educators who will provide instruction not only in the center itself but also in the surrounding small town centers. Wherever feasible, the special services facility will be associated with a local educational institution, both physically and philosophically.

Changes in the process of change

Attitudinal shifts on the part of both consumers and health workers will provide a powerful force for change in the health system as well as in the process of education. Increasingly consumers will assume accountability for their own care, will know what constitutes quality care, and will demand it. Providers will be more aware of cultural needs and concerns of clients, of the individual accountability of each provider, and of the collaboration necessary to make changes and to provide quality care—accessible and acceptable to the clients. Evaluation and research will generate and support change in the education of health care workers, as well as in the system of health care delivery. The following will be new sources and areas of evaluation and research in education:

1. Evaluation by students. Students in significant numbers will serve on all faculty committees, which will make recommendations about student life and about their preparation as health care workers. The students will have the opportunity to feed into the system their evaluation of proposed actions or decisions before they are implemented.

2. Evaluation of teaching. Regular evaluation by students, peers, and outside consultants will judge the effectiveness of each faculty member's teaching. Effective teaching will be a most important component in making decisions on salary increments.

3. Evaluation of learning and content. Each school will retain outside, impartial evaluators to survey the products of the system (that is, their own graduates) at a reasonable time beyond graduation, to ascertain their attitudes toward the quality and relevance of their education. Those who have employed the products of the system will evaluate the quality and scope of their employee's learning.

4. Research. Those institutions sponsoring health-related research will become more concerned with research on the delivery of health care in various types of settings—especially those outside the hospital—and on the cost effectiveness of various approaches.

5. Research on teaching techniques. Schools and colleges producing health care workers will actively seek funds from all sources to experiment with innovative and efficient methods of teaching. More experiments involving control groups will be mounted. Funds will be provided to allow teachers to experiment with new teaching tools. Successful teaching techniques employed by the military and by industry—techniques such as those used by the United Airlines Center in Denver—will be explored for possible application.

6. Councils of the Future. Every institution of health education will establish and maintain a "Council of the Future," in the sense proposed by Toffler in his book, *Future Shock*. These councils, consisting of students, faculty, practitioners, and consumers of health care—individuals and agencies—will brainstorm freely, even wildly, about the future, making predictions, drawing up plans, and initiating change. They will draw on all the resources of research for their thinking and feed back their conclusions into all the components of the system. They will have the authority to implement experimental programs based on their predictions, thus helping their institution to "invent the future."

• • •

To create the necessary changes in this nation's health system, energies must be focused toward changing education. This is a task too important to be left solely to professional educators. Each person concerned with health care has a role to play in the process and direction of change in the educational system, as well as in the delivery of health care. Education and practice must join in establishing and maintaining an efficient health system that meets the health needs of all American citizens.

The decision makers, the policy formulators in the present health system, and the consumers all can be change agents to create the health system of the future. The personnel of every health agency—both professional practitioners and community members—must continually interface with educators. They must participate in planning the content and process of education, in teaching students at educational institutions, and in evaluating education. Their input and involvement in the educational process is essential. At the same time, each of the health agencies must offer its facilities as a laboratory for the onsite education of health workers. The agencies will feed ideas into the educational system, and the educational system, through its students and faculty supervisors, will feed ideas into the agencies. By working together through such a symbiotic relationship, both educational institutions and health agencies will generate the changes in the health system that have been outlined above.

Toffler, in *Future Shock,* states that the inability to speak with precision and certainty about the future is no excuse for silence. Health care providers, legislators, planners, and consumers must heed the alert!

SUGGESTED READINGS

American Association of State College and Universities, Resource Center for Planned Change: A future creating paradigm: a guide to long range planning from the future, for the future, Washington, D.C.: 1978, The Association.

Bell, D.: The coming of post-industrial society: a venture in social forecasting, New York, 1973, Basic Books, Inc.

Boulding, K. E.: *Toward the year 2000,* Publication No. 132, Boulder, Colo., 1971, Social Science Education Consortium, Inc.

Cornish, E.: The study of the future: an introduction to the art and science of understanding and shaping tomorrow's world, Washington, D.C., 1977, World Future Society.

Elliott, J. E., and Kearns, J. M.: Analysis and planning for improved distribution of nursing personnel and services: final report, Publication No. HRA 79-16, Hyattsville, Md., 1978, U.S. Department of Health, Education, and Welfare.

Fowles, D. G.: Some prospects for the future elderly population, Washington, D.C., 1978, Administration on Aging.

The Futurist: a Journal of Forecasts, Trends, and Ideas about the Future, Washington, D.C., World Future Society. (Bi-monthly.)

Gingras, P., ed.: National conferences, Publication No. HRA 77-3, Bethesda, Md.: 1976, U.S. Department of Health, Education, and Welfare.

Gray, R., and Sauer, K.: Nursing resources and requirements: a guide for state-level planning, Boulder, Colo. 1978, Western Interstate Commission for Higher Education.

Health, Futures Conditional **5**(3): Entire issue, 1977.

Kodadek, S., ed.: Inventory of innovations in nursing, Publication No. HRA 77-2, Bethesda, Md., 1976. U.S. Department of Health, Education, and Welfare.

Kriesberg, H. M., et al.: Methodological approaches for determining health manpower supply and requirements. vol. 1: Analytical perspective, Washington, D.C., 1976, Robert R. Nathan Associates, Inc.

Kriesberg, H. M., et al.: Methodological approaches for determining health manpower supply and requirements. vol. 2: Practical planning manual, Washington D.C., 1976, Robert R. Nathan Associates, Inc.

Lee, P. R., LeRoy, L., Staleup, J., and Beck, J.: Primary care in a specialized world, Cambridge, Mass. 1976, Ballinger Publishing Co.

Lum, J. L. J., with Leonhard, G.: Panel of expert consultants: final report, Boulder, Colo., 1978, Western Interstate Commission for Higher Education.

Mott, P. D., King, S. R., and Gavett, J. W.: A simplified method for approximation of shortages of rural physicians. Public Health Rep. **92**(4): 322-325, 1977.

Perelman, L. J.: Growth and education: a strategic report to the Rockefeller Brothers Fund, Boulder, Colo., 1974, Western Interstate Commission for Higher Educaton.

Toffler, A.: Future Shock, New York, 1970, Random House.

2

The emerging role of the pediatric nurse practitioner

Jan Tenney and Diane Synhorst

HISTORICAL PERSPECTIVE

The emerging role of the pediatric nurse practitioner is best viewed in perspective by considering certain recent trends within our health care system. The nurse practitioner, like the physician's assistant, represents an innovation in health care delivery. Each of these roles was developed in an effort to increase the number of primary health care providers.

In the mid-1960s, a shortage of primary care physicians seemed imminent. Many new physicians were choosing to enter specialty areas, while a maldistribution of physicians providing primary care was already present. It appeared that the demand for primary health care services would soon exceed the supply of providers. The threat of such a development caused members of the health care field to search for sources from which potential providers might be pulled and quickly trained in primary care. Two groups of potential new providers were identified—registered nurses and medical corpsmen returning from Vietnam.

Underlying assumptions of the new health care provider movement were (1) that appro-priately trained nonphysicians could manage many commonly encountered health problems, thus helping to free the physician's time and expertise for the management of more complicated disorders, and (2) that persons with previous experience within the health care system could be trained quickly and relatively inexpensively to assume primary care roles, thus helping to prevent the overall cost of health care from becoming prohibitive.

Through the efforts of early proponents of these new roles and the cooperation of physicians, the concept of nonphysician health care providers has begun to gain recognition and acceptance among both recipients and traditional providers of health care. Research describing and evaluating the new health care provider roles has been generated at a rapid pace. These new providers have begun to adapt their practices to meet existing and developing health care needs. Some have chosen to increase the depth of their knowledge and skills through association with specialists while others have continued to concentrate on primary care and health maintenance.

ORIGIN OF THE PEDIATRIC NURSE PRACTITIONER CONCEPT

The pediatric nurse practitioner (PNP)* concept was first introduced by Silver and Ford at the University of Colorado in 1965.[1] They recognized that there was an insufficient supply of prepared personnel to meet the increasing demands for effective child health care. Silver believed that registered nurses were the only large group of nonphysician health professionals who could be prepared quickly to help improve the quality and accessibility of care of our child population.[2] Through the joint efforts of the University of Colorado College of Nursing and College of Medicine, a 4-month educational program, consisting of intensive pediatric theory and practice, was designed to prepare registered nurses with baccalaureate or master's degrees to assume PNP roles.[1]

Early studies of program graduates indicated that these PNPs were able to manage a high percentage of pediatric ambulatory care either independently or in collaboration with pediatricians. One survey of parents who had experienced the services of a PNP-pediatrician team indicated that 94% approved of this joint approach and 57% believed that such joint care was better than the care received from a physician alone.[3]

With the early success of Colorado's PNP program, interest in the new role grew and additional PNP programs were initiated across the country. In 1969 representatives of the American Academy of Pediatrics (AAP) and of the American Nurses' Association (ANA) Maternal Child Practice Division began a series of joint meetings to establish educational guidelines and a scope of practice statement for the PNP. The product of these early meetings was a statement published in 1970 entitled "Guidelines on Short-Term

---

*May also be referred to as a pediatric nurse associate (PNA).

Continuing Education Programs for Pediatric Nurse Associates."[4] The Joint Statement[5] identified the overall goal of PNP educational programs to be that of providing graduates with the knowledge and skill necessary to assume direct and responsible professional roles in ambulatory child health care. To meet this goal educational programs were to prepare graduates to perform such functions as securing health and developmental histories, conducting basic physical and developmental assessments, providing anticipatory guidance in problems of child rearing, recognizing and managing specific minor childhood conditions, and making independent nursing decisions as well as collaborative decisions with physicians.[5]

EDUCATIONAL PROGRAMS

Formal educational programs for PNPs follow the basic guidelines proposed in the Joint Statement. The statement recommends that programs be developed under the sponsorship of accredited collegiate nursing programs and that program development be a collaborative effort between the Department of Pediatrics and the Department of Nursing. Only registered nurses are to be eligible for entrance into the programs. A minimum of 4 months' educational experience consisting of classroom work, clinical practice, and work experience is recommended.[5]

Although basic guidelines have been established for PNP programs, variations are still present in areas such as program length, inclusion of preceptorships, and curriculum. Concern exists among educators and practicing PNPs in regard to program funding, establishment of appropriate standards, provision for continuing education, and development of an accreditation process for educational programs.[6] A few educators advocate the incorporation of nurse practitioner training into existing baccalaureate nursing programs. However, the issue as to whether or not such an educational innovation is appropriate has yet to be resolved.

As of 1974 there were 50 formal educational programs for the preparation of PNPs. Of these 50 programs, 42 awarded certificates at the time of completion. PNP training coordinated with master's degree programs started in 1972 and comprise the remaining formal programs.[7] Although there is a push toward formal educational preparation of PNPs, there are still a number of PNPs prepared through on-the-job training. At present it is estimated that there are 4,000 formally trained PNPs across the country; the number of informally trained PNPs is unknown.[8]

CERTIFICATION

Soon after the publication of the Joint Statement, attention turned toward the development of a certification procedure for PNPs. In 1973 the National Association of Pediatric Nurse Associates and Practitioners (NAPNAP) was formed independently by a group of PNPs for the purpose of helping nurse practitioners improve their quality of infant and child health care. The NAPNAP identified as one of its major tasks the development of a PNP certification program.[9]

Around this same time the AAP and ANA were also developing a certification program for PNPs. A major point of contention between the AAP and ANA was over which agency should exert the most control over the certification process. The ANA believed that the major responsibility should lie with nursing and that a qualifying examination should be prepared by the ANA in consultation with the AAP, rather than its being prepared with equal participation by both agencies. The AAP believed that it should have equal input into the development of the certification examination. In January of 1974 the AAP's executive board announced its decision to dissociate itself from the ANA Certification Program for the Pediatric Nurse Practitioner

in Ambulatory Health Care and revealed its intention to develop a certification procedure in consultation with agencies other than the ANA.[4]

The first PNP certification program to be developed was under the direction of the ANA. The ANA certification program requires a number of months to complete. The process consists of assessment of knowledge through written examination, demonstration of clinical practice through descriptions submitted by candidates, and endorsement by colleagues.[10] The written examination is offered each year. After successful completion of all phases of the program, PNPs receive a certificate and are listed in the *ANA Directory of Certified Nurses*.[11]

In addition to the ANA's certification program, there now exists a separate PNP certification program cosponsored by the AAP and NAPNAP. Representatives of these two organizations, along with nurse and physician faculty members, first met in 1974 to discuss development of a program for entry level certification of PNPs. These representatives believed that it was important to establish a board of nurses, pediatricians, and faculty members that could develop a nationwide certification procedure. Thus the National Board of Pediatric Nurse Practitioners and Associates was formed in 1975. Thereafter test committees were appointed to devise a national qualifying examination. Test items were developed by PNPs and pediatricians with the assistance of the National Board of Medical Examiners.[9]

The National Board of Pediatric Nurse Practitioners and Associates offered its first national qualifying examination in February, 1977.[9] The examination has since been offered on a yearly basis. Candidates who successfully complete the examination are awarded certificates of achievement and are listed with the National Board of Pediatric Nurse Practitioners and Associates. Their names are also sent to state boards of nursing and medicine, to nursing and medical associations, and to the NAPNAP and AAP.[8]

SCOPE OF PRACTICE

In practice the PNP functions as a primary care provider in the health care delivery system. The practitioner assesses the child's health status and promotes the child's psychosocial, developmental, and physical well-being. As a result of professional education and clinical experience, the PNP is able to employ a wide variety of skills in her practice. These skills include making physical and developmental assessments through appropriate examination techniques, discriminating between normal and abnormal findings and determining what findings require collaboration or referral to other health professionals, recognizing and managing a variety of common childhood illnesses, facilitating effective communication between families and health care providers, providing anticipatory guidance to parents in aspects of child rearing, and participating on an equal and collaborative basis with other members of the health care team.[12]

The PNP role includes clinical responsibilities that extend beyond the scope of traditional nursing practice. The PNP retains her overall nursing focus of health care promotion. Yet, through additional education and experience, she expands her technical skills and knowledge base so that she is able to make more comprehensive nursing judgments. The PNP assumes a direct and responsible role in preventive child health care and serves as an advocate for the child within the community.

All PNPs have certain common goals. However, if one observes various PNPs in action, it becomes apparent that each PNP's practice is unique. There are numerous factors that influence variations in practice. Among these are the individual PNP's personality characteristics, previous clinical experiences, knowledge base, educational preparation, and existing interprofessional relationships. Perhaps the most influential factor in a PNP's practice is the clinical setting in which she functions.

Most commonly PNPs are employed in ambulatory pediatric care settings such as private pediatricians' offices, health maintenance organizations (HMOs), outpatient clinics, state health departments, and community health agencies. PNPs usually become involved in health care supervision and the minor illness management of normal children. Recently, however, PNPs have begun to be employed in ambulatory specialty clinics and tertiary care settings where they deal with children having specialized health problems.

To illustrate the differences in functions as related to clinical settings, the practices of two PNPs in dissimilar settings will be described.

The first practice is that of a PNP working within an HMO. Employed within the HMO are pediatricians, obstetricians, family practitioners, internists, a radiologist, nurse midwives, family counselors, a nutritionist, a health educator, nurses, physician's assistants, and a PNP.

The PNP works with a pediatrician as a collaborative member of a child health care team. She and the pediatrician share a caseload of patients and work from a joint daily schedule. Patients range in age from birth to 16 years of age. The PNP functions as a primary care provider in the health supervision of well children and adolescents as well as in the management of minor illnesses and common childhood problems. The pediatrician assumes major responsibility for the assessment and management of those patients with more complicated problems and for handling emergency situations. Some patients evaluated by the PNP are managed independently while others are managed in collaboration with the pediatrician. The pediatrician is always available on site for consultation with the PNP in regard to patient care concerns. Parents are familiar with the team approach and may specify which care provider they prefer to see. On occasion the PNP independently conducts well child care clinics for those children whose parents request her services.

The PNP performs a wide range of functions in the area of child health supervision. She elicits health and developmental histories and makes physical and developmental assessments. She plans and implements routine immunizations, provides anticipatory guidance for parents in certain aspects of child growth and development, and counsels parents in regard to minor child-rearing problems. The PNP uses developmental assessment tools, such as the Denver Developmental Screening Test, to test children with suspected developmental delays. She devises sensorimotor stimulation programs for children when appropriate and arranges for necessary follow-up. In collaboration with the pediatrician the PNP refers children to outside agencies or to other health professionals within the HMO when more involved diagnostic work-ups are needed or for the management of specialized problems.

A portion of the practitioner's responsibilities includes telephone triage and counseling in minor problems as well as telephone follow-up of ill children. She also participates in the supervision of, and delegation of tasks to, ancillary personnel. She assists the health educator in planning the in-service education of the nursing staff regarding care and management of children. On occasion the PNP serves as a preceptor for nurse practitioner students and provides clinical experiences for undergraduate nursing students interested in the PNP role. She also assists the pediatric staff in the selection and generation of a variety of parent education materials.

The second practice is that of a PNP employed within a university-affiliated developmental disabilities center. The center provides a wide range of diagnostic, evaluative, and residential services for children and young adults with special problems. Such problems include mental retardation, cerebral palsy, meningomyelocele, convulsive disorders, learning disabilities, and a variety of other handicapping neurological conditions. Patients and their families may be self-referred or referred by professionals within the community.

The PNP functions as a member of an interdisciplinary team consisting of a pediatrician, medical social worker, nurse, occupational therapist, physical therapist, speech pathologist, audiologist, psychologist, and PNP. The team provides outpatient evaluations and recommendations for handicapped children from birth through 3 years of age. Each time a child is seen in the outpatient clinic, he receives a team evaluation, a problem management plan, and recommendations for follow-up. Individual team members are responsible for input into those aspects of the child's care that are related to their particular areas of expertise. Once a child's initial evaluation and management plan have been completed, he is periodically reevaluated by the team to monitor his progress and to provide continued guidance for his family.

Within the team the pediatrician and nurse practitioner are primarily responsible for identifying each child's health needs. Such needs may include not only those related to the child's disability but also those related to his general health supervision. The PNP elicits health and developmental histories and performs physical examinations on every child. The pediatrician may not see each child at every visit but is available for consultation and reviews all records and care plans formulated by the PNP. Although the specific focus of a child's visit to the outpatient clinic is his particular handicapping condition, his overall health status must also be assessed.

Therefore the PNP includes well child care and minor illness management among her services.

The PNP serves a dual role of interdisciplinary team member and team coordinator. When the team establishes a diagnosis for a new patient, the PNP provides emotional support for the family members and helps them to gain an understanding of the child's condition and its implications to his overall needs. She integrates input from individual team members, explains the team's assessment and suggested management plan to the family, and assists in the implementation of the plan. She identifies community resources that may provide supportive or educational services to the family. She is also responsible for communicating the team's findings and recommendations to the child's primary care physician and other professionals involved in his care. In performing these functions the PNP assumes a major role in maintaining continuity of care for the child as well as his family.

An important part of the PNP's practice is parent education. She provides individual instruction for parents in the practical management of their handicapped child's physical and emotional needs and conducts nutritional counseling when necessary. She also produces informative materials regarding various developmental disabilities. In addition to her responsibilities within the outpatient clinic, the PNP provides consultant services to pediatric acute care facilities. She assists in case finding, discharge planning, and formulating nursing care plans for children who have developmental disabilities. She also participates in the in-service education of hospital nursing staff on topics related to the management of handicapped children.

In comparing the practices of these two PNPs, several differences are readily apparent. The first relates to the types of patients seen. One PNP deals with basically normal children from birth through early adolescence. The other concentrates on handicapped children under 3 years of age. A second difference involves the type of team approach employed. Although the first PNP utilizes the services of other consulting health professionals, it is she and the pediatrician who comprise the basic child health care team. The second PNP functions within a large interdisciplinary team, in which the services of each team member are an integral part of child care management. The areas of expertise are somewhat different for each practitioner: one serves as a primary care provider in health supervision and management of minor illness; although the other participates in primary care, her major focus is on health problems secondary to a child's handicapping condition.

Despite the variations in practice resulting from different clinical settings, these two PNPs have certain functions in common. Both assume a major responsibility in the identification of child health care needs. They both participate in counseling, whether it be in relation to common childhood problems or to special problems secondary to a handicap. Each PNP also plays an important part in parent education. Both practitioners combine the utilization of advanced nursing skills of physical and developmental assessment with the more basic nursing skills of assessing the psychosocial needs of children and their families. Collaboratively with other health professionals, each PNP works toward the major goal of maintaining each child she sees in a state of health that is optimal for him.

NURSE PRACTITIONER RESEARCH

With any innovation in the health care field, whether it be a new role or a new clinical method, research is important in the evaluation and future development of that innovation. Spitzer points out that before nurse practitioners and other new health providers become a permanent part of our health care delivery system, their roles must undergo the scrutiny of evaluative research.[13]

Spitzer identifies seven basic stages within the evaluative research process:

1. Determining a need for the innovation—in this case, for the nurse practitioner role.
2. Determining the safety and effectiveness of the new role.
3. Assessing the quality of care provided by the new practitioner once sufficient documentation of safety and effectiveness has occurred; quality of care studies usually consist of comparing the new provider's performance to established standards of care.
4. Assessing role efficiency; for a new role to be practical and lasting, it must be efficient either to providers or recipients of health care.
5. Demonstrating that health professionals, as well as health care recipients, are satisfied with the new practitioner role.
6. Determining the extent to which transfer of function from traditional provider (physician) to new provider (nurse practitioner) has occurred.
7. Surveying on a long-term basis, which may help to identify problems or benefits of the role that were not apparent during the initial stages of evaluation.[13]

In light of Spitzer's seven stages of evaluative research, it is possible to identify certain stages of research that have been approached in the nurse practitioner literature and some that require further documentation.

The nurse practitioner developed out of an apparent need for more primary care providers. Once nurse practitioners began to function within various clinical settings, studies that focused on competence of practice were generated. Early study designs varied widely and many such studies involved a relatively small number of patients and nurse practitioners. However, a few trends are apparent. The care provided by nurse practitioners in the areas of child health care supervision and assessment of minor illness is comparable to that provided by pediatricians.[14-16] A high degree of agreement has been reported between physical assessment findings of PNPs and pediatricians.[17] Such study results tend to support, at least indirectly, the safety and effectiveness of the nurse practitioner role.

In assessing nurse practitioner competence, early studies have touched on quality of care evaluation. Assessing the overall quality of care provided by nurse practitioners—or physicians for that matter—is an arduous task. Researchers continue to attempt to devise appropriate criteria and valid measurement techniques for quality of care assessment. There is a good chance that nurse practitioners provide increased health education, anticipatory guidance, and attention to the psychosocial needs of patients. Such services may well make the difference between good and excellent health care. Yet objective evaluation of such services and their effect on overall quality of care remains extremely difficult.

Efficiency studies per se have not been done on the nurse practitioner role. However, that nurse practitioners carry out a wide variety of independent functions within child health supervision is implied in many of the early studies on competence. Recently researchers have begun to realize the importance of analyzing cost factors in nurse practitioner education and utilization. Some of the studies that have been conducted have investigated the educational cost of preparing PNPs[18-19] and the potential for income generation[19] as well as the effect of PNP utilization on health care costs to the patient.[16] All of these factors are important in determining the cost effectiveness and cost benefits of nurse practitioner services. Thus far research findings seem to indicate that PNP utilization within private or clinic settings is economically feasible; yet a need exists for more definitive research.

Evaluation of provider and client satisfaction with the nurse practitioner role has been approached indirectly through studies on acceptance. PNPs as primary care providers are fairly well accepted by parents,[3] and the degree of acceptance seems greater among parents who have had more acquaintance with PNP services.[20,21] Physician acceptance of the PNP role varies somewhat according to the samples surveyed. In general physician acceptance is high, particularly among those physicians who have worked with nurse practitioners.[22-25]

The extent to which transfer of function has occurred is implied in studies that describe actual functions performed by PNPs.[22,25,26] Most PNPs maintain a common central core of activities, including basic physical and developmental assessment, management of minor illnesses, parent education, and counseling. Variations in the degree of utilization are wide. Some PNPs appear to be underutilized, either not performing functions for which their increased education has prepared them or staying "locked into" the performance of routine nursing tasks. Others have extended their range of new functions even beyond that which was included in their formal educational programs.

As the nurse practitioner role continues to develop and more nurse practitioners are incorporated into practice settings, both the impetus and the opportunity for more sophisticated and well-controlled research studies have occurred. Studies in competence, acceptance, and utilization continue to be important. In addition, studies in cost analysis and quality of care assessment are necessary to fill in obvious gaps of information.

The nurse practitioner role has existed for more than 10 years. Now may be the time for researchers to begin to approach the final and perhaps most important stage of evaluation— that of long-term surveillance. Has the nurse practitioner made an actual impact on the health care delivery system, and if so, what is the nature of this impact?

GROWING PAINS

Role development of the nurse practitioner has been fraught with a few difficulties that might aptly be termed "growing pains." Some of these difficulties are shared with fellow new health care providers and others are unique to nurse practitioners.

Physicians have long been considered the chief decision makers within our health care system and the only health professionals skilled in the diagnosis and management of illness. As a result of the new health care provider movement, nonphysician personnel have assumed a number of functions previously held within the exclusive domain of medical practice. It is not surprising, then, that this movement has met with some resistance among a number of traditional providers and recipients of health care services.

To those of us in clinical practice, whether we be nurse practitioners or other new health care providers, evidence of such resistance may be present. Although the actual number of physicians and patients who are resistive to our roles is small, the negative attitudes that they present may be a source of frustration. As nurse practitioners, it has been our experience that resistive attitudes on the part of physicians and patients are usually temporary. By continuing to provide the high-quality health care of which we are capable, we and other new health care providers are often able to convert negative attitudes to positive ones.

The nurse practitioner, unlike other new health care providers, is firmly entrenched in the foundations of traditional nursing. In her expanded role she is a newcomer to the field of primary care. Yet as a nurse she is a familiar and generally well-accepted member of the total health care system. The fact that the nurse is well known within the present system may facilitate the ease with which she expands her role. However, the term "nurse" also carries with it a certain stereotype, which may make role expansion difficult. The nurse has for generations been typically viewed as the physician's handmaiden. The fact that most nurses are women and most physicians are men, combined with the fact that the classic pattern within our society is one of male dominance, tends to reinforce this stereotype.

Nearly every nurse practitioner, particularly in the early phases of her role, is likely to encounter a few intrapersonal conflicts. Bates points out that it is not unusual for the new nurse practitioner to undergo one or a series of "identity crises." One such crisis may center around how the nurse practitioner views her role in relation to that of the physician. Having assumed a variety of previously medical functions, the new practitioner may wonder if she is a valuable care provider in her own right or merely an assistant to the physician.[27] The nurse practitioner may initially become quite involved in the utilization and development of her new skills, sometimes to the temporary exclusion of her more basic areas of nursing expertise. This may further add to feelings of identity confusion.[28] As a nurse the practitioner's emphasis has been on the comfort and support of patients. Yet in her expanded role she places additional emphasis on making skilled assessments and decisions in patient management. This apparent discrepancy between the roles of nurse and nurse practitioner may form the basis for another so-called identity crisis.[27]

Bates also views the physician who works with the nurse practitioner as having to resolve a few intrapersonal conflicts. Having been taught to make independent decisions on the basis of his own clinical evaluations, the physician may not be comfortable in relying on the clinical judgments of the nurse practitioner. He may also have difficulty in sharing his more rewarding patient relationships.[27] He may even perceive the nurse practitioner as a competitor.[29] This combination of factors may make it impossible for the physician to relinquish any part of his role to a newcomer without experiencing a certain amount of identity confusion.

During a new nurse practitioner's period of adjustment the importance of peer group support cannot be overemphasized. By keeping in contact with other nurse practitioners, the new practitioner helps to avoid professional isolation. Nurse practitioners across the country, realizing the importance of professional and peer support, have begun to organize into regional groups. Some of these groups are independently formed while others are affiliated with national organizations. Within such nurse practitioner groups ideas and concerns can be shared and current issues of common interest discussed.

Conflicts involved with the nurse practitioner role can be resolved, but resolution requires effort on the part of the practitioner and those with whom she works. Once initial role reorientation has occurred, the nurse practitioner may find substantial rewards in her practice. Eventually the successful nurse practitioner becomes able to transcend her initial overemphasis on newly acquired skills so that she is able to integrate them with her preexisting nursing skills into a well-balanced professional approach.[28]

Many nurse practitioners and physicians feel that as a team they can provide more comprehensive and accessible care to patients. Opportunities to teach and learn from each other are increased. Within a new sort of collegial relationship nurse practitioners and physicians may share the burdens as well as the rewards of clinical practice.[27]

The nurse practitioner role is high in

intrinsic job satisfaction factors such as job creativity, importance of role, use of one's skills, and interesting nature of the work.[30] Nurse practitioners are likely to command higher salaries than traditional nurses, enjoy increased status, and experience more gratifying patient relationships.

While the difficulties within this new role are significant, they are for the most part temporary. The positive aspects of the role are also significant and are by far more sustaining. Once successful resolution of conflicts has occurred, the nurse practitioner and those with whom she works are likely to experience feelings of satisfaction from collaborating as a team in the provision of high-quality health care.

CURRENT ISSUES

The pediatric nurse practitioner role is one around which several issues are presently focused. One of these issues is national certification. Certification is important in ensuring the public high-quality health care from PNPs, as well as in lending greater credibility to the PNP role. Much progress has already been made in the area of PNP certification; yet work remains to be done. At present the certification of PNPs is conducted on a voluntary basis but eventual mandatory certification is anticipated. The unfortunate rift between the AAP and ANA over philosophical differences has resulted in the development of two separate certification procedures for PNPs. It is hoped that continuing efforts on the part of these two organizations will result in a single national certification program that is acceptable to both pediatricians and nurses.

A second major issue surrounding the PNP role, as well as that of other nurse practitioners, is the legal scope of practice. Nurse practitioners, by virtue of their being registered nurses, are licensed to practice professional nursing. Their practice is largely governed on a state-wide basis. Individual state nurse practice acts establish education, examination, and licensing requirements and define the functions of the professional nurse in both general and specific terms.[31] Registered nurses may legally perform those functions held to be within the realm of professional nursing as stated in individual nurse practice acts. In determining the legal scope of nursing practice, since the two are closely related, both nurse and medical practice acts must be viewed. If the nurse and medical practice acts within a state are not consistent in their references to nursing, the legal scope of nursing remains indistinct.

The nurse practitioner has assumed many functions that previously have been within the exclusive realm of medical practice. A discrepancy has become apparent between traditional nursing functions delineated in existing nurse practice acts and new functions being assumed by nurse practitioners. As a result many states have attempted to revise their nurse practice acts so that the nurse practitioner role is afforded clear legal sanction.[32]

Specific types of revisions have varied from state to state, and none seem completely satisfactory in providing clear definitions of the expanded nursing role.[32] Revision of nurse practice acts often requires appropriate revision of medical practice acts so that continuity is maintained. This entire legislative process is complicated and time consuming. However, it would seem that the process is a necessary one if the nurse practitioner role is to be legally viable.

Since the nurse practitioner entered the scene a decade ago, there has been a gradual change in the focus of health care. What has developed is a tendency to view health care needs in the light of health maintenance and prevention of illness rather than merely in the light of disease management. A push toward physical fitness has occurred. People are more aware of the advantages of proper nutrition. A "back to basics" attitude has taken hold, perhaps contributing to a renewed interest in natural childbirth and breast feeding, as well as to the upsurge of family practice and midwifery specialties. National media campaigns to educate the public in aspects of preventive health care have resulted in a more knowledgeable and perhaps more critical group of health care recipients than ever before. People are no longer satisfied to be free of illness; they want to be healthy.

The grim physician shortage, predicted as recently as 1970, has not occurred. On the contrary, it appears that a physician surplus is more likely. It would seem, then, that the original stimulus for the development of the nurse practitioner role is no longer present. Despite this fact the value of nurse practitioners in health maintenance, patient education, and attending to psychosocial needs of families is becoming apparent. It is these aspects of health care that our present society has begun to recognize as important in health care services. Although nurse practitioners were initially developed to increase accessibility of care, physicians and patients are realizing that nurse practitioners often contribute components that previously have been missing in primary health care.

Will nurse practitioners become permanently assimilated into our health care system? Now, while physician supply is increasing, is the critical period during which the answer to this question will be decided. The answer lies in the performance of existing nurse practitioners, research on role effectiveness, and evaluation of quality of nurse practitioner care.

REFERENCES

1. Silver, H. K., Ford, L. C., and Stearly, S. G.: A program to increase health care for children: the pediatric nurse practitioner program, Pediatr. **39:**756-760, May 1967.

2. Silver, H. K.: A blueprint for pediatric health manpower for the 1970's, J. Pediatr. **82:**149-156, Jan. 1973.

3. Day, L. R., Egli, R., and Silver, H. K.: Acceptance of pediatric nurse practitioners, Am. J. Dis. Child. **119:**204-208, March 1970.

4. Schorr, T. M.: A difference in child care, Am. J. Nurs. **74:**433, March 1974.

5. American Nurses' Association, Division on Maternal and Child Health Nursing Practice, and American Academy of Pediatrics: Guidelines on short-term continuing education programs for pediatric nurse associates, Pediatr. **47:**1075-1079, June 1971.

6. Dunn, B. H.: President's message: a voice for PNP/A faculty, Pediatr. Nurs. **4:**59, July-Aug. 1978.

7. Sultz, H., Henry, O. M., and Carrell, H.: Nurse practitioners: an overview of nurses in the expanded role. In Bliss, A., and Cohen, E., eds.: The new health progressionals, Germantown, Md., 1977, Aspen Systems Corp.

8. American Academy of Pediatrics: News and comment, Evanston, Ill., 1978, the Academy.

9. McAtee, P., Zurflush, P., and Andrews, P.: Certification: a progress report, Pediatr. Nurs. **3:**26-27, Nov.-Dec. 1977.

10. American Nurses' Association: Certification programs of the American Nurses' Association Division on Practice, 1978-1979, Kansas City, Mo., The Association.

11. American Nurses' Association, Division of Maternal and Child Health Nursing Practice: Certification as a pediatric nurse practitioner, publication code CR-26 3M, Kansas City, Mo., 1978, The Association.

12. American Nurses' Association: Scope of practice for the pediatric nurse practitioner, publication code MCH-7 1M, Kansas City, Mo., 1977, The Association.

13. Spitzer, W. O.: Pediatric nurse practitioner, N. Engl. J. Med. **298:**163-164, Jan. 19, 1978.

14. Chappell, J. A., and Drogos, P. A.: Evaluation of infant care by a nurse practitioner, Pediatrics **49:**871-877, June 1972.

15. Hoekelman, R. A.: What constitutes adequate well-baby care? Pediatrics **55:**313-326, March 1975.

16. Burnip, R., et al.: Well-child care by pediatric nurse practitioners in a large group practice, Am. J. Dis. Child. **130:**51-55, Jan. 1976.

17. Duncan, B., Smith, A. N., and Silver, H. K.: Comparison of the physical assessments of children by pediatric nurse practitioners and pediatricians, Am. J. Public Health **61:**1170-1176, June 1971.

18. Hoekelman, R. A.: Pediatric nurse practitioner: analysis of potential training and utilization in New

York State, N.Y. State J. Med. **72**:1991-2000, Aug. 1, 1972.

19. Yankauer, A., et al.: The cost of training and the income generation of pediatric nurse practitioners, Pediatrics **49**:878-887, June 1972.

20. Breslau, N.: The role of the nurse-practitioner in a pediatric team: patient definitions, Med. Care **15**:1014-1023, Dec. 1977.

21. Mackay, R. C., Alexander, D. S., and Kingsbury, L. J.: Parents' attitudes towards the nurse as physician associate in a pediatric practice, Can. J. Public Health **64**:121-132, March-Apr. 1973.

22. Bullough, B., et al.: Pediatric nurse practitioners in the work setting, Pediatr. Nurs. **3**:13-18, Nov.-Dec. 1977.

23. Kahn, L., and Wirth, P.: An analysis of 50 graduates of the Washington University pediatric nursing practitioner program. Part 4: Perceptions and expectations of physicians supervisors, Nurse Pract. **3**:27-31, Jan.-Feb. 1978.

24. Lawrence, R. S., et al.: Physician receptivity to nurse practitioners: a study of the correlates of the delegation of clinical responsibility, Med. Care **15**:298-310, Apr. 1977.

25. Yankauer, A., et al.: The outcomes and service impact of a pediatric nurse practitioner training program: nurse practitioner training outcomes, Am. J. Public Health **62**:347-353, March 1972.

26. Wirth, P., Storm, E., and Kahn, L.: An analysis of the fifty graduates of the Washington University pediatric nurse practitioner program. Part 1: Scope of practice and professional responsibility, Nurse Pract. **2**:18-23, July-Aug. 1977.

27. Bates, B.: Physician and nurse practitioner: conflict reward, Ann. Intern. Med. **82**:702-706, May 1975.

28. Anderson, E. M., Leonard, B. J., and Yates, J. A.: Epigenesis of the nurse practitioner, Am. J. Nurs. **74**:1812-1816, Oct. 1974.

29. Bates, B.: Nurse-physician dyad: collegial or competitive? In Three challenges to the nursing profession: selected papers from the 1972 American Nurses' Association Convention, Publication NP-42, Kansas City, Mo., 1972, American Nurses' Association.

30. Bullough, B.: Is the nurse practitioner role a source of increased work satisfaction? Nurs. Res. **23**:14-19, Jan.-Feb. 1974.

31. DeAngelis, C., and Curran, W. J.: The legal implications of the extended roles of professional nurses, Nurs. Clin. North Am. **9**:403-409, Sept. 1974.

32. Hall, V.: The legal scope of nurse practitioners under nurse practice and medical practice acts. In Bliss, A., and Cohen, E., eds.: The new health professionals, Germantown, Md., 1977, Aspen Systems Corp.

3

Maintenance, prevention, and promotion

changing public and private sector views of individuals'
responsibility for personal health

Donald M. Watkin

The provision of health care is far from an exact science. The cost of acquiring evidence to support or to deny the validity of many of the hypotheses dealing with plans for the delivery of effective and affordable health care has been estimated to be astronomical, primarily because parameters of the success or failure of health care delivery hypotheses have such huge variances in human populations that study groups of enormous size would require investigation over many years.[1,2] In the absence of statistically acceptable scientific tests of hypotheses, society is left with the unenviable issue of how to select for implementation one or more unproved hypotheses. The alternative—the status quo—is unacceptable from the humanitarian, the economic, or the political point of view.

Confronted with an issue demanding answers, society has only one option, namely, to use the utmost prudence in choosing the hypotheses for implementation.[3,4]

In most of life's ventures prudence when exercised by highly motivated, well-trained, charismatic leadership usually pays off. Certainly in socially oriented programs like health care delivery, nothing succeeds like success.[5] However, the parameters quantifying success among the American people may be anything but scientific. The measurement of success or failure of adult-oriented health care policies is hampered by a dearth of scientifically acceptable methodology. For example, among adults there are few parameters with the precise end point and limited time frame of infant mortality. Hence popularity becomes one of the most prominent indicators of success.

The popularity of a concept in the health field may rest on many vaguely defined factors. Among these are accessibility of the physical location where the concept is being implemented; its acceptability to those it serves; its applicability to their specific needs, real or perceived; its safety, that is, its freedom from hazards or side-effects; its cost; its cost-effectiveness; and its effectiveness, something that often can be measured only in retrospect.

Self-responsibility for personal health is exactly this type of scientifically unproven but potentially effective (based on a prudent evaluation of the information that is now

29

available) concept.[6] It produces no measures of success or failure for instant evaluation. However, it does have universal accessibility (with the exception of fetuses, infants, very young children, and others who may be completely helpless and whose responsibility for personal health must be assumed by surrogates). It certainly has wide applicability. Potentially it also has acceptability, safety, low cost, and cost-effectiveness. In other words, self-responsibility for personal health has the necessary ingredients for popularity. Realization of many potentials of the concept will depend on the people who implement it and the methods they use.

The essential ingredient of popularity—whether of the personalities of the leadership or of the concept per se—has an ephemeral quality. The popularity and therefore the success of self-responsibility for personal health will depend on the caliber and the capacities of those who implement the concept as well as on the methodology, techniques, and communications skills they use in that implementation.

DEFINITIONS
Maintenance

As a concept health maintenance is applicable to all from recently conceived fetuses throughout life to centenarians (assuming, of course, that surrogates play their appropriate roles when indicated). It implies optimizing any level of health status through the judicious application of available knowledge. In terms of self-responsibility (and that of surrogates), health maintenance comprises not only prevention and promotion but also the seeking out of, and compliance with, those levels of health care advice required to optimize health status. Bringing health maintenance to and keeping it at optimal levels demand a greater understanding of the health industry than most nonprofessionals have today. The proper roles of nurses and their

assistants, pharmacists, nutritionists, therapists, social workers, and the variety of physicians must be comprehended. The right of patients, relatives, friends, and physicians themselves for consultation must be appreciated.

Prevention

The concept of prevention is applicable in various formats to all human beings. It implies the prudent application of available information and technology with a view toward avoiding absolutely (for example, in cases of accidents, drug or hormone overdosages, poisonings, suicides, electrocutions, and burns) or deferring the development of genetically ordained or unavoidable, environmentally caused diseases. As an overall objective prevention seeks to avoid or defer disability or disease, enabling mankind's standard survival curve to move toward higher survival percentages at older ages.

Promotion

Health promotion is a concept that applies to all. It includes both maintenance and prevention,[7] but it goes beyond them. Health promotion assumes a positive, constructive attitude toward health. It seeks to establish life-styles that will obviate diseases by anticipating them—not by their early detection after they have gained a foothold—and that will reduce disabilities from accidents by eliminating their causes. It furthers self-responsibility for early disease detection and for accident prevention. It advances compliance with established medical regimens prescribed for specific indications.

CHANGING PERSPECTIVES: CONFRONTING THE REALITY OF COST
Health professionals

Not long ago health care was viewed as a field so complex that only doctorate-level practitioners could assume responsibility for its management. As the health field became even more complex and the time of physicians more scarce and costly, allied health professionals began to assume authority over certain areas of health promotion—an authority gladly delegated by physicians. These allied health professionals included nurse clinicians, physicians' assistants, psychiatric social workers, psychologists, pharmacists, nutritionists, and therapists. The effectiveness as well as the cost-effectiveness of health care attributed to such delegation have resulted logically in the next step, namely, general agreement by all health professionals that persons must assume ever-increasing responsibilities in the promotion of their own health. This agreement has been accompanied by constant reinforcement of the precept that education is the first line of defense against disease and disability and also the vanguard of all efforts to promote health.

Public sector

Health professionals employed in public agencies long have been aware, at least in theory, of the necessity for diffusion of authority, the need for more and better education, and the requirement that ultimate responsibility for personal health be borne by individuals. However, there have been too few public-sector health professionals facing too many problems demanding resolution in too short a time. The result has been the practice of crisis medicine, that is, giving priority only to resolving the most pressing of immediate problems. The combined onslaughts of the frustrations created by bureaucracy, of political pressures, and more recently of demands for lower taxes have required public-sector health professionals to focus more and more on the practice of crisis medicine for the solution of immediate issues. Education has been a casualty,[8] and therefore the concepts of health promotion and self-responsibility for personal health

have been seriously disabled if not made totally inoperative. The situation has been aggravated by the continuing low pay schedules for most public-sector personnel and the practice of cutting personnel rosters through attrition. Hence, even though public health agencies should and could play leading roles in promoting health through education and the associated shift toward self-responsibility for personal health, what is happening in the public sector serves as a serious deterrent to the implementation of constructive concepts well known to all public-sector health professionals.

Private sector

Most health professionals in the private sector have placed little emphasis on health promotion and on education that advances the cause of self-responsibility for personal health. In general the private sector has stressed the diagnosis and treatment of complaints associated with existing disease, disability, or accident. While some screening is undertaken, this is usually performed as part of the differential diagnosis of the presenting complaint. Notable exceptions to these generalizations may be found among pediatricians and some obstetricians whose professions have for many years emphasized and practiced all that is implied in health promotion.

The reasons for lack of emphasis on health promotion and education in self-responsibility in the private sector are threefold:

1. Tradition has it that these are responsibilities of the public sector.
2. Private health professionals function in a system in which time is extremely valuable—so valuable that only top-priority matters receive time allotments. Demand for instruction in health promotion and self-responsibility is low; hence the supply of person-hours allotted to such matters is proportionately low.

3. The costs to private practitioners for health promotion and education in self-responsibility in the absence of public demand are too high. The public has shown itself unwilling to pay for programs designed to obviate something that has not yet and (to any specific individual) may never happen. Third-party payers such as insurance companies and even government-subsidized financing schemes have shown no willingness to assume responsibility for paying the bill.

A variant from the traditional fee-for-service format of private health care delivery has developed in this decade, namely, the health maintenance organization (HMO).[9,10] Precursors of the present generation of HMOs such as the Kaiser-Permanente Medical Care Program have flourished for many years, and the Kaiser plan in particular interprets its data as indicating success in health maintenance, defined in terms of keeping patients from needing high-cost hospital care.[11] The vast majority of HMOs, however, were demonstrations immediately preceding, or were developed as a result of, the passage of the Health Maintenance Organization Act of 1973. At present the HMOs are primarily closed-panel group practices that agree to meet the demands for the health care of patients who pay a fixed fee in advance for a broad range of services. The demands imposed are almost exclusively for curative medicine, which the consumers also demand be delivered at low cost. The concepts of maintenance, prevention, and promotion have been subordinated to the point of virtual extinction by concerns about financing, organizing, and administering the delivery of medical care services.[12]

In present HMO operations, subscriber demand for low-cost curative medicine has led to states of chronic understaffing. This in turn has necessitated the HMO's "playing catch-up," since the time, personnel, and funds are not available to promote health or educate subscribers in self-responsibility. All resources are used in "catching-up" with the diagnoses and treatments of existing diseases.

WHAT OF THE FUTURE?

As a start, the bad news must take priority; without any doubt rough times are ahead for the proponents of health promotion and education in self-responsibility. The combination of rising costs for health care and public rebellion against the high costs of government at all levels have compelled some of the strongest advocates of across-the-board health care (including health promotion) to back off from originally held positions. These include leaders in the bureaucracies and the legislative and executive branches of government, in unions, in professional organizations, and in academia. Meanwhile the public continues to be inundated with ads and fads that promise the restoration of health but that in reality often foster only the wealth of the promoters. In fact, within the health industry, controversy has erupted regarding the ethics of incentive bonuses for providers' encouraging disease prevention as a means of controlling the costly utilization of health care services.[13,14]

The bad news of the present sets the stage for a cautious appraisal of the good news. As noted above, health promotion and surrogate responsibility or self-responsibility have been long-standing and well-accepted doctrines among pediatricians and obstetricians. Fluoridation has protected the teeth of many Americans for more than three decades. An impressive reduction in cardiovascular disease mortality and morbidity rates since 1966 has occurred while the American public has been taking a greater interest in weight control, physical exercise, the hazards of smoking, and the dangers associated with uncontrolled high blood pressure.[15] Perhaps most significant is the decision of the Canadian Department of National Health and Welfare to increase emphasis on human biology, environment, and life-style and to limit expansion of the costs of health care organizations.[16,17] An improved Canadian life-style has received the greatest attention, and its promotion has received the largest increases in funding.[18] In the United States vigorous campaigns have been initiated against staggering odds to restrict the use of tobacco and to require higher standards for safety of and lower levels of potentially toxic emissions from products of the motor vehicle industry. While other bits of good news could be added, these examples suggest that some progress has already been made and that more can be achieved with suitable input to the social-economic-political-scientific agglomerate that makes up this nation, indeed the world.

Assuming that progress can be made, society must place in order of priority its greatest needs. Certainly foremost among these is *consensus*.[19] This collective opinion must be shared by far more than a majority of health professionals; it must be shared also by leaders of government at all levels, by leaders of industry, and by the ultimate consumers themselves.

Consensus in any one of these groups, let alone in all of them together, has never been achieved in the past and will not be achieved in the future without another top-priority need: *leadership*.[6] Leaders must be well informed, believable, impeccably honest and charismatic. They should regard health promotion and education in self-responsibility for personal health as the ingredients of the salvation of mankind—as well they may be. They must be willing to devote endless amounts of time and energy to the cause of overcoming obstacles that inevitably will be strewn across the path to successful implementation. Not all leaders will emerge from

the ranks of health professionals. Nonetheless, those who do not will lean heavily on health professionals for information and for advice on how to proceed. Hence health professionals will be in critical roles in getting the movement toward consensus off the ground.

The task of health professionals and of all leaders in the movement will be far easier if priority is given to a third major need: timely *evaluation* of all measures undertaken. As pointed out previously, resources to show scientifically with unquestionable statistical proof that health promotion and education in self-responsibility for personal health are effective and cost-effective clearly are not available. However, this in no way suggests that nothing in the way of evaluation should be done. It should be the responsibility of every health professional to collect, organize, and interpret whatever information can be collected during the course of project and program development and continuation. If the collection of data is well planned and their interpretation conducted in an unbiased manner, the results of such evaluations will at least provide the bases for prudent decisions on future strategy. Should they be favorable, they may be used effectively by the leadership in gaining consensus. Should they not be favorable, they may be used to demonstrate the integrity of the program's management and its determination to find new and better methods that will lead to the desired objectives.

The nation and the world are presently stalemated in resolving the problem of health maintenance and promotion. With time running out, the issue is not how to break the deadlock but rather how fast the needed consensus can be attained. Indeed, time is of the essence because, in lieu of consensus derived through rational negotiations and discussions, political and economic forces will seize authority and impose solutions.[20] A deliberately aggressive but nonetheless prudent approach—supported pari passu by prudent evaluation of interim results—would seem to offer the best solution at this time.

Regardless of how aggressive an approach is used, there is no doubt but that considerable time will be required. Since the changing of life-styles[21,22] and the induction of a new (for many) sense of self-responsibility for personal health are involved, reason alone will not prove omnipotent. The large numbers of cigarette-smoking health industry personnel, of drug users in positions of responsibility, and alcoholics among highly educated executives document this fact. However, an outstanding characteristic of the latter half of this century has been the time implosion. Experience previously mentioned with the declining mortality and morbidity from cardiovascular disease since 1966 shows what can be done without major planning in little over a decade. With the implementation of policies characterized by aggressive prudence, measurable success conceivably may be achieved in as little as 5 years. Since nothing succeeds like success, even that interval may be reduced in duration if results promulgated during that half decade provide adequate thrust for the campaign.

EPILOGUE

All health professionals have vital roles to play in forwarding the concepts of health promotion and education in self-responsibility for personal health. However, no group is more prominent in its significance to the cause than that of community nurses. Their closeness to the people with whom they work daily gives them the auras of confidants who can be approached with no vestige of fear on the entire spectrum of health-related concerns. Important also, community nurses are in a position to obtain the initial and follow-up data essential to the evaluation process.

While most nurses rightfully assume that they are already performing beyond reasonable expectations, the question may well be asked whether their performance might be improved qualitatively with greater measurable results among the people they serve for the same or even less quantitative effort. If nurses look inward, they may observe that, as individuals, they are not always practicing what they preach to their patients. They may find also that there are several mission-related areas in which the information base derived from their education, training, and experience is deficient. The deficiency may lie well beyond the conventional parameters of nursing in such fields as nutrition, pharmacology, physical medicine, political science, and economics. Once aware of what is lacking, nurses may fill the gaps by reading, course work, and field trips and by consulting with other professionals who may even be serving the same constituency. They also may serve themselves as well as other professionals by engaging whenever possible in teaching activities. Needless to say, they should take advantage of the opportunity that contact with their students provides for furthering their own education.

In terms of their role in the evaluation process, nurses who have not already done so should become familiar with the problem-oriented medical record (POMR) system. This widely used system provides an ideal means for collecting data in a format that can be used not only for resolution of ad hoc patient care problems but also for evaluation, teaching, and providing the ammunition with which to persuade the ultimate consumer to adopt progressive ideas.

Qualitative changes in daily routines may assist community nurses and all other health industry personnel to become more productive. Much of such increased productivity may be derived from devoting less time to relatively meaningless procedural controversies and more time to meaningful personal contact with patients and community leaders.

The concept of self-responsibility for personal health is here to stay. While controversy still rages over the time frame in which irresponsible patients should be expected to become accountable for their behavior, economic pressures have placed the burden of proof on those who maintain that professional ethics require continued devotion of time, effort, and resources to the maintenance of the relatively few who have the potential for, but fail to exercise, self-responsibility.

The concept of health promotion has yet to mature as a national institution. However, as the success of self-responsibility for personal health care becomes more evident, public appreciation of and demand for the concept of health promotion will rapidly further its maturation. The opportunity created by such growing demand must be seized by professionals in the health industry. Failure to do so will leave the concept open for exploitation by quacks, faddists, and commercial interests. The present fiscal crisis in health care may be the long-awaited spark igniting an explosion of public demand for and support of the efforts of health professionals to advance health promotion as an effective as well as cost-effective means of crisis resolution that is applicable to all from before conception to death, after long, happy, and productive lives.

REFERENCES

1. Ahrens, E. H., Jr.: Report of the diet-heart review panel of the National Heart Institute, Monograph No. 28, New York, 1969, American Heart Association.
2. Ahrens, E. H., Jr.: The management of hyperlipidemia: whether, rather than how, Ann. Intern. Med. **85:**87-93, 1976.
3. Breslow, L., and Somers, A. R.: The lifetime health-monitoring program: a practical approach to preventive medicine, N. Engl. J. Med. **296:**601-608, 1977.
4. Bassuk, E. L., and Cerson, S.: Deinstitutionalization and mental health services, Sci. Am. **238:**46-53, 1978.
5. Watkin, D. M.: Logical bases for action in nutrition and aging, J. Am. Geriatr. Soc. **26:**193-202, 1978.
6. Watkin, D. M.: Personal responsibility: key to effective and cost-effective health, Fam. Community Health 1:1-7, 1978.
7. Watkin, D. M.: Aging, nutrition and the continuum of health care, Ann. N.Y. Acad. Sci. **300:**290-297, 1977.
8. Shabecoff, P.: Cutbacks proposed for U.S. health aid, the New York Times, December 3, 1978, pp. 1, 38.
9. Bates, B.: Nursing in a health maintenance organization: report on the Harvard Community Health Plan, Am. J. Public Health **62:**991-994, 1972.
10. Lum, D.: The health maintenance organization delivery system: a national study of attitudes of HMO project directors on HMO issues, Am. J. Public Health **65:**1192-1202, 1975.
11. Smillie, J. G.: Operation of Kaiser-Permanente Program (correspondence), N. Engl. J. Med. **297:**63, 1977.
12. Davies, D. F.: Is HMO a euphemism? (correspondence), N. Engl. J. Med. **291:**312, 1974.
13. Giest, R. W.: Sounding board: incentive bonuses in prepayment plans, N. Engl. J. Med. **291:**1306-1308, 1974.
14. Egdahl, R. H., Taft, C. H., and Linde, K. J.: Method of physician payment and hospital length of stay (editorial), N. Engl. J. Med. **296:**339-340, 1977.
15. Levy, R. I.: Statement of Robert I. Levy, M.D., Director, National Heart, Lung and Blood Institute. In McGovern, G., Chairman: Diet related to killer diseases, II. Hearings before the Select Committee on Nutrition and Human Needs of the United States Senate, February 1-2, 1977, Committee Print No. 83-693 0. Washington, D.C., 1977, U.S. Government Printing Office.
16. Lalonde, M.: Address by the Honorable Marc Lalonde, Minister of National Health and Welfare of Canada, Pan American Conference on Health Manpower Planning, September 10-14, 1973, Ottawa, Canada, Scientific Publication No. 279, Washington, D.C., 1974, Pan American Health Organization.
17. Lalonde, M.: A new perspective on the health of Canadians: a working document, Government of Canada, Ottawa, April, 1974, Catalog No. H 31-1374, Ottawa, 1974, Information Canada.
18. Lalonde, M.: Beyond a new perspective: Fourth Annual Matthew B. Rosenhaus Lecture, 104th Annual Meeting of the American Public Health

Association, Miami Beach, Fla., October 17-21, 1976, Am. J. Public Health **67:**357-360, 1977.

19. Garrahy, J. J., and Boe, J.: Roles of the National Governors' Association and the National Conference of State Legislatures in the coalition of public interest groups seeking cost-containment (letter to the editor), Washington Post, December 2, 1978, p. 18.

20. Greenberg, D. S.: Washington report: health "reform" massacre on Capitol Hill, N. Engl. J. Med. **299:**1199-1200, 1978.

21. Belloc, N. B., Breslow, L., and Hochstim, J. R.: Measurement of physical health in a general population survey, Am. J. Epidemiol. **93:**328-336, 1971.

22. Belloc, N. B., and Breslow, L.: Relation of physical health status and health practices, Prev. Med. **1:**409-421, 1972.

PART TWO

Family life-styles today

☐ It is essential that the community health nurse understand the dynamics of today's changing family structures, changing life-styles, and all the forces from within and without that are continually impacting these evolving structures and life-styles.

Equally important is the community health nurse's understanding of and sensitivity and responsiveness to the client's cultural heritage, which determines his or her weltanschauung.

As social psychology has demonstrated, people are in constant psychosocial interchange with their cultural milieu. Through the socialization process an individual learns a system of cultural meanings, values, beliefs, and patterns of living and develops a personality and a specific way of viewing the world. An individual cannot be understood apart from an understanding of that person's social and cultural background.

Chapter 4 presents Chen-Louie's original and most insightful view of cultural interactions and the health care implications of these interactions for persons of bicultural heritage. Her conceptual framework is a practical, useful analysis of the structure of interactions among differing groups and individuals.

In Chapter 5 Jordheim ably describes alternative life-styles and family structures that have undergone rapid and radical changes in the past two decades.

Meagher, in Chapter 6, points up the need for health care professionals to become aware of the complex interactional processes involved in divorce. This awareness is essential for understanding and intelligent, effective intervention in helping clients through the divorce process and subsequent problems of coping with the stressors involved in being a single parent.

In Chapter 7 Cross gives us a clear, concise discussion of child abuse that points out the need for collaborative efforts between community health care professionals and emphasizes the need for objective evaluation and research of this growing problem. The material will help readers increase their understanding and improve their ability and skills in detecting potential and actual child abuse situations.

An insightful paper contributed by Chulada, Chapter 8 updates for the reader the progress in family planning efforts in recent years and the programs that have been evolving throughout the nation. Among the challenges cited by the author are the need to expand services, to obtain adequate funding for programs, and to prepare adequately educated health care personnel to provide services. Also cited as needs in family planning are the development of improved contraceptive methods, expanded public education and outreach programs, and increased funding, through federal and private sources, of local agencies and organizations. The writer further calls for more competent management of programs in the field of family planning.

37

4

Bicultural experiences, social interactions, and health care implications

Theresa T. Chen-Louie

WHO ARE THE BICULTURAL PEOPLE?

When I think of a bicultural person, I immediately have the image of an immigrant who has grown up in one culture and has been transplanted into another. Along with the set of values and attitudes he has, he adopts the culture and customs of the new land. On the other hand, there are bicultural people who are natives of the land in which they live. They have their set of customs and values, and outsiders who come to trade or invade their land bring in their attitudes and culture. Whether or not the natives will accept the outside culture will depend on the political status of the outsiders and/or the usefulness of the new culture to the natives. As an example, the native Americans were colonized and their culture was systematically discounted by the invaders. When the white culture was thrust upon the native Americans through education and health care while their land was confiscated, there was a passive resistance to adopting the white culture. This is in sharp contrast to the European immigrants who have come to this country to find a new livelihood. They have been absorbed into America's expanding frontier and developing labor market; and further,

they had a common achievement goal. It was more natural for the European immigrant to adopt the new culture for it was more akin to their own. The degree to which they retain their Old World values depends on their economic and survival exigencies.

The treatment of the Asians, blacks, and Mexicans and Hispanics has been systematic discrimination and stratification. They are relegated to devalued occupations, restricted from acquisition of property, and excluded from immigration. The dominant society knows little about their culture and when you ask people to identify the cultures with which they are not familiar, they will single out the Asian, Hispanic, black, and occasionally the American Indian. By the same token, you may ask a black, American Indian, Hispanic, or Asian the culture with which he is not familiar and chances are he will indeed name a minority culture before he will the "white, American" culture. How do you account for the fact that European white ethnics are considered not very different from American culture? American Indians have been in this country longer than white settlers and blacks have been here at least as long; yet neither heritage is familiar to the nation as a whole.

White and nonwhite have taken it for granted that the white culture of the developed nations is dominant to that of the Third World.

CONCEPTS RELATED TO BICULTURISM

Anthropologists have been foremost among those calling attention to our cultural differences. Some broad concepts that are drawn from their literature are cultural shock, ethnocentrism, acculturation, assimilation, value discrepancies, and value imposition.[1] They caution the health workers to be sensitive to the role that culture plays in the life of people. To introduce technology into undeveloped countries, they suggest a principle that can be applied to any kind of change in bicultural situations: to institute change in an established culture one must find out about that culture and identify something that it has in common with the principle of the proposed change. It is important that the health worker be in tune with the customs and values of the client; to build rapport with a client from a different culture, we need to reach the client, which includes looking for communication cues to cross-cultural values and customs.[2]

Sociologists focusing on families, groups, and institutions have given health workers these frames of reference, which may be helpful in analyzing behavior: families of differing cultures and groups of differing races, stratification of different cultural groups in society, as well as the economic and political stratification of minorities by institutions.[3] Some of the sociopsychological concepts that these frames of reference bring to mind are prejudice, discrimination, alienation, anomie, and conflict.[4-6]

NEED FOR OPERATIONALIZED CONCEPTS FOR HEALTH WORKERS

The behavioral concepts listed so far deal with different cultures on a macroscopic level. These concepts and theories have not come to grips with the power issues in human relationships vis-à-vis cultural differences. Both individual and institutional racism are still based on a conflict model and fail to express the nuances of power struggles, that is, the "topdog" and "underdog" statuses and their consequences in interactants' reflected self-appraisals. Furthermore, as observer and participants of daily interaction, a health worker needs to have a handle on operationalized concepts in order to deal with the day-to-day pluses and minuses of face-to-face encounters. To help develop a sensitivity toward another culture, we need to have some knowledge and overall understanding of the historical, social, and cultural experiences of the people. We must identify the groups of bicultural people who are experiencing the most poignant and oppressive experiences, because they are under greater environmental stresses than other groups. Finally, we need to develop closer interaction with these bicultural groups. We do not necessarily have to know the minute details of cultural differences. It is far more important to know how to treat people who are different—people whom we too often unintentionally consider "less" than we are.

When bicultural speakers share their cultural differences, their central message is "Treat us as individuals." Behavioral scientists advocate the comparison of cultural differences as a stepping stone toward recognizing people's cultural uniqueness. It is interesting to listen to bicultural speakers identifying cultural differences for the audience. They get highly charged and tell the audience that it is not health workers' ignorance of cultural diversity that hurts them; it is how they treat bicultural people, discounting them, that infuriates them. The caution we can draw from this is that we may think that just being aware of the differences will sensitize us. Rather before we can get a handle on sensitive caring, we must identify our behavior, our interactive processes and communication, which discount cultural diversity and therefore individual dignity.

In this chapter I will cover the concept of biculturism and its historical evolution as well as the phenomenon of bicultural experiences and their implications for the nursing profession.

DIFFERENTIATING TERMS RELATED TO BICULTURISM

The term "bicultural groups" implies that the groups straddle two cultures, life-styles, and sets of values. Since bicultural can imply an ethnic or racial mixture, let us first review the differences among ethnicity, race, minority, and subculture.

The members of an ethnic group possess a common ancestry, a sense of historical and cultural uniqueness. Their social and cultural heritage is passed on from generation to generation. They may share a common linguistic, national, racial, and/or religious origin.[7,8]

Race is a biological term, and a racial population results from past breeding patterns. The group members thus share distinguishing physical features—for example, skin color, hair type, and facial features—and genetic traits such as blood grouping, hemoglobin variation, and serum enzymes.[9] Ethnic and racial groups may overlap: for example Chinese and Japanese Americans are one racial group; Chinese Buddhists and Japanese Buddhists can also be considered one ethnic group, if Greely's definition of ethnic group is used.[10] In a single ethnic and racial group, the biological and cultural similarities can reinforce one another. The group that is mixed both ethnically and racially may have specific racial features and therefore its members are identified more readily by their physical characteristics than by their unique cultural patterns. By maintaining a biological and sociocultural distinction as well as a shared sense of solidarity, the ethnic and racial group may become isolated from the dominant cultural group. A bicultural group can be an ethnic group or a combined ethnic and racial group; the second culture of the bicultural group, of course, is the dominant culture of the society. A minority group is so designated because of its limited access to power in a society; at the same time the group is assumed to have inferior traits and undesirable characteristics.[6,11] And a bicultural group is definitely a minority in the society. Bicultural groups therefore share a common ancestry and a unique culture through history as they pass on their cultural heritage. The group may also share common physical features and genetic traits. Subcultural groups may be part of either a dominant or a minority group: they may share both ethnic and racial characteristics with the larger group of which they are a part. Because of the uniqueness of their life situations, however—their philosophy perhaps, their ideology, or their age, gender, or social class—they share a common culture different from that of the larger cultural group, which includes both the dominant and the minority groups. Thus we see that these groups, like adolescents, the poor, or prison inmates, have their own subcultures.

BICULTURAL GROUPS VERSUS MINORITIES

As is apparent, bicultural groups encompass many different groups, each of which has a common ancestry, and all have come into contact with another culture. In the United States there are many bicultural groups. Each bicultural group is considered to be a minority within the country's total population. However, many eastern and southern European groups share certain biological characteristics with the Anglo-Saxons and other northern Europeans. Although they have retained their cultural integrity, many have made inroads into the political and economic sectors and thus are considered part of the dominant group. The chasm created by cultural, political, and economic inequality remains unbridged between the dominant group and the Third World minority groups.

The fact that we are using "bicultural" and "bilingual" to refer to Third World minorities instead of just "minority" reflects a more humanistic approach. It implies a respect for and an acknowledgment of the culture of the immigrant or the minority group. During the 1960s people in human services urged workers to be sensitive to prejudice and discrimination. In the 1970s and 1980s we have been more inclined to consider the cultural rights of minorities, to have an awareness of bicultural life experiences. Our attitudes have been going through a subtle change as the Third World minorities have been developing sociopolitically in this country. At the same time, sociocultural theories have gone through successive stages of evolution, as is discussed below.

THEORETICAL EVOLUTION IN BICULTURISM

The social sciences in America have their origin in Europe, and theorists have been imbued with the European world view. The early American social scientists viewed their discipline from the white man's perspective. It is only in the last decade that we have seen theoretical analyses that are indigenous to the multicultural society of America. In the past, theories dealing with bicultural experiences focused on the status of immigrants, dominant/minority group conflicts, and value discrepancies; white and nonwhite theorists studied the problems of the minorities as well as their deviant behavior from the point of view of a normative white culture. Only within the last decade or so have nonwhite social scientists articulated the academic racism within the social sciences and postulated theories based on minority experiences.[12,13] Examples of theories on biculturism, ad-

dressed below, show the changing focus from assimilation, to theories oriented toward pathology, to victimization and paternalism, and finally to cultural identities.

Assimilation

In the latter part of the nineteenth century, the influx of European immigrants and black slaves were plunged into the expansion of a frontier economy and the promotion of industrial and urban growth. The story of the immigrants was hard work and long hours in the land of opportunity, but they would experience success and become a part of America. Americanization, however, was never really to include the blacks, the native Americans, and to some extent, the Chicanos and Asians.[14,15] Parks developed a theory of the race relation cycle. According to him, when dominant and minority groups come into contact, their relationship and interactions are characterized by competition, accommodation, and finally, assimilation.[16] Implicitly the goal is toward integration. The idea of the "melting pot" was that the multicultural groups would coexist in a more or less integrated society. Assimilation presupposed conformity to the norms of the majority white values, and the disappearance of the cultural heritage of the minorities as they took on the customs and values of the larger society. It never occurred to the dominant groups that ethnic and racial groups would want to retain their cultures. Neither has the dominant group been aware that through their own cultural ideology and Protestant heritage, they are proponents of individualism based on dominance and control, competition and appropriation. They have therefore perpetuated the cultural disparity.[17]

Pathological orientation: social deviance

The melting pot theory did not stand the test of reality. As social scientists observed the plight of minorities, they came to label the phenomenon as pathological. Focusing their research on the low-income minorities, they explained that the problem with racial minorities stemmed from the disintegration of families, for example, broken families, premarital promiscuity, illegitimacy, juvenile delinquency, perpetual unemployment, and welfare dependency.[18-20] Disorganized families lead to social disorganization and community disintegration. As they have with the germ theory, scientists have isolated the causative agent for these problems; they have found it to be the minority culture itself, which manifests itself through laziness and lack of motivation, in short, the welfare culture. Behaviors that are unlike the ideal, white, normative behavior are considered deviant. Thus mental health workers are inclined to label bicultural patients as sick and their family patterns as pathological.[21,22]

Victimization and paternalism

Scholars who use the dominant group as a referent with which to compare them see minority groups as deviant; those who focus on the minority experiences perceive the historical, political, and economical determinants as leading to the subjugation of minority groups. Blauner, in recent years, observed Western colonization of non-Western people throughout the world. He found a parallel in the United States: the domination of the Third World—and the black experiences in particular—amounts to domestic colonialism. The labor systems in this country destroy and weaken the culture, even the communal ties of people of color. Racial stratification, domination through class, and economic exploitation all work toward efficient control of the minorities and economic profit for the majority.[12] This theory explains the fact that the plight of the minorities is rooted in other than their intrinsic familial or personality problems.

The pathology-laden theories were rein-forced by the traditional response from the dominant society to the minorities—the rescue approach. From the settlement houses and charities of the pre-Roosevelt years to the full-scale welfare institutions of the New Deal and the War on Poverty of the Johnson era, the political reality has been to help the disadvantaged. The response to the effects of domestic colonialism has been paternalism, not unlike the way a good master treats his slave. While dollars were being poured into deprived areas to bring them up to code, we continued to find a prevailing racial privilege and cultural domination.

Cultural identities

Bicultural scholars and writers have been searching for their cultural identities although there are no specific codified theories advanced as yet. Trapped by the assimilation theory and the illusion of white supremacy, people of color have been viewing themselves as the dominant culture had led them to believe—that they are in fact inferior. When they examine the realities of their self-concept, their own appraisals have become filled with self-hatred.[23-25] In the meantime, some Black social scientists have offered another type of literature highlighting the strengths of their people.[26] "Black is beautiful" is a cultural and political slogan that has awakened other bicultural minorities to reexamine their cultural identity. The consensus emerging from the bicultural literature is that, as long as the economic and social status of the minorities continues, the experience of alienation will continue. The focal issue is that survival under adverse conditions must be brought forth and duly acknowledged as an unassailable strength of the people.[27] For example, in a family with a dishwasher father and sweatshop sewer mother, the focus is not only on the family scene where the parents are not present or the children are without supervision. Amidst the frustrations of poverty and oppression, the children must take on the spiritual strength of the toiling parents in order to acquire the necessities for survival. The family's value lies not only in what they learned in the old country: their heritage is the unique bicultural heritage distilled from their experiences and social status in this country.

Bicultural identities derive from a blending of values from various cultures, particularly those that are learned from the primary group settings as well as from contact with a different culture, for example, from either the dominant group or other minority groups. There is a dialectical relationship of the values that are accepted; sometimes they are in consonance and sometimes at dissonance. Beyond the accepted values, there are other values that may impinge on the person. Sometimes the person is swept up in the trends; at other times he selects to be apart from the pressure and hazard and the consequence of being buffeted by them. In the process of value incorporation, there can be either harmony or conflict or both, which in turn are affected by external events, sociopolitical movements, and/or the community's bicultural orientation as well as by the degree of cohesiveness of the primary groups. As many bicultural social scientists have pointed out, the conflicts arising from bicultural people's struggle within the sociopolitical realities and their coping with racism are greater than their value discrepancies of Old World versus New World differences.

DEGREES OF BICULTURAL IDENTIFICATION

Bicultural people may be aware of their cultural identities. On the other hand, if their life experiences are involved with much struggle for survival, their sense of bicultural identity is certainly not in the forefront. Their primary concerns are the urgency to survive and constant battles with oppressive frustra-

tions. Based on the assimilation model, stages of acculturation may be identified; thus the typology of assimilation. The traditional person is secure in Old World values and hence experiences less conflict. The marginal man is trapped in the conflict of ambivalence. He accepts neither Old World nor New World values and is himself accepted by neither group. The bicultural person is supposed to work out his loyalties and come to a new identity.[28,29] The limitation of such a typology is that it contains too few variables in the process of adaptation.* As I pointed out earlier, one's bicultural identity is an evolutional process with forward and backward movements and static moments as well. The blending of values may create consonance as well as dissonance within the person. There are many considerations along the evolution of their bicultural identities.

Early in this century the economic and occupational opportunities were proliferating as the country was expanding industrially. The country's resources were able to meet the demands of the workforce. There was a place and function in the society for the immigrants; they inherited the land and its opportunities and became adapted to the ways of this country. During this same period Third World immigrants and former slaves were the labor force that built the country. Racism deprived them of the opportunity to gain a higher sociopolitical status. The movement to Americanize immigrants, especially after World War I, followed the ideal of the assimilation model.[30] Interestingly, until the 1950s

---

*Cultural values of the Old World and the New World are not the only variables affecting bicultural people. Culture is not an unbroken continuity: history, racism, politics, economics, and media are a few macroscopic variables that come into play. Ben Tong enunciated many caustic criticisms against simplistic analysis in "A Living Death Defended as the Legacy of the Superior Culture" (Amerasia 2:178-202, Fall 1974).

and 1960s even minorities considered themselves to be "assimilated"; they denied experiencing prejudice.* Not until the 1970s, when separate bicultural identity was recognized, did people acknowledge that they were different, that they were discriminated against but were basically praiseworthy. In the past three decades of relative peace and technological advances, we gradually have come to realize the ultimate limitation of our resources. Job and capital are and will be limited, and the competition between white and nonwhite will become more intense; the success of one will lead to the exclusion of the other. While the struggle for civil rights has made some headway with a mandate for school integration and affirmative action in employment, a beginning backlash has ensued in the name of "stop busing" and accusations of "reverse discrimination." The development of bicultural identities is influenced by these political currents. Just as the reverberation of "Black is beautiful" spurred racial consciousness and bicultural identification, so, too, the blockage in civil rights progress may indeed leave its mark.

There are different variables in the consideration of bicultural identities: (1) chronology or duration in the country, (2) language facility, (3) location of residence in relation to ethnic population concentration, (4) educational and economic opportunities, (5) neighborhood conditions, (6) bicultural services available in the community, (7) cumulative racist encounters, (8) primary group cohesion, and (9) self-concept and its function of culture retention.* There are different degrees within each variable; each variable has its continuum with stages and conditions (Table 1). For example, the language facility continuum moves from "non-English-speaking" toward "learning English" at one end. On the other end, there is "English-speaking only"—the native-born bicultural person who may be oriented toward the mainstream culture. The continuum does not necessarily represent a movement from conditions that are blocking to conditions that are enhancing bicultural identities. A bicultural person may be on different points of the continuum at different times. The different points on the continuum serve to show the complexities of bicultural identities. In other words, the variables are not correlated in a linear fashion, that is, the reader cannot read across the page and connect all of the first conditions listed in each variable and arrive at a conclusion about bicultural identity. The variables listed in Table 1 include those that are related to cultural as well as to social, economic, and environmental variables. Duration in the country is no longer an index of acculturation and assimilation. One person may represent the tenth generation in this country but may have been raised in an environment not conducive to bicultural identity; he may be unemployed and may not articulate well to the larger culture. Another person may be a first-generation immigrant who is a highly sought nuclear physicist even though he possesses limited English-speaking ability. In the section on cultural enrichment, the reader may get a

---

*Many bicultural people claimed to be "Americans" while they were treated as foreigners. A prime example was Senator Daniel Inoye: a decorated soldier, he was treated as a "Jap"—a story he repeated in conferences and on television. In my survey of Chinese American identities in 1966, most of my respondents claimed that they were "Americanized" and were "not discriminated against."

---

*Koshi listed eight continua of cultural variables affecting practitioners'/clients' perceptions and responses. The continua purportedly alleviate the tendency to treat individuals as a group entity. Koshi's variables do not, however, deal sufficiently with bicultural people's identities and experiences with racism. (Koshi, P.: Cultural diversity in the nursing curricula, J. Nurs. Ed. **15**:14-21, March 1976.)

Table 1. Cultural continua with variables affecting bicultural identities

Duration in country	Language facility	Residence and ethnic concentration	Educational opportunity	Economic opportunity	Neighborhood condition
Recent immigrant	Illiterate	Separated from dominant group	School values and teaching incongruent with reality experience	Unskilled	Run-down neighborhood; crime ridden, with economic stagnation
First generation; immigrated during adulthood	Non-English-speaking	Ghetto with high concentration of same cultural group	Truant or dropout	Skilled but skill not marketable	Congested; insufficient housing and dense populations
First generation; immigrated during childhood	Learning English; finding difficulty in retention	Breaking into exclusive dominant-group residences with no other bicultural groups	Bilingual education with encouragement to learn about own culture	Highly skilled but language deficit	Government supported; plans for rejuvenation
Second generation	Has mastered English	Semi-integrated residence with few residents of same bicultural group	Remedial education for non-English-speaking pupils	Skilled but market is discriminatory	Tourist showcase with active commerce
Third generation	Bilingual abilities	Integrated residence with multicultural groups	Integrated education; acknowledges contribution from minority culture	Skilled and employed	Active commerce owned and operated by same cultural group servicing community
Later generations	English-speaking only			Highly sought technical skill	Safe integrated neighborhood with cooperative community members

better sense of the application of the variables.

Bicultural life-style

I have previously discussed the myth of the melting pot. Immigrants from a different culture transplanted to a new land may share some common experiences in terms of culture shock, value discrepancies, and discrimination. For the sake of survival they may be keenly aware of their national or racial pride and of a need for achievement, for keeping in

Bicultural community services	Racist encounter	Self-concept	Primary group cohesion	Function for culture retention
Absence of human and cultural services except debt/credit services (loan shark, pawn shop) | Has places for worship | Cultural preservation services: ethnic media (newspaper, radio, television), ethnic school, folk medicine | Bilingual; health and social welfare services | Advocacy services (legal services); affirmative action services against discrimination	Dominative racist encounter | Aversive racist encounter | Cultural racist encounter within these institutions: legal (including penal system), educational, and occupational	Low self-concept; despair; apathetic | Low self-concept; self-hatred | Conflictual; ambivalent | Self-esteem, valuing culture	No sense of belonging | No stability in family | No peer or other reference group | Sense of caring in family or reference group expressed nonverbally | Sense of cohesion in family or reference group | Miscegenation: from in-group rejection to acceptance | Acceptance and cohesion in integrated reference group	For survival, retaining old culture, or evolving pattern by necessity (single-female household or family working as one economic unit) | Culture retention to counteract alienation | Culture retention to preserve family or group cohesion | Sharing of culture with others who appreciate it | Disseminating cultural values

close contact within the family and kinship system, and for gravitating around the ethnic community. As their economic opportunity and occupational status changes, their mobility and separation from the ethnic community may give a semblance of "assimilation." Their life-styles may alter with socioeconomic and ecological changes; for example, having obtained middle-class status, they provide themselves with the goods and services they can now afford. The assimilation model explains that these people would indeed be acculturated. It does not explain the reality that these people do not give up their bicultural identities; nor are they usually freed from racial discrimination. They may have unique bicultural experiences in spite of their middle-class life-style. On the other hand, the life-style of the immigrants may tend to be closely linked with the goods and services provided by the bicultural communities. Again, depending on the immigrant's position in regard to the different variables described above, he may indeed have a life-style more comparable to his corresponding social class.

If life-style differences are based more on social class and material availability, how are the bicultural people different from the people in the mainstream culture? The differences evolve from their cultural enrichment as well as from their persistent struggle against racism.* One may say the former is their support system; the latter, their perennial problem. A review of the variables that affect bicultural identity will point up cultural enrichment as well as deprivation as a result of racism.

Cultural enrichment

A bicultural neighborhood provides essential cultural services to the people. The ethnic concentration of bicultural community services, education, and occupational opportunities may enhance one's bicultural identity and cultural enrichment. However, the effects on bicultural people may not always be helpful. I will use San Francisco as an example to illustrate the cultural effects of Chinatown.

The Chinese population in San Francisco has increased to approximately 10% of the city's total population.[31] Not only is there a Chinatown in the city, but there is also a large residential area that is gradually being occupied by Chinese. A new commercial district has developed for the residents who find Chinatown too far to go for their goods and services. Chinatown continues to be rich in culture and community services. Those who live in Chinatown can mingle with their own ethnic group. There are many ethnic newspapers, bookstores, and grocery and herb stores. There are several Chinese theaters as well as Chinese radio and television programs. Chinese-financed and Chinese-owned businesses serve both the local residents and non-Chinese. Families continue to keep Chinese festivals while the lunar New Year is billed as a tourist attraction promoted by the city and the Chinese Chamber of Commerce. There are multiple bilingual churches including those of the Buddhist, Protestant, and Catholic denominations. Bilingual education in the public schools and in ethnic schools in the afternoons after regular school provides some cultural heritage for the young. There are many bilingual health and welfare services for the non-English-speaking residents that utilize government-sponsored income maintenance and housing programs. Furthermore, there are bilingual legal services and affirmative action advocates to defend immigration and racial discrimination cases. Chinatown is a vigorous bilingual bicultural community. Those who encounter overt or covert racism are more likely to find helpful support in such a community. Those who cannot compete in the dominant labor market can find menial, though often exploited, occupation within the business community. Those who cannot find work within or outside of the community, for example, the youths

---

*Bicultural experiences include the blending of popular culture and one's own cultural enrichment along with interracial struggles. Cole sees black culture as consisting of three components: American mainstream (material culture, values, and behavioral patterns), minority sense (continued need to detect hostility for self-protection), and blackness (the unique inputs of being black with all of the cultural heritage that African and American entails). (Cole, J.: Culture: Negro, black and nigger, Black Scholar 1:40-44, 1970.)

who drop out of school, are alienated. They have not sought support within the available services; indeed they terrorize and extort from the merchants instead.

Immigrants find a great deal of support within the community to enhance their survival and ease their transition to this country. Many middle-class business and professional people have found occupations within the community, which keeps them in close contact with the culture; their life-style, however, may be middle class. They might have moved to other residential districts but they continue to work in the ethnic community. The alienated youths, on the other hand, have not been able to utilize the environmental options to enhance their self-concepts and cultural identities.

Compare the bicultural community of Chinatown with the small bicultural Mexican-American population in Richmond, California. There is no visible ethnic community there except for a few grocery stores that carry some ethnic food. Newspapers and books must be purchased from Mexican-American communities elsewhere. There is one social agency serving Spanish-speaking people. The scope of the service is limited by the lack of bilingual personnel. Health and welfare services are available only in the white community, and the workers there have no bilingual capabilities. Even though bilingual education has been mandated, there are not enough bilingual teachers to provide the needed education. Then, too, the school district's administrative concern is with revenue cuts, program eliminations, and mainstreaming rather than with bilingual education for a small number of students. There is little bicultural exposure in the local community. People do not have the environmental option and cultural enrichment that the San Francisco Chinatown residents do. In such a community the preservation of Mexican culture will have to be generated through the family network.

There are also fewer supportive services for the immigrants' survival. Isolated Spanish-speaking professionals work in a community controlled both economically and politically by white, English-speaking people. The people there encounter greater frustration and more racial strife. Their lack of a sense of ethnic solidarity does not enhance their bicultural identity.

The family is a primary source for cultural continuity. Customs and values are cultivated on a day-to-day basis without the members' even being aware of the fact. Ethnic food preferences and taboos; the use of herbs, if any; health beliefs and practices; customs for courtship, marriage, birth, and dying; gender role; and child rearing are carried out. Morals, religion, work values, achievement, time, and relation to nature and society are infused into daily practices and parental admonitions. A sense of privacy, territoriality, interpersonal etiquette, and communication patterns are generated first within the family network.

Today bicultural families, except those that are newly transplanted, are sharing more characteristics with the rest of the society. Families are becoming more mobile, although adults resist mobility and remain in old neighborhoods. Families are becoming smaller with fewer extended members. Both parents work, and the mother is less a central nurturing person and more an operating head of the household. Other relatives may enter to partake in the socialization of the young. Family roles are not as rigidly defined as in early immigrant days. They are more open and equalitarian. Family members may be more involved with reference groups so that the family spends less time together as a social unit. Although family members may be geographically distant, they can be called upon as back-up support during emotional and financial crises.[32]

Along with bicultural personal identities,

families are changing and adapting. Cultural values do not disappear but are blended with prescriptions found in the popular culture to become new forms. Bicultural people who are in similar socioeconomic statuses as their counterparts in the dominant culture share many common values and life-styles. The degree of their cultural value rentention is dependent on customs practiced within the families. They may have no political ties with their native countries. However, when any domestic or international affairs involving an ethnic or national confrontation with the major culture occurs, bicultural people are put into a suspicious position. Witness the Japanese-Americans' internment during World War II.

The old country may lose meaning at one time, only to gain new meaning at another. Today a fifth-generation ethnic may travel to the old country to search for his roots because cultural meaning has taken on a new perspective. One's old-world culture is therefore not a concrete entity that melts away as one lives in the new country for generations. Environmental, socioeconomic, and political import impact cultural identities more than the assimilation model has intimated.

Problems with racism

Preference for one's race is called racism, while preference for one's own ethnic group is labeled ethnocentrism. White racism has another dimension: power, that is, control and influence over the other races. Jones defines it thus:

Racism results from the transformation of race prejudice and/or ethnocentrism through the exercise of power against a racial group defined as inferior, by individuals and institutions with the intentional or unintentional support of the entire culture.[33]

Kovel differentiates two types of racism: the dominative and the aversive. The dominative racist is one who demonstrates openly his racial hatred and acts out his bigoted beliefs. The aversive racist tries to be polite, correct, and cold to avoid interracial contact. He does not act out overtly his belief of his own racial superiority.[34] The aversive racist can espouse liberal causes and yet does not really treat members of other races as equals. Jones points out yet another type of racism: cultural racism in which the racial superiority is institutionalized in the culture. Institutional racism includes established laws, customs, and practices that systematically reflect and produce racial inequality. Institutional racism is a major force that perpetuates racism by transmitting cultural values and socializing individual racists. Institutions are racist whether the people who maintain such practices have racist intentions or not. For instance, school admissions and frequently job openings are based on test scores. Yet tests can be culturally biased against minorities. The practice of using Anglo tests, for example, is a form of cultural racism. Bicultural people encounter cultural racism continuously. It is the most insidious and most difficult type of racism to deal with because it is deeply embedded. It creeps up without reason and often unintentionally. On such an occasion the majority member may be embarrassed while the minority member feels awkward, if not angry and frustrated. The problems of bicultural people stem from the unequal distribution of resources and power in the society and are linked to various forms of racism. Yet identifying the racist issues can lead to still more conflict, for instance, provoking the anger of American white ethnics. Nor does it negate the struggle that Third World bicultural people must constantly face. Cultural racism is pervasive and extends into all aspects of daily living, including the health care system; the most profound consequences are found in the economic, educational, and legal domains.

Within the health care system, bicultural people encounter insensitivities to their personal dignity as well as to their health needs. There is a lack of bicultural and bilingual health care workers. Should they be admitted to the health professional schools, they may find that the educational content is biased; that the institution fosters racist practices and that instructors and students also are frequently racist. They find both racist clients and co-workers within the health care system. The problem is that as well intentioned and "humanistic" as health workers and institutions claim they are or want to be, cultural racism is so pervasive that they have taken racism for granted. However, bicultural people are keenly aware of their being depersonalized in the health care system.

As health care workers we need to recognize our own racism in day-to-day practice. In the following section we will examine interactional racism with examples derived from the health education or health service institutions—teacher/student, student/student, and health professional/client interactions.

Phenomenon of discounting

The predominant interactive process of racism is discounting. Discounting expresses one's ethnocentric or racist attitudes through the communication process, attributing the "one-up" position to one's own or group and assigning the "one-down" position to the bicultural person or group. The discounting of bicultural persons may be effected through direct communication or indirect comment. Discounting can communicate dominative, aversive, or cultural racism. When discounting takes place in a face-to-face encounter, the relationship derived from the interaction is that of distrust, and the stage is set for offensive and defensive acts. The problem for the bicultural person is that power statuses are unequal within society—an inequality

that will filter through to the interactional scene.

There are a number of subprocesses in the phenomenon of discounting and each has its corresponding type of racism:

1. Degrading (dominative racism)
2. Despising (aversive racism)
3. Depersonalizing or stereotyping (cultural racism)
4. Disguising (aversive racism)
5. Condescending (cultural racism)
6. Fearing (aversive racism)

In all of these processes the communicator sends messages that do not enhance the other's self-concept. If the communicator is commenting about the bicultural third party, the appraisal is overtly or covertly negative. Communications like these actualize racism.

Degrading is communicating overtly that the bicultural person is definitely inferior and unworthy. Black health workers are particularly familiar with degrading remarks directed against them:

"Don't touch me with your black hands!" a patient tells the nurse. There are many patients who specify that they do not want "colored" nurses to take care of them. Some will not take medicine from bicultural nurses.

A nursing instructor comments: "I know who would complain about not getting their assignments or important information—the Black students, because they're always late to their clinical!"

A white nurse's aide reports that the patients' families consult her about the patients' condition instead of talking to the black registered nurses or to the black head nurse on duty.

The preceding examples show that overt dominative racism can be a conscious expression (as in the first case), the result of careless rumors thought to be based on fact (as in the second case), or a remark made unmindfully (as in the third case). Degrading messages frequently call forth anger in the recipients.

Despising is communicating covertly that the bicultural person is inferior or intolerable. This form of communication is very common, as it is closely linked to ethnocentrism.

"Don't get hysterical. You Latins are so emotional." says a health worker to the client.

"Those Indians must have lied. Everyone who came in to see the patient claimed to be a sister or brother. There were a dozen of them!" comments a nurse.

"Don't go to the herbalist or witch doctor; they're quacks!" recommends a nurse to the client.

A liaison nurse making a referral to the public health nurse reports the multiple health problems of a young Black client and ends with a comment that if the patient were not Black she would probably not be in "such a mess."

One nursing student comments to another about their peer, "I don't know what Leona is saying half the time; she has such a heavy accent. How can anyone ever understand Filipino English?"

A nursing instructor confides, "I have this Chinese student I don't know how to deal with. She won't say much. She's so passive aggressive."

A nursing supervisor asks a Korean nurse repeatedly, "Now do you understand me? Are you sure you understand?"

The problem with the process of despising is that the communicator seems to express vaguely some concern on the one hand but prejudice on the other. The receiver of the message feels uncomfortable and cannot quite legitimately come back with a counterattack because of the quasi-good-intentioned double message.

Depersonalizing or stereotyping is addressing a bicultural person as though that person had no personal identity. The message is that a bicultural person is just a clone of the rest of the group.

As a Chinese nursing instructor, I have been called "Taiko" many times by colleagues and secretaries, including a black secretary. Taiko is a Japanese-American who had been teaching a few years before I arrived on the scene.

Nurses interviewing patients make assumptions such as, "Do you go to see herbalists?" "Do you eat rice every day?" "Do you live with your mother-in-law?" "I know that the Mexicans have a lot of beans in their diet. Do you like beans?"

Stereotyping is a negative act, for example, imposing a characteristic on a bicultural person who may not possess that characteristic. For example, one may assume that a Chinese immigrant would get a great deal of support from his relatives, since ethnics are known to be "clannish." Or, American Indians "have problems with alcoholism"; any disheveled Indian may be suspected to be intoxicated.

Health workers are urged to learn more about the cultural diversity of their clients. The hazard of a little knowledge is that, when applied and generalized, the communicator is actually placing preconceptions on the bicultural person. As I have pointed out before, there are varying types and degrees of bicultural identities. Having the physical characteristics of a racial or ethnic group does not make one a carbon copy of the rest of the group.

Disguising is sending a message by using symbols or metaphors that have both positive and negative connotations. The communication appears ostensibly to be positive or even complimentary. It may, in fact, be so intended. However, because of the negative stereotyping of ethnics, the message conveys an unsavory aspect to the receiver. The sender may or may not be aware of the consequence. He may even consider it humorous. The bicultural receiver, having been in the one-down position in multiple situations, is particularly sensitive to the negativity and does not appreciate a joke at his expense. Such a double message is difficult to deal with, especially since part of the message is hidden or implied. The receiver would be considered defensive or ungracious if he should remark about the subtle offense. The sender can always insist that there is no negativity intended or implied.

Like the Asian elementary students whom their teachers love because they are "good in math" and have "excellent manners," Asian nursing students are know to be "quiet" and "conscientious."

Making small talk with Asian patients, a health worker comments, "I just love to go to Chinatown and eat in the noisy native restaurants." Health workers are heard to like Chinese patients for they are so "compliant" and Japanese patients for they are "stoic and don't complain."

A male patient once commented to me that he was glad to see me and that he really "missed" his "Lotus Blossom." My student nursing friends nicknamed me "sexy Susie Wong." The American images of Chinese women portrayed by the media are limited to quaint beautiful sex objects.

In all of the above examples, the message senders overtly expressed compliments. The symbols they used in these cases indicated a lack of praiseworthiness; nor would they be likely to apply those same symbols to themselves. The underlying racism was disguised. However, the bicultural person would know and feel the discrepancies in the double messages. The message sender may protest that the bicultural person seems to "look for" negativity. But then only if one has been oppressed would one sniff out the disguise without having to look for it.

The next two communication processes frequently take place indirectly; that is, comments about the persons are not made in front of the bicultural persons. They are aversive and cultural racist processes. In the condescending process the message sender may not want to embarrass directly the bicultural person. In fearing, avoidance attempts are made to create greater distance and thus ensure the "safety" of the message sender.

Condescending is communication whereby the message sender conveys pity, sympathy, or disdain. The focus of the message is on the abject and degrading position of the bicultural person. The disadvantage and the harsh reality may in fact be very frustrating for the bicultural person. However, having his handicap highlighted only accentuates his oppressed status, thereby making it more frustrating for him. Pity and sympathy are common, almost automatic reactions. We find a parallel example in the disabled person: one is apt to feel sorry for their limited function. Disabled people, however, do not want to be reminded of their dysfunction and to be pitied. Likewise the bicultural person would not like to have his sense of dignity overshadowed by his disadvantage.

My student community health nurses frequently react to the obvious lack of educational and occupational opportunities for low-income black families.

"I feel sorry for the young black men hanging out at the corner stores. They never had the education I've had and can't move on," commented one student.

Another student who worked the night shift said, "When I get off early in the morning I see these black young men loafing around already. I really feel sorry that they never had work opportunities."

Non-English-speaking immigrants are often working at jobs that no other members would assume—sewing, fruit picking, dishwashing, laundering, and so forth. Observers of their lot are apt to comment more on their unfortunate lives than on the workers' endurance and fortitude.

Sometimes it seems to lie beyond health workers' comprehension that their clients could have grown up and never experienced economic stability in their families. They do not seem to care to "get ahead." They want to upgrade their lots but easily find many roadblocks, for example, not following through with job training or job hunting because there was no "transportation." On the other hand, achievement-oriented people would have taken the bus to reach their destinations! When a health worker or student nurse has put in a great deal of energy to get referrals and resources for a client, and the client presents multiple trivial "excuses" as to why he did not follow through, the health worker's emotion may range from initial pity and sympathy to anger and frustration to final dismay.

Fearing is communicating avoidance caused by certain vague anxieties or mild to extreme discomfort experienced by the message sender. The message receiver can sense the anxieties and lack of trust. He may respond with ridicule or disregard, or he may provoke further discomfort. He may ignore the message and set up a mutual aversion. The basis for the fear again is ethnocentrism and cultural racism.

Some student nurses reported their experiences in an economically depressed neighborhood: "They stared at us. There were many people just sitting out on their porches or standing at the corner stores. They just looked and looked . . . made us really uncomfortable."

One Asian nurse reported that a white nurse had asked her to go along with her to some home visits in the black neighborhood. "I'm scared to go alone," she added. Yet the incident was not openly reported or discussed with the supervisor. The fear was concealed.

Attempting to obtain some information about herbal medicine, a white nurse felt very "strange" going to the Chinatown herb shops. No one seemed ready to talk to nonnatives. The language barrier was definitely a problem. The mutual aversion was so strong that she was able to obtain little information.

Fear of nonacceptance along with the fantasy of physical assault blocks effective communication. Under situations of cultural disparity, the more one concentrates on the differences, the greater one fears rejection, unfriendliness, and even "violence." There may be a physical threat, but it is a racist notion to connect a particular ethnic group with crime and physical assault without any supporting evidence.

BICULTURAL HEALTH CARE INTERACTIONS
Discounting in health care

Discounting is not limited to racist situations. It takes place in other interactional scenes where there are power imbalances. My purpose for highlighting discounting is twofold. First of all, although it occurs often racism is not often addressed in the health care field. My intent is to reiterate its importance and at the same time attempt to desensitize any accompanying emotionality. Second, discounting demonstrates clearly how ethnocentrism and racism are expressed in our communication. It points out how and where bicultural people are not treated with dignity and respect. We are repeatedly admonished to examine our values, attitudes, and life-style as we work with different cultural groups.* With the interactional examples that illustrate discounting, we can more easily identify how our prejudices are expressed.

As discounting is part of a cultural style through which the dominant group communicates with bicultural people, one finds many examples in the health care system. I have presented only a handful of illustrations in this chapter. The purpose of focusing on discounting is to show that while there are

---

*Branch refers to the sensitization process as "personal reeducation," that is, participating in cultural awareness courses; examining personal beliefs, attitudes, and behaviors; and engaging in continuous dialogue with bicultural people. (Branch, M.: New approaches in nursing: ethnic humanism views. In Branch, M., and Paxton, P., eds.: Providing safe nursing care for ethnic people of color, New York, 1976, Appleton-Century-Crofts.)

indeed conflict and power imbalances in these situations, there is no room for "blaming." The creation of cultural racism is a collective effort. Individuals are not to be blamed, though individuals do have the responsibility of treating bicultural people with respect in each situation, especially when rendering health care. When you are aware of being defensive, reflect on your own role. Do you perceive others as blaming you? Are you blaming yourself? Do you wish that your culture could be shared as much as you have made an effort to explore and thus share the bicultural health values and attitudes?

Having an image of the different types of discounting makes it easier to identify similar discounting occurrences in ourselves and others. Do not be dismayed that we stumble into discounting all the time. From now on observe bicultural responses to your discounting. How do people handle themselves when their dignity is violated? Are they suspicious and hostile? Are they apathetic? Do they in turn discount the fact that they have been affronted? How would you respond if you were discounted?

Toward cultural enlightenment

Racism is a fact of life. We realize that the historical roots of cultural racism are deep-seated. In our attempt to humanize health care, we also aim to reduce our racist attitudes. What we discover is that our racism recurs insidiously. There are, however, stages of enlightenment in our struggle to reduce racism. To begin, we must accept our deep-seated racism whether it is conscious or not. As we cannot divest ourselves from our culture, we certainly will find racism emerging in our values and attitudes. It is important that we identify and acknowledge it.

In our encounters with bicultural people we should begin to widen our own perspective by exploring the other culture, observing the other culture on its own merit, and comparing and contrasting that culture with our own. We must watch for the pitfall of judging the other culture by our own cultural norms. We must not expect or subtly coerce our counterpart to adopt our culture and be assimilated into it. If we should observe any behavioral discrepancies, that is, characteristics in the other culture that are not valued in our culture, we should explore their origin. Are the characteristics indigenous to the cultural values or are they a result of cross-cultural interaction? For instance, how do we explain that many low-income black families are headed by women? What are the influences from the African matrilineal kinship system? What is the role of the American welfare system that awards aid to families with dependent children only if the male is absent, and not if the male is present but could find no job to support his family? To cope with survival and the system, the families continue to be headed by women.

Moving on in our development of cultural sensitivity, we will begin to identify the cultural strengths of the other culture. We will gradually understand that many "negative" characteristics may be the consequence of the group's adaptive mechanisms in a racist society. The final stage is to learn from the other culture a wisdom that may enrich our own lives and culture. For instance, many healing practices handed down empirically in the various cultures may indeed broaden our healing knowledge. Learning the other cultural practices will contribute to our own healing perspectives, and in many cases, to the understanding of the energy system now espoused by holistic health practices.

Bicultural health care: the nurse's role

In the nurse/client interaction the nurse is not only alert to the discounting process but to many other aspects as well. Nurses and health workers often feel a certain insecurity about "not knowing very much about a certain culture." They know that bicultural people are different, and might like to know some of the basic patterns of bicultural behavior. In addition, it is useful to pay attention to one's cross-cultural communication. Since there are many texts that address cross-cultural communication, I have only covered racism in communication.[35, 36] However, I will briefly summarize some patterns of bicultural behavior in health care.

Bicultural health behaviors may not differ from dominant health care behaviors as much as one might think. There are indeed some common denominators:

1. Care receivers want their health needs taken care of promptly. Long waiting and rigid scheduling may therefore discourage clients from seeking care, especially those who have many role responsibilities. Low-income families are known to seek care in a crisis; by the same token middle-class male wage earners are inclined not to seek health care until they are incapacitated for work.

2. Health care consumers want practitioners to respect them. Perfunctory treatment will discourage their trust in the practitioner; clients want to be sure that the doctor knows the cause of illness and is comprehensive and conscientious in making the diagnosis.

3. Clients want an explanation of the cause of their illness and the rationale for the treatment.

4. The cost of health care should be within one's ability to pay. This is not always the case. Nonetheless, if the fee for service is too high and the client is not treated with respect, the practitioners are suspected of being too commercial and self-serving.[37, 38]

5. The efficacy of treatment is measured by the disappearance of symptoms, as opposed to the cost, that is, the doctor's fees and the cost of drug and laboratory work. The duration of healing, for example, is taken into consideration. If there is no perceivable progress in spite of continuous treatment and mounting medical bills, clients will give up or turn to other practitioners.

The following bicultural behaviors may be different from those of the dominant group:

1. Bicultural people may have specific concepts of health and illness that are different from the rational scientific concept. Bicultural clients want a very clear "scientific" explanation of illness causation; at the same time their own explanation is just as valid, and certainly should not be discounted as "superstitious."

2. After some exposure to the rational scientific concept, the bicultural concept of health and illness may be drawn from a blending of Old World and New World culture. Such integrating of various ideas now becomes the bicultural knowledge base.[39, 40]

3. Bicultural people may have medical and healing options indigenous to their cultural health system in addition to the rational scientific medical system. The probability of using folk medicine is increased when there is a vigorous ethnic community where indigenous medicine is available.

4. There is a pragmatic approach in the selection of folk versus scientific health systems. People the world over have both Western medicine and their own folk medicine but have come to rely on scientific medicine for acute illnesses.[41, 42] In the case of long-term and nonacute illness, where lingering symptoms are not cured by scientific medicine or effectively controlled by indigenous medicine, bicultural people have the option of trying both.

The degree to which any bicultural individual may exhibit these behaviors will depend on their bicultural identity as well as on their situational "lay-referral" system. The variations that may account for the differences are discussed in the previous section. One cannot predict that all bicultural people will fit into a preconceived model.

A WORD FOR THE NURSE

It is interesting to note that the use of the term "bicultural" indicates a sensitivity to and acknowledgment of the culture of the alien who in the past would have been led down the road of assimilation. Acknowledgment of biculturism legitimizes cultural retention. Bicultural experiences in this country are closely associated with power imbalances, ethnocentrism and racism. The pervasiveness of cultural racism can be seen in the social theories about bicultural people—theories evolved from assimilation, social deviance, and victimization to the formulation of bicultural identity.

Nurse anthropologists have generally recommended that nurses explore unfamiliar cultures and at the same time examine their own values, attitudes, and life-styles; they will gain sensitivity through the process. Bicultural nurses have described the cultural differences and have asked their colleagues to accept the clients as individuals along with their cultural differences. Few writers have asked health workers to examine the cross-cultural interaction per se to increase cultural sensitivity. I have explained the differences between ethnocentrism and racism. Ethnocentrism may lead to group conflict; racism creates inequality and continually puts the bicultural people in the one-down position. It seems clear to me that, to promote good nurse/client relationships, the nurse needs to be aware of her role in perpetuating the unequal status of bicultural people. Discounting accounts for operationalized racism in communication. My experiences lead me to conclude that concrete examples of racist communication will heighten the nurse's awareness of similar inequities. No one is exempt from racist values. Do not be discouraged or defensive about your racist propensity. As you watch your discounting process you will be greatly humbled each time you acknowledge your racism.

In assessing cultural differences consider the many social, economic, and environmental concomitants, along with the cultural variations. It is impossible for health workers to be acquainted with each of the various cultures. However, it is useful to know the key indicators and to look for answers. Once you embark on the road to cultural exploration, you will find many fascinating aspects, and your own perspective will become broader. Reflection of your own life-style and values will lead to a greater self-knowledge. Acceptance and tolerance of the differences of bicultural people may lead to a more accepting attitude toward yourself. In humanizing the health care of the bicultural people, the nurse is humanized in the process.

REFERENCES

1. Leininger, M.: Transcultural nursing: a promising subfield of study for nurses. In Reinhardt, A. M., and Quinn, M. D., eds.: Current practice in family-centered community nursing, St. Louis, 1977, The C. V. Mosby Co.
2. Hall, E., and Whyte, W. F.: Intercultural communication: a guide to men of action, Hum. Org. **19:**5-12, 1960.
3. Shibutani, T., and Kwan, K. M.: Ethnic stratification, New York, 1965, Macmillan Publishing Co., Inc.
4. Allport, G.: The nature of prejudice, Reading, Mass., 1954, Addison-Wesley Publishing Co., Inc.
5. Rose, P.: They and we: racial and ethnic relations in the U.S., New York, 1974, Random House, Inc.
6. Levine, R., and Campbell, D.: Ethnocentrism: theories of conflict, ethnic attitudes and group behavior, New York, 1972, John Wiley & Sons, Inc.
7. Rose, A.: Race and ethnic relations. In Merton, R. K., and Nisbet, R., eds.: Contemporary social problems, New York, 1961, Harcourt, Brace & World, Inc.
8. TeSelle, S., ed.: The rediscovery of ethnicity, New York, 1974, Harper Colophon.
9. Damon, A.: Race, ethnic group and disease, Soc. Biol. **16:**69-79, June 1969.
10. Greely, A.: Why can't they be like us? American ethnic groups, New York, 1971, E. P. Dutton.
11. Makielski, S. J.: Beleaguered minorities, San Francisco, 1973, W. H. Freeman & Co., Publishers.

12. Blauner, R.: Racial oppression in America, New York, 1972, Harper & Row, Publishers, Inc.
13. Kagiwada, G.: Confessions of a misguided sociologist, Amerasia **2**:159-164, Fall 1973.
14. Gordon, M.: Assimilation in American life, New York, 1964, Oxford University Press.
15. Zander Vander, J.: American minority relations, New York, 1972, Ronald Press.
16. Park, R.: Race and culture, New York, 1952, The Free Press.
17. Van den Berghe, P. L.: Race and racism, New York, 1967, John Wiley & Sons, Inc.
18. Cattell, S.: Health, welfare and social organization in Chinatown, New York, 1962, Community Service Society of New York.
19. Moynihan, D. P.: The tangle pathology. In Staples, R., ed.: The black family: essays and studies, ed. 2, Belmont, Calif., 1978, Wadsworth Publishing Co., Inc.
20. Leighton, A., and Leighton, D.: Character of danger, New York, 1963, Basic Books, Inc., Publisher.
21. Muensterberger, W.: Orality and dependence: characteristics of southern Chinese. In Rohein, G., ed.: Psychoanalysis and social sciences, New York, 1951, International Universities Press,Inc.
22. Sue, S., and Sue, D.: The reflection of cultural conflict in the psychological problems of Chinese Americans, paper presented at the First National Conference on Asian American Studies, Los Angeles, April 1971.
23. Surh, J.: Asian American identity and politics, Amerasia **2**:158-172, Fall 1974.
24. Tong, B.: The ghetto of the mind: notes on the historical psychology of Chinese America, Amerasia **1**:1-31, Nov. 1971.
25. Watanabe, C.: Self expression and the Asian American experiences, Asian American Review, Spring 1972, Berkeley, University of California Ethnic Studies, pp. 10-20.
26. Nobles, W.: Africanity: its role in Black families. In Staples, R., ed.: The black family: essays and studies, ed. 2, Belmont, Calif., 1978, Wadsworth Publishing Co., Inc.
27. Billingsley, A.: Black families in white America, Englewood Cliffs, N.J., 1968, Prentice-Hall, Inc.
28. Kerckhoff, A. C., and McCormic, T. C.: Marginal status and marginal personality, Soc. Force **34**:48-55, 1955.
29. Sue, S., and Sue, D.: Chinese American personality and mental health. In Tachiki, A., et al., eds.: Roots: an Asian American reader, Los Angeles, 1971, University of California Asian American Study Center.
30. Hartmann, G.: The movement to Americanize the immigrant, New York, 1948, Columbia University Press.
31. Department of Health Education and Welfare: A study of selected socio-economic characteristics of ethnic minorities based on the 1970 Census. Vol. II. Asian Americans, DHEW Publication No. (OS) 75-121, Washington, D.C., July 1974, U.S. Government Printing Office.
32. Mindel, C. H., and Habenstein, R. W.: Ethnic families in America, New York, 1976, Elsevier North-Holland, Inc.
33. Jones, J. M.: Prejudice and racism, Menlo Park, Calif., 1972, Addison-Wesley Publishing Co., Inc.
34. Kovel, J.: White racism: a psychological history, New York, 1970, Pantheon Books, Inc.
35. Lynch, L. R.: The cross-cultural approach to health behavior, Rutherford, N.Y., 1969, Fairleigh Dickenson University Press.
36. Samovan, L., and Porter, R.: Intercultural communication: a reader, Hartfort, Connecticut, 1972, Wadsworth Publishing Co., Inc.
37. Hayes-Bautista, D.: Para jugzar 1 doctor, unpublished master's thesis, 1971, University of California, San Francisco.
38. Herrera, T., and Wagner, N. N.: Behavioral approaches to delivering health services in a Chicano community. In Reinhardt, A., and Quinn, M., eds.: Current practice in family-centered community nursing, St. Louis, 1977, The C. V. Mosby Co.
39. Chen-Louie, T.: The pragmatic context: a Chinese American example of defining and managing illness, unpublished dissertation, 1975, University of California, San Francisco.
40. MacLean, C.: Traditional healers and their female clients: an aspect of Nigerian sickness behavior, J. Health Soc. Behav. **10**:172-186, 1969.
41. Logan, M. H.: Humoral medicine in Guatemala and peasant acceptance of modern medicine, Hum. Org. **32**:385-395, 1973.
42. Colson, A. C.: The differential use of medical resources in developing countries, J. Health Soc. Behav. **12**:226-237, 1971.

SUGGESTED READINGS

Conily, P.: Racism: the ever-present hidden barrier to health in our society, Am. J. Pub. Health **66**(3):246-247, 1976.
Glittenberg, J.: Adapting health care to a cultural setting, Am. J. Nurs. **14**(12):2218-2221, 1974.
Glittenberg, J.: Guidelines for cross cultural health programs, Nurs. Outlook **21**(10):660-664, 1973.
Marshall, D., et al.: Attitudes toward health among children of different races and socioeconomic status, Pediatrics **46**:422-425, 1970.

Richek, H. G.: A note on prejudice in prospective professional helpers, Nurs. Research 19:172-175, 1970.

Stotsky, B. A., and Dominick, J.: Mental patients in nursing homes. Part 4: Ethnic influences, J. Am. Geriatr. Soc. Jan. 1969.

Watts, W.: Social class, ethnic background and patient care, Nurs. Forum 6:155-162, 1967.

White, E. H.: Giving health care to minority patients, Nurs. Clinics N. Am. 12:27-40, March 1977.

5

Alternate life-styles and the family

Anne E. Jordheim

The American family—father, mother, and children—has undergone radical changes within the last two decades. Although 90% of all American children are still brought up within a family, with at least one biological parent, in 1977 the Bureau of Labor Statistics showed the following:

Of all American households 19% fit the traditional family, in which the father works and the mother stays home to take care of the household and one or more children.

Of all American families 18% consist of two working parents and one or more children.

Of all American households 30.5% are made up of married couples without children or with children no longer at home.

Of all American families 6.8% are headed by single parents—6.2% by women, 0.6% by men.

Of all American households 28% have a single person as the head who lives either alone or with related and/or nonrelated persons but without children.

The greatest single factor to influence modern family life is that 56% of all working-age women either work outside of the home or are in the process of seeking employment.

Today Americans are espousing more alternate life-styles than ever before. The reason is that the traditional family system no longer seems to meet the needs of all modern men and women. Young people especially are anxious to explore new and alternate life-styles and to form new and exciting relationships.

Divorce is no longer considered a failure and disgrace. In some circles it is praised as a courageous act, the cessation of a nonfunctioning marriage, leaving the partners free to try again or to try different life-styles.

Cohabitation—used here in the sense of two persons of the opposite sex living together without a legal marriage—is on the increase and is more readily accepted even by the older generation.

Children born outside of marriage no longer bear the same stigma as in former days; neither do their mothers.

A strong liberal trend permeates the nation. Although a conservative backlash attempts to combat most new and alternate life-styles, the changes seem to be here to stay.

Also, there are obvious changes in the kinship system, which tends to be less meaningful than ever before. Rarely does one find three generations living together these days except in a few recently immigrated ethnic groups.

The urge for autonomy by the young and the much-publicized generation gap have been detrimental to many less educated, conservative parents and their better educated, liberal children, who no longer understand each other, leaving scars not easy to heal.

Paradoxically, many young people leave conformity to try something new, only to find another kind of conformity as part of the alternate life-style they choose.

Peer group attachments versus kinship contacts create conflicts in all generations. Old people, though often in social isolation, may prefer to live among their peers as they do in retirement homes and golden age villages. Young people traditionally have preferred the campanionship and advice of their peers rather than their elders. Middle-year persons, however, are frequently squeezed between the demands of their growing children and aging parents, usually with an increase in financial burdens, thus restricted of the freedom to establish their own life-styles, which they might prefer to enjoy with their peer group rather than with relatives.

Since the nuclear family no longer is the ideal for which everyone strives, modern family life specialists have been forced to broaden their concept of the family. As many alternate life-styles evolve, or are brought out into the open the new definition of family must include a personal commitment to and concern for the alternate family, as has been practiced within the traditional family.

The following definition of the modern family is a composite of the expressions of several experts in this field: The *family* is a relationship community of two or more persons coming from the same or different kinship groups, either by birth, choice, or both. A person joining this family affirms the relationship consciously and is accepted on the basis of who he or she is and what he or she

can contribute to the group. Each person shares the responsibility for supporting, maintaining, and enriching this family unit.

MONOGAMY

It is not possible to write about alternate life-styles without investigating modern monogamy, which is still considered the foundation of our society. One man and one woman committed to each other and legally married has been and still is to many people the ideal relationship.

However, changes within modern monogamy may threaten either partner, especially the modern division of roles. Where formerly only men worked and supported the family, now women are sharing this responsibility in increasing numbers. Where formerly housework and childrearing were a woman's function, now men participate in these activities in increasing numbers. Roles have become blurred and democratized. It was formerly taken for granted that the husband would come home tired from work to a dinner cooked by his wife. In not so few families these days the wife comes home tired from work to a dinner cooked by her husband. Socioeconomic pressure on the average American family has made it a necessity for women to become wage earners. To many this means the difference between poverty and a satisfactory life-style.

The question frequently asked is: Is monogamy feasible in a society where two people may be married to each other for more than 50 years? Not too long ago, when life spans were shorter, such marriages might have lasted 15 to 20 years. Of course some monogamous couples weather all storms within such a close relationship and survive, closely cemented and deriving great satisfaction and pleasure from each other; others may have come to a compromise and understanding; yet others merely exist side by side because for some reason they wish to stay together, although mutual love and affection no longer exist. Nearly half of all American marriages end in divorce; there are no statistics about how many of these were monogamous relationships.

Interestingly, young people marry later today than ever before. They wish to select their life partner carefully, since many of them still expect an exclusive and permanent relationship within marriage.

Alternatives to monogamous marriage have always been available, especially to the rich. At the end of the twentieth century, many persons in the United States can choose their own life-styles and human relationships regardless of religion, color, gender, socioeconomic status, political affiliation, affectional preference, and/or ethnic background. According to the previously mentioned definition of the modern family, almost everyone can ultimately also choose his or her own family.

COMMUNES

Communes in American history date back to the time when religious orders were established to participate in opening up this vast new continent.

A great variety of communes have been founded during the last two decades. Many of them have failed. Religious communities have had a better survival rate than most, as have highly structured, well-financed, usually autocratically run communes that have met the needs of young people searching for a secure, well-regulated, protected life-style. Work and income are usually shared, and if both men and women are present, monogamy is the only condoned relationship.

Secular, loosely organized communes often go through a series of fad stages and are discontinued because of disagreements of the division of work, financial inadequacies, and sexual promiscuity. Women in such communes are often forced into precisely the traditional roles they wanted to get away from.

Since the commune has been substituted for the kinship system—the family—it has provided young people (and some older ones as well) with a new sense of experience, experimentation, freedom (often an illusion), and a way to "find themselves" as persons.

At this time more religious than secular communities or communes can be found in the United States. Aside from Catholic and Protestant religious communities, the Mennonites, Mormons, Hutterites, and others are known for their communal life-styles.

For example, the Bruderhof (Brothers' Farm) of New York State, a German-origin Protestant commune, derives its income from manufacturing and selling wooden educational toys that are widely used in nursery schools. All labor and income are shared. Men work in factories, on the farms, and in grounds and building maintainance. The women stay home, caring for house, children, and sometimes older members of the family. Monogamous marriage is not the only approved choice: single, celibate persons are also accepted. Leadership comes from one family and is passed from father to son.

The children of the community are of prime importance. The Bruderhof runs its own grade school; it publishes children's books and songs, makes records and musical instruments for children, and encourages arts and crafts in its expertly run kindergartens. Life in this commune seems to rotate around a kind of sturdy, devoted, uncomplicated family life no longer known to most American homes.

It is predicted that in the future fewer communes will be founded; fewer people will feel the need for this kind of shared life, not because the American family has become stronger but because the United States is developing into a more introverted, egotistical nation. Americans would rather live alone or in a less demanding relationship than a commune, where privacy is at a minimum and where the individual out of necessity is considered less important than the group.

HOMOSEXUAL FAMILY

Households headed by one or two gay parents are by no means uncommon in the United States. Although definitive data are not available, there appear to be far more lesbian mothers (with or without a female partner) than there are gay fathers raising children.

Since there are more male homosexuals, husbands more frequently espouse a gay lifestyle in addition to an otherwise traditional marital relationship, usually on a part-time basis, with or without the wife's knowledge. The Kinsey Institute for Sex Research found that 20% of male homosexuals interviewed had been married at least once and that 44% of those had one or more children. (It is supposed that a larger number had fathered children both in and outside of marriage).

It is not within the scope of this book to discuss the total spectrum of homosexuality; however, some facts affecting the family must be mentioned. All of these facts have been documented through research done by some of America's foremost social, behavioral, and medical scientists.

Of all American males 10% have overt homosexual relations while married.

Same-sex orientation does not mean that the gay man or woman does not wish for children; nor does it mean that he or she is not fond of children.

There is no single group called "homosexuals"; there is, however, just as with heterosexuals, an infinite variety of behavior patterns, personality structures, and functions.

Societal pressure is the reason why gay persons may enter into a heterosexual marriage relationship and remain "in the closet" with their homosexual relationship. If they decide to come out, an understanding could be reached with their usually, though not always, heterosexual spouse before inevitable anguish and distress result. Although the many changing patterns in marriage, family, and intimacy are acknowledged, to suddenly discover that one's mate has a same-sex preference is undoubtedly devastating. However, some wives take this in stride, perhaps because of love, ego, and social reasons, though most often it is because they are trapped with small children and in need of the husbands' paycheck. The rare family, whether or not there has been a divorce, accepts the father's or mother's gay lover into its midst.

Very complex psychological involvements are always present; for example, as the gay partner's acceptance of his or her sexual orientation increases, so does self-esteem and self-identity.

Sexual orientation, whether heterosexual or homosexual, does not indicate that the person cannot be a responsible, reliable, devoted, loving, and able parent.

There is no scientific evidence that children of gay parents are likely to become gay; most homosexuals are the children of conventionally heterosexual parents.

Fitness for parenthood should be judged by the caliber of the parent, not by his or her sexual orientation.

Researchers find it difficult to interview lesbian mothers, whether they are divorced or not, because these mothers fear having their children taken from them as has happened in some states.

Foster care agencies in cities such as New York and Philadelphia have, without fanfare, placed gay teenagers whose heterosexual foster parents could not deal with them into selected homes of well-adjusted gay male couples. Contrary to the fears of the skeptics, a father-son relationship developed. The teenagers thrived with people who had problems and life experiences similar to their own and were able to accept them completely.

When heterosexual parents discover that their son or daughter is gay, often they disown them and cut them off from any family relationship—so necessary a support system for any person, and more so for those struggling with their sexual identity. Most larger cities now have a Parents for Gays organization where help is available to work through the problems of accepting a gay son or daughter.

It may be difficult for any person, even a nurse, who has not yet come to terms with her own sexuality, to relate to and understand the homosexual family. Unless she is sure she can handle the situation she should consult an expert either for help in learning about human sexuality or for actual assistance in helping the family.

Anyone entering family-oriented community nursing must be equipped to work nonjudgmentally with patients of all sexual orientations, with patients whose attitudes and behavior may be different from her own.

SINGLE-PARENT FAMILY

The problems of the one-parent family and the divorce process will be discussed in detail in Chapter 6; however, since many people choose to be single parents, they espouse an alternate life-style.

Within the last 10 years there has been a 50% increase in families headed by a single person, usually a woman. According to the 1977 Bureau of Labor Statistics, 75% of these mothers are wage earners. Since not all single mothers are divorcees or are separated from their husbands, children are increasingly reared in households without a male role model.

In some ethnic groups the mother's boyfriend, father's girlfriend, or a relative may substitute and take on a parent role. Single parents may have one, many, or serial monogamous relationships with persons of the same or opposite sex. Experts in family life are not certain what effect these alternate life-styles have on children. Some find them beneficial to children while others think they are detrimental. All agree, however, that a child will become a better adjusted adult if he lives in a home with one loving parent than if he lives with two parents who hate and despise each other.

Difficulties often arise when the child is brought up by a stepparent with or without the help of the biological parent. Neither is it easy to merge two single families with his children, her children, and, perhaps later, their children. However, more and more families dare to take this difficult step and seem to succeed in adjusting to the problems of a larger family with several sets of parents and stepparents.

From this omnigenous family a new kinship system has been created, the result of breaking up and re-forming new marital unions. As a consequence extensive and complex alliances occur between divorced persons and their respective families, sometimes reaching into several generations. Since new and old relatives change with each divorce, a wide variety of interpersonal relations are created, some not very meaningful, others retained and cherished for years, perhaps even for life.

If parents with children divorce and remarry, "step-relatives" soon abound, including as many as eight grandparents. Two and more divorces are not uncommon nowadays. Therefore, with the confusing array of relatives and step-relatives, such emotions as love, hostility, indifference, rejection, acceptance, and loyalty may result. A man and woman can easily "progress" from monogamy to serial monogamy (or polygamy) and thus on to the omnigenous family—and not only through legal marriages and divorces. In some ethnic and other groups omnigenous relationships exist through human bonding outside as well as inside of marriage.

Because an increasing number of divorced couples feel that as civilized individuals they ought to remain friends, and many do, an omnigenous family may soon be one of the more popular alternate life-styles in the Western world.

The drawbacks can be clearly identified, although the advantages may be similar to those of an extended family. Children no doubt can benefit from love given by many relatives as well as by having to relate to a variety of persons. As long as friendly and rational interaction is maintained within the omnigenous family, well-adjusted children may be the result of this type of family constellation.

NONTRADITIONAL FAMILY

While group marriage is nontraditional, it is by no means a new form of alternate lifestyle. Since most group marriages consist of one husband and two or more wives, we need only to look into history to find such families. However, group marriages are illegal in the United States. In such marriages sexual sharing is taken for granted; such sharing may lead to jealousies and eventually to the break-up of the relationships. These marriages are sometimes compared to marathon encounters in their seriousness and intensity, especially if children are involved. The complexities of interaction, even if the partners all relate equally well to each other, are conflict ridden with problems difficult to solve. If one partner, usually the man, is the dominant person in the marriage, and if the wives and respective children are financially dependent on him, some means of conflict resolution has to be found. This usually means separating the families. Few group marriages consist of one woman and two or more men.

The question arises at this time: If medical science is capable of fertilizing a human egg in a test tube and implanting it into a uterus, could the group marriage of the future be a husband, a wife (legal or not) with nonpatent fallopian tubes or an unhealthy or no uterus, and a wife (not legal) with a healthy uterus into which the first wife's fertilized ovum will be implanted? Then the child might truly belong to all three partners. This question could become reality because we have the technology to accomplish it, though we have no idea what the possible psychological implications would be.

According to the 1977 U.S. Census Bureau, 47 million heterosexual couples cohabit—a sevenfold increase within the last 7 years. Although in some states, after as few as 3 years of living together, the couple acquires common-law status, in other states this legal classification does not exist. In these states the couple has no rights to each other's property, health insurance, and/or other benefits. They are legally two completely separate entities even if they share a bed, home, and life.

In 1977 about 60% of those who cohabited were younger than 30 years old, a statistic now moving upward to an older age group. Approximately one third of all persons living together were previously divorced, and because they had experienced failure in marriage now wished to explore one or many relationships before contemplating a new marriage.

Although the duration of cohabitation is considerably shorter than that of marriage in the United States, the cohabiting life-style is very similar to that of marriage. The role division and sharing of household chores is fairly traditional, with women carrying responsibilities far beyond those of the men. Cohabiting couples may be as committed to each other as married couples; however, they obviously have more freedom to end the relationship than married persons do. The end of cohabitation may be equally as painful as divorce.

The 1978 generation of young heterosexual persons finds even cohabitation too constricting. They may enter a relationship with a sexual commitment, but meet at her or his "place," spending only weekends rather than every day together in order to preserve their independence and privacy. Thus the sometimes trapped feeling of cohabiting is eliminated and the enforced absence may make their "hearts grow fonder".

Many other types of nontraditional marriages can be found in this country. Divorced couples cohabiting without remarriage has become popular as have long-distance marriages, in which both partners work in different cities and get together only on weekends and during vacations.

"Nonparenthood," couples choosing not to have children for various reasons such as interference with careers or a sense of social responsibility, is on the increase.

Often forgotten are parentless families in which an older sister or brother holds together and brings up a family; they do exist.

The extended family is, of course, not new, except that nowadays nonrelatives may also be a part of this alternate family constellation.

Nuclear dyads who do not consider themselves a part of a commune or group marriage espouse a life-style in which two or more couples share a house, work, and money but otherwise have privacy. Sometimes single persons are also included in this family. Friendship and mutual support are expected, but sexual relationships are approved only within each couple.

Very new are "rooming-together" families, for example, a divorcee and her children and a divorced man to whom the divorcee is not married but is only a platonic friend; both adults date others outside the home if they wish.

In many parts of the country, single persons—women mainly but also men—may adopt children, thus founding a family.

Single women who do not wish to marry but want a child may either ask a special friend to be the father or be artifically inseminated by a physician and thus not know who the father of the child is. These women also create a family in this way; they may be lesbians and live with another woman or they may be heterosexual and live alone or with others.

Golden age families are found in adult villages and possibly old age homes, where groups of old people live together, share their work and finances (and maybe sex), but mainly wish to be of mutual support and enjoy each others' companionship.

Finally, same-sex unrelated families reside together—friends or relatives or both—for the purpose of saving money and avoiding loneliness. As an example a group of elderly Protestant ladies—all professional women—who pool their money and share the housework, but work during the day and volunteer at night and on weekends in the community where needed, using their extra money for benevolent activities such as sending city children to summer camps in the country, helping the hungry of the world. Each woman has her own studio apartment. Only dinner is eaten together in a large dining room. This family has no leader; every person is equal; all have the same voice in the decision-making process.

"Neogamy" is also an alternate life-style—a bonding between two persons, especially of older age, who establish a relationship to meet intimacy and/or sexual needs. Since nonmarried, older women by far outnumber nonmarried, older men, neogamy may also be the bonding between two women or a younger man and older woman.

Many older Americans live in social isolation and poverty. Some may wish to marry but cannot do so for financial reasons, since one partner may lose an income. Cohabitation is therefore rapidly increasing among senior citizens. Closeness, affection, and companionship may be more important to some older persons than sex, although they may also have sexual needs, especially if they have lived in a long-time sexual relationship and are physically and psychologically healthy.

COLLEGE COLLECTIVES

"Living together" is common in college communities, and in some colleges men and women live in the same dormitories. For many young people this seems to be highly acceptable, although it disturbs most parents. Living in the same dormitory does not necessarily mean cohabitating; neither does "living together."

The college "collective" is a recent arrangement that alleviates the financial difficulties that most students encounter. A group of students of both sexes rent a house, share work and money, and are mutually supportive but usually date outside the collective. Often members of the group find each other because of a common religious identification. There may be a Catholic house, a Methodist or Episcopalian house, a Jewish house, and/or others.

Eyewitness reports tell of the brotherly and sisterly affection dominating such houses, which of course precludes any sexual relationships. The students save money in this way, meet persons they enjoy, and encounter a quasi-family situation that may be an improvement over dormitories, living alone in a room, or even their own home environment. The fact that members of the college collective are peers enhances this alternate life-style, which young people seem to prefer in certain colleges and universities.

The collective is generally governed by an elected council of students; dictatorship or autocracy is unacceptable as are students who do not contribute their share of work and money to the group.

OCCASIONAL OR TEMPORARY FAMILY

Many life situations demand adaptation to a substitute kinship system. The occasional or temporary family usually consists of persons who are voluntarily or involuntarily thrown together by controllable or uncontrollable circumstances.

A retired person living with a family whose members are not blood relatives; a foster child being brought up by parents other than his own; a professional ·group "living together" for any length of time, for example, on a trip or during a conference; persons on a religious retreat; battered wives in a shelter for women; alcoholics or drug addicts in a rehabilitation center or half-way house, inmates in a prison; chronically ill patients in a hospital ward; the staff in a place of work; buddies in war—these occasional families may have a profound effect on the person who is a part of such a group.

Nursing students living in a dormitory and spending most of their waking hours together can also be called an occasional or temporary family.

The significance of the occasional family is to be found in the support system—founded on friendship, affection, and love—which provides an unforgettable life experience. Identification with the group is so strong that it can be therapeutic and revitalizing, which is why rehabilitation often takes place in groups. The occasional family becomes the backbone for anyone who is mentally or physically ill and/or socially rejected. Friendships—human bonding—originating in such an environment often last a lifetime.

ROLE OF THE NURSE

The role of the nurse when dealing with persons living alternate family life-styles is only difficult if she cannot find her own niche in contemporary society. The nurse herself may espouse an alternate life-style. No doubt all of the categories described in this chapter cover a variety of persons with different vocations, jobs, and/or professions.

Whether or not the nurse lives in a traditional family group should by no means influence her professional goals and functions in community nursing. A nonjudgmental, empathic, warm, and caring attitude can be found in all walks of life. The community health nurse must strive toward these human qualities as a basis for good nursing, health counseling, and human relations.

It is the nurse's responsibility to encourage and promote, to help and heal. It matters not whether the patient lives in a relationship the nurse cannot comprehend or would not choose. Although a liberal, open-minded approach to family-centered nursing may present personal conflicts for some nurses, they simply must ignore it, overcome some of their prejudices (so often learned in childhood), and establish interpersonal relations with their patients on a humane level.

If the nurse has difficulties with this she should seek help from a good friend, counselor, psychologist, or psychiatrist. If she cannot care for patients without judging and being distressed by their alternate life-style, she should get out of community nursing.

Religion, color, gender, age, race, socioeconomic status, political affiliation, affectional or sexual orientation, ethnic background, chosen life-style—none of these matters to a sensitive person in family-centered community nursing. Only the person and helping him or her cope with illness—whether mental, physical, or social—are of importance.

If a nurse's life-style is uncomplicated, satisfying, and happy, this does not mean that changes cannot occur to suddenly place her in an alternate situation. Such a change in life-style may be the result of extrinsic circumstances or may be voluntarily chosen through a rational decision making process. This may place the nurse "on the other side of the fence," now becoming the receiver and acceptor of family-centered nursing, as well as the provider.

In the life of a family there are phases that require careful nurture and negotiation.

The nurse, as provider or consumer, may have to participate in maintaining and reestablishing family relationships during her life cycle. She may have to clarify and restructure role expectations and functions within the family. Above all, the nurse may wish to promote an affirmation of freedom for all family members, so that they may redefine and alter their role expectations throughout their lives.

The family-centered community nurse thus realizes that this development process is a continuing growth experience dependent on meaningful relationships within the traditional or alternate family at every age of human experience.

SUGGESTED READINGS

Clauton, G., and Downing, C.: Face to face to face, New York, 1975, E. P. Dutton & Co., Inc.

Dressler, P., and Avant, R.: Neogamy in older persons, Alternate Lifestyles, 1:1, February 1978.

Fish, S. L.: Becoming partners, Alternate Lifestyles, 1:4, May 1978.

Humphreys; L.: An interview with Evelyn Hooker, Alternate Lifestyles, 1:4, May 1978.

Libby, R. W. and Whitehurst, R. N.: Marriage and its alternative: exploring intimate relationships, Glenview, Ill., 1977, Scott, Foresman & Co.

Mallan, L. B.: Young widows and their children: a comparative report Social Security Bulletin, Washington, D.C., May 1975, U.S. Government Printing office.

Miller, B.: Adult sexual resocialization, Alternate Lifestyles, 1:4, May 1978.

Mowery, J.: Systemic requisites of communal groups, Alternate Lifestyles, 1:4, May 1978.

National Gay Taskforce: Gay parent support packet, 80 Fifth Ave., NY 10011 (1975).

Pickett, R. S.: Monogamy on trial, Alternate Lifestyles, 1:4, May 1978.

Silverstein, C.: A family matter: a parents' guide to homosexuality, New York, 1977, McGraw-Hill Book Co.

Tiger, L.: Omnigamy: A new kinship system, Psychol. Today, July 1978.

U.S. Department of Labor: Women who head families: a socioeconomic analysis, Special Labor Force Report 190, Washington, D.C., June 1976, reprint from Monthly Labor Review.

Yllo, K. A.: Non-marital cohabitation, Alternate Lifestyles, 1:1, February 1978.

6

Separation, divorce, and subsequent coping problems of single-parent families

Margaret A. Kessenich Meagher

The *Statistical Abstract of the United States, 1977,* stated that the rate of divorces per 1000 population was 5.0%. In 1975 the rate per 1000 women 15 years and over was 20.3%. The median duration of marriages was 6.5 years and the median age of divorce in the first marriage was 30.2 years for males and 28.1 years for females. There were 1.08 children involved in each divorce.[1] In Denver, Colorado, in 1979 the divorce rate was three out of every four marriages.[2] To understand these alarming statistics and to aid the people that they represent, we need to examine the causes, processes, and consequences of divorce.

LOVE, MARRIAGE, AND DIVORCE

We must first look at the marital relationship, its basis—love and family—and the impacts change have on it. I have borrowed my concept of love from Erhard Seminar Training—better known as est. Love is allowing myself and my partner the space to be who we are and who we are not. Love may or may not include marriage. Marriage, as distinct from love, is a formal living situation in which two people are committed to work out their joint efforts in living. The emotional commitment varies with each type of marital contract, and the contract can be between any two partners, regardless of sex. The essential part of the contract is the agreement in living, not the sex of the partners. Basically then marriage involves your doing your thing, me doing my thing, and particularly us doing our thing.[3] This is necessary so that each person can grow, the couple can grow, and the family can grow. We must grow to affirm and realize ourselves. Mutual growth, as individuals and as a couple, is the goal of marriage.

Children are not the goal of a marriage; they may or may not be involved. If children are involved in the marriage, the interplay exists between you doing your thing, me doing my thing, us doing our thing, them doing their thing, and all of us doing our family thing. The contract involving children becomes very complicated and is directly related to stresses causing divorce (see Fig. 1).

Normally the idea of the family as the center evolves at the onset of family development—the birth of the first child. Making the

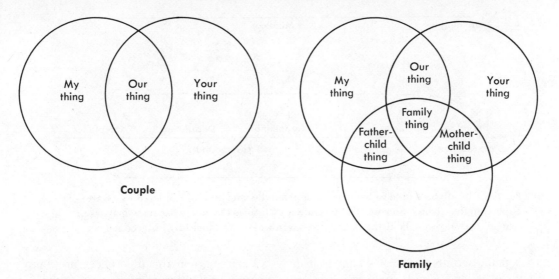

Fig. 1. The family thing frequently takes up the greater percentage of the our thing and takes up space from the your thing and the my thing.

family the central focus of a marriage can cause problems, although this emphasis frequently prevails in the United States. For instance, when each child is born the energies of you, me, and us shift to the child and family. With the addition of children less emphasis is placed on us, and the couple frequently neglects their relationship (Fig. 1). This loss of energy underlies marital discord.

Strong family demands drown out the marital relationship; the marital process deteriorates; individual and marital growth are arrested; and the marriage contract between the two adults disintegrates. If each partner can continue individual growth and if together they can sustain the marital relationship, they can cope with any crisis and grow in their relationship. Without individual growth the relationship will die. Death of a relationship does not necessarily mean divorce. Many couples spend their lives in a stable but unsatisfactory marriage. Consequently they do not grow in their living situation; indeed they frequently lose contact with themselves.

But a shift of energies often creates maturational and situational life crises that may lead to divorce. These crises can be identified in the divorce process.

DIVORCE AS LIFE CRISIS

Marriage is a formal process of coupling and divorce is a formal process of uncoupling. As defined by Bevis[4], processes have three characteristics: (1) inherent purpose, (2) internal organization, and (3) infinite creativity. The inherent purpose of the divorce process is to separate and terminate the existing marital contract. The internal organization of the divorce process involves viewing the divorce on a continuum having a beginning, a middle, and an end (see Fig. 2). It begins with the first urgings of separation on either party's part and ends with the development of a single life-style for each. The middle of the divorce process encompasses all of the phases of the grief process as well as the problems of an identity crisis and the resulting adjustments to independent living. The infinite creativity of divorce is the emergence of

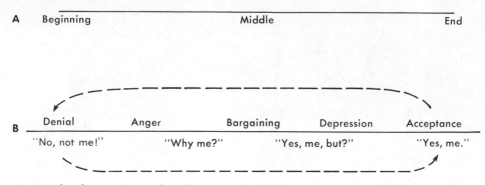

Fig. 2. A, The divorce process has a beginning, middle, and end. **B,** Kübler-Ross's stages of grief applied to the divorce process. There is no set pattern as to when what stage may occur. They may all thread throughout the entire divorce process. The final stage is acceptance.

two separate adults, each of whom is in a growth place and is able and willing to be independent, and both of whom are capable, if there are children, of continuing co-parenting functions.

A person experiencing divorce also experiences a life crisis. Aguilera and Messick[5] have defined crisis as a turning point. Divorce is such a turning point. It can be a time of growth. People can either stumble through it or they can use it as an opportunity to change.

A crisis may be maturational or situational. A maturational crisis is part of the normal growing process—puberty, for example. A situational life crisis can range from a job change to a car wreck to a heart attack. Either a situational or a maturational crisis may spark a divorce, and the divorce will always produce a situational crisis; it may or may not produce a maturational crisis. If one partner is ill and the marital contract is unfulfilled, the crisis is situational. If one person has grown away from the other, the crisis is situational for the one who has grown away and both situational and maturational for the other partner. Divorce causes job changes, moves, adjustments to new surroundings, and contacts with new people. These are situational crises.

Usually when the differences are simply maturational, the partners are grown up enough to move away from each other without feeling devastated, and the maturational differences are easily resolved. When the couple experiences both situational and maturational problems, the divorce process is much more complicated and it is a painful life experience. The maturational and situational crises both create change, with which the couple may be unable to cope; frequently they both experience severe loss and grief.

GRIEF PROCESS AS PART OF DIVORCE

Grief is a part of divorce because divorce is no different than any other loss process. Grief is an emotional process that, along with its various phases and stages, has been reviewed in the literature.[6-13] There are clearly three stages: (1) shock and disbelief; (2) the working phase, or phase of developing awareness (or crying phase); and (3) the resolution, or restitution, stage.

Most authors discuss phases and stages of grief in response to a death. I apply them to the death of a relationship—to divorce. Kübler-Ross talks about the five stages of grief in response to a death. She identifies (1) denial, (2) anger, (3) bargaining, (4) depression, and (5) acceptance. A combination of the above can be used in a grief diagram involving the divorce process, and the process can be seen on a continuum as diagrammed in Fig. 2.

In a divorce, loss may be anticipated when a partner first thinks of separation or divorce; both partners may also experience loss in the period just before the filing of the divorce papers. The actual loss is when the divorce is final and independent living begins.

The divorce process, however, can be more painful to experience in our society than a death. Death usually is an accepted loss; divorce is not. We ritualize the departure in death: when someone dies, people gather around, send food, and try to comfort the grieving relatives. In a divorce there is no funeral, no flowers, no food, and no ritualized grief. Many times the divorced find themselves alone and "celebrating" the divorce from a lonely place. The divorced person is isolated. Married friends no longer invite them out as often as they did before the divorce, and long-time friends may cease to recognize either partner when they are no longer a couple. With divorce there is social disapproval, isolation, and frequent avoidance of any aspect of the process by those around the divorcing person. People in the throes of divorce experience more than the loss of the partner: they experience also the loss of friends and family. The problems a person experiences, then, are the loss of a support system as well as the loss of the partner. The more hostile the divorce is, the more society avoids the predicament. This avoidance increases the difficulty of the change from the married to the unmarried status.

REASONS FOR DIVORCE

Within the difficulties of coupling, the panics of crisis, and the pain of uncoupling, one can find recurring patterns that can be iden-

tified as the more immediate causes of the divorce:

1. Inability of people to talk with each other
2. Poor skills in active listening
3. Fear of closeness
4. Outgrowing of the relationship
5. Not allowing time for our thing
6. Neglect of your or my thing in a relationship

Another immediate cause is the rise of the women's movement. The women's movement has had a liberating effect on divorce. Women no longer have to suffer through an unhappy marriage or see marriage as the only life-style option for them. In addition, the no-fault divorce frees many people from the destructive blame of divorce. Now two people can split feeling better about themselves and each other. Many people in the public eye have been divorced and are divorcing. People see public models for the divorce process every day in the news and in everyday living. Generally divorce is more widespread and certainly it is more acceptable now than it was 10 years ago.

DIVORCE AND CHILDREN

More than 913,000 divorces were granted in the United States in 1973. One million children were probably affected by these divorces.[14] These children are frequently pawns in a situation that is so traumatic that no one fully recovers. The children are usually caught between two fighting adults; they are the real losers in a divorce.

In 1976 Barbara Walters hosted an NBC-TV special, *Children of Divorce*. Walters and her guests talked of the emotional impact that divorce has on children and the confusion the process holds for the child who has not been prepared for the shock. Even if the child is prepared, the realization of the separation and the resulting change in life-style becomes a major adjustment. Some children feel guilty about the breakup. If the resulting divorce is precipitated by arguments about the child, he may feel responsible for the breakup. He may also feel a vague sense of guilt or feel that he has contributed to the divorce. No matter how the child interprets the divorce, it is painful for him.

Depending on the type of divorce and the resulting custody situation, the child may become the victim of the process. The degree to which he is victimized is in direct proportion to the amount of unresolved anger there is in the relationship that is being severed.

Frequently married couples split and the problems in the relationship remain. The degree to which the parents allow their problems to rotate around the child will determine how much the child will become the victim and/or will be used in the situation. Sometimes the child ends up being the one getting divorced! If the child is of school age, he frequently experiences more absence and separation than the adults do. Parents often place the child in a care center in order to facilitate their working. The child then experiences not only a divorce but also an increased absence of one or both parents. The resulting change in life-style is proportionate to the life-style change in the parents' lives. The child is frequently more isolated from the parents, or is farmed out more to sitters, and is forced to fend for himself. The child of a divorce also often gets caught up in the feeling of distance created between the divorcing partners and learns not to get close to people. The more OK the divorce, the more role modeling the child sees for establishing closeness and appreciating differences in others. As long as the splitting couples separate from an OK place, they avoid putting the child in the middle of their differences. The child will survive the divorce process feeling better about himself and will be able to establish close relationships. If a couple is able to continue co-parenting with warmth

and concern for the child, the child will develop a close relationship with each partner and learn to get what he needs from each parent.

As soon as the couple is sure of the split and plans are formalized, the child should be included and should be given data as to how the divorce will affect him. Limits are set on the private life of the couple, however. Negative details should be left out. If problems resulting from sexual expression are areas that have contributed to the divorce, the child should not be included in the data. This information belongs to the couple alone.

The more the couple can resolve their anger in the divorce process, the less trauma the child will suffer and the more options there will be for an OK divorce. If the anger is unresolved, however, the child too frequently becomes the victim of the divorce process. The degree to which the divorce process is filled with anger and old resentments the more problems there will be in working out the custody. The more adult the partners have acted, the more effective the parenting has been and, of course, the smoother the continued parenting will be.

Krantzler talks about divorce as the healing process of change;[15] this healing process can occur only in an environment that nurtures a sense of okayness for each person involved.

How does one resolve the anger in a divorce process?

1. Identify the anger rackets. A racket is sometimes a substitute feeling. For example, many couples radiate anger rather than sadness or fear. This anger is a racket and the underlying feeling is fear. Demonstration of this anger is usually a product of old unresolved angers. The anger stamps are collected and built up over the years and are used to bring on a negative relationship or at least to continue keeping it alive.

2. Decide to give up the anger. A couple

can decide to give up all of the anger if they want to and are willing to.

3. Work out the anger in therapeutic settings. A couple can help to stop the negative feelings from building up and breaking up the relationship.

4. Avoid spreading the anger to everyone you meet. Limit your "rage phase" to the appropriate person or at least to a safe setting. Do not take out angry feelings on the children just because they are handy.

5. Work out physically. Exercise is a healthy way to channel pent-up anger.

The more anger that is given up, resolved, or worked out during a divorce, the better the chances are for successful joint custody and the healthy co-parenting that results from the successful ending of a relationship.

There is no set, healthy pattern for the child to maintain in grieving the loss of separated parents. It is unhealthy if the child shows no reaction. A child grieves over a divorce just as his parents do. The process is as vivid and as painful for him as it is for the adults. The child will work through the same five stages of grief—denial, anger, bargaining, depression, and acceptance. At least if he is acting out, he is expressing his feelings. Usually, the child who shows no reaction fears abandonment. When working with a child, look for fear and guilt, which may be blocking his expression of grief. Frequently the parents are so busy with the divorce process and its problems that they neglect the child.

The most healthy response from the parent to the child is to reassure the child that he will get what he needs. Teach the child early to ask for what he needs. Knowing he will get what he needs will make the child feel secure. A child needs to know he is loved and wanted, even if it isn't in a setting to which he is accustomed. He needs to have a place at each parent's home to call his own. He needs to know that each parent is still a parent and that each parent's home is the child's home. The child needs to feel stability and routine; the sooner these are developed the better it will be for him. Stability and routine should characterize where the child stays, when he comes and goes, where he goes, his school, and what sitter he will be with. If the child is old enough he should be given a number to call so he can reach a parent at any time. The child needs to feel a sense of "okayness" and not to feel responsible for the relationship between the couple. The child needs simple information as to what is going on between the parents. It is not okay to spring the divorce on the child.

The damages to the child in the divorce process are as follows:

1. The child may be neglected.

2. The child may be the object of the adults' frustration.

3. The child may be used by one parent to blackmail the other.

4. If the child has not been taught to ask for what he needs, he may use withdrawal to fill his time.

5. The absence of one parent and the increased stress on the single parent with whom he lives may leave the child outside of the daily routine and throw him into a harried environment.

Some rules for single parenting have been derived from several workshops and from Goldberger:[15A]

1. Be yourself. Avoid victimizing the child and placing him in a one-down position.

2. Talk to your co-parent in an adult manner. Negotiate around the child's care.

3. Do not place the child in the middle of your hassles.

4. Provide for the child to contact the other parent during a parent's visitation time.

5. Do not make the child a target for your anger.
6. Do not "bad mouth" the other parent in front of the child.
7. Create a sense of okayness for the child. Respect his privacy and the other parent's privacy.
8. Include the child in your social life.
9. Include yourself in the child's life, that is, the child's play life and the child's school life.
10. Allow the other parent to become involved in the child's school life.
11. Do not mold the child into the role of the absent spouse.
12. If you are unable to do the above, seek professional help.
13. See that the child has a place of his own at each parent's home.

PROBLEMS OF CUSTODY

When children are involved in divorce, custody planning enters the picture. Many times primary custody of the children goes to one parent. However, I believe that if the divorce can be an OK process, the custody of the children should be joint. Both parents can continue to be parents. The court battles can occur over the financial aspects of the divorce situation, not over the children. Let the children be free! Even if the lawyers recommend primary custody, joint custody should be preferred for all who remain adults in a divorce process.

Joint custody is more work for the couple, for the lawyers, and for the therapists. But it is worth the effort to the child so that the child does not become the victim of a win-lose situation. Primary custody is a win-lose situation. Because of couples' inability to negotiate child custody, child stealing has become a predominant problem in the United States.

Unfortunately many couples are not able to separate the issues of old anger from the marital relationship, and therefore they work out their old angers and resentments in a final, devastating battle over custody. The eventual outcome is that all who are involved in the process are losers; the custody battle leaves scars on the entire network of the people involved in the divorce process.

KIND OF DIVORCE

Through my work I have identified six kinds of divorce. The first kind I call a *contract divorce*. In a "contract divorce", two people are able to sit down together and work out an OK situation. Both parties realize they have grown apart and see divorce as an option. The children present no real problem, although they do present some problems in daily living and co-parenting. This continuing parenting is done from a concerned place, and the children are involved. The parents are clear about their roles and are receptive to problem solving with the children's input. Usually people in a contract divorce do not seek help and rarely are seen as a couple. One partner may seek help around an individual problem he or she is having with individualization. This usually lasts a minimal time period and the person moves quickly through the divorce process.

The second kind of divorce is the *shocker-shockee*. In the "shocker-shockee" divorce, one partner has no idea what the other partner is up to. The first time the second person knows about it is when the divorce papers are served. That person is shocked and stunned. In this divorce situation the party initiating the divorce proceedings is well into the divorce grief process—usually into the third phase, resolution. The shocked party experiences a lag in the divorce process and is usually in the first phases of grief—shock and disbelief. The imbalance between the two partners is great and this usually leads to a painful divorce process. In the shocker-shockee type of divorce, the couple often have had dysfunctional communication from the very beginning. They also most frequently lack skills or concerns for active listening and generally have developed a mass of anger and are unwilling to negotiate most issues. Withdrawal from problem solving in each partner has been predominant throughout their marriage. Custody battles may or may not be a part of the divorce.

The third type of divorce is called the *female battered*. In the "female battered," the woman has been the brunt of the man's expression of his emotions. The man has existed at the expense of the woman, at least emotionally. Frequently she seeks help and begins to build a new self-worth. As this growth occurs, she no longer hides the pain or submits herself to the suffering or "victim position"[16] with her husband. Once she realizes she has sufficient strength to escape the relationship, she files for divorce. He usually objects to the incident with threats. If he does object, the transaction between the two could be lethal.

Games[17], a series of ulterior transactions with a predictable feeling outcome (payoff) may escalate. A first-degree game is usually simple and can be seen at a cocktail party ("My car is better than your car"). In a second-degree game, the couple close the windows so the neighbors will not hear the yelling. In a third-degree game, there is physical abuse of some kind, possibly even homicide or suicide.[18]

If games escalate between two people and the two are not willing to stop, the best intervention is separation (with a restraining order, if necessary). This is one of the most difficult divorce processes for a therapist because of the game situation and the usually uncooperative male partner. Conflict resolution is slow and painful if it occurs at all. Frequently the focus is on the woman and her growth. The counselor may or may not see the man. If he is willing to see someone, it is

best for him to see another clinician to avoid the formation of a triangle and the perpetuation of third-degree games between the partners.

The fourth type of divorce process is the *male battered*. For years he has taken verbal, if not physical, abuse from the woman. Outwardly he may appear to be the strength in the relationship but inwardly she runs the show and controls him. With this type, as with the female battered, the couple is rarely seen as a couple because the relationship is so destructive. The most successful intervention in individual therapy is to work with the partner who seeks help first. If the other partner is willing to be seen, a referral to another clinician is in order.

The fifth type of divorce is the *willing and unwilling partner;* after a process of a month to a year, the parties often agree to part. Communications are more open and direct, with less physical injury. This couple resorts to closing the windows prior to "discussion." Their level of game playing hurts, but consists of predominantly second-degree games. In this situation a couple may or may not be in therapy together. Usually the couple is more receptive to change and more often welcomes divorce as a growth process. This may not occur initially, but usually the agreement to work and to grow through the divorce takes place later in the growth process.

The sixth and most lethal divorce I have seen is in the "willing and unwilling partner" who resort to third-degree games. This type of game involves physical injury and may end with the partners killing each other. Usually these people are so entrenched in their dependence on each other that any attempt to break off threatens them with abandonment, and they panic. The partners are not whole people and fear functioning on their own, much less developing a whole new lifestyle for themselves. Usually, if they are receptive to counseling, the sessions are minimal. Once the partners are confronted with patterns and predominant functions, they flee in anger. The anger masks the fear each has to be a separate person and independent of the other.

Sometimes one person may muster enough strength to seek help, and usually I work with that person to complete the conflict of separation and individualization. The treatment period is long and stormy, marked by ambivalence and frequent reconciliations. The cycling and recycling of the marriage may occur from 1 to 4 years before the person finally makes the final break to the unmarried stage and begins to develop an independent life.

LIFE AFTER A DIVORCE

There is life after divorce. If the process has been creative and healing, the partners will come out as whole people and will be able to function independently. They will be able to reestablish satisfying life goals and find new ways of living without each other. Continued parenting will evolve if the couple has children. The ex-partners will be able to separate their parenting roles from their previous marital relationship. They will, however, have the problems of single-parent families.

COPING PROBLEMS OF SINGLE-PARENT FAMILIES

The coping problems of single parents begin at the onset of the divorce process when the couple begins to discuss the issue of separation. At this time the issue of custody of the children arises. If it is an OK divorce, custody will not be an overwhelming issue. If the divorce is drenched in anger, the issue will be paramount. The question of who will have the children and who will take responsibility for their growth and development is uppermost.

Once the couple has decided the issue of custody and has separated, the post-divorce period involves coping with being a single parent. It is not easy for either party. Working out the mechanics of taking the children here and there gets complicated. With joint planning the problems are fewer, however. A primary custody situation with uncooperative parents can be draining, time consuming, and exhausting. Frequently the process takes 3 to 6 months just to work out new life patterns after separation. If the co-parents (or parent) accept the responsibility without becoming victims, the children will have a fairly healthy adjustment.

Frequently, however, fathers at this point reassess their commitment to their children, shifting to a concerned parent, a less concerned parent, or an absent parent. If the father decides to accept custody or joint custody, he undergoes a major change in his life. In our society women still take primary responsibility for the planning of child care. A man is usually not programmed to deal with the details of making a household work; however, some fathers do. His adjustment usually takes about a year, and it demands dedication, effort, and practice in selflessness. He needs to learn to develop a sense of enlightened self-interest. This is the task of a single parent with primary custody. All single parents experience a painful process in combining single life, parenting, work, and the mechanics of living.

The central issue in divorce seems to be custody. When there are no children, the couples then hassle over the dog, the cat, or the bedroom set! In all situations, if the two discuss the problems of custody in a mature manner, the process is a lot less painful and far more productive. Following decisions on custody, then, the task is to manage the children and cope with the unresolved angers without letting feelings interfere between the lives of the split couple and the children.

Another problem that needs coping with is when the child asserts himself regarding a need for the other parent. If it is an OK situation and the possibility is real, every effort should be made to arrange for him to be with the other parent.

All of the coping problems can be lumped under life-style adjustments. The mechanics of daily living are a problem when there are two parents at home and they are cooperative; they become an even greater problem when one parent is absent. Child care is a problem from the child's as well as the parents' point of view. The child needs to adjust to decreased time with parents (especially if the child is less than 10 years of age). The parents cope with the search for responsible, loving care givers and the expense of employing them. This can add several hundred dollars to the monthly expenses, depending on the number of children involved and, of course, their ages.

Again, coping with the anger generated through change and loss is a paramount adjustment. It is intensified when the parents have not resolved or channeled old angers between themselves. In these situations the child eventually becomes the victim of the divorce process. Children end up between the parents and receive no parenting. Coping with anger is no easy task, especially if the divorce has not been a clean one. There is no way to measure the pain and the anger for all involved when an angry divorce just ruminates and never resolves itself.

The parents need attention, too. Coping with all of the activities, work, and adjustments is no easy task. Many times the parents end up without their own needs being met. The anger cycle begins again and the person ends up depressed.

There are no words to describe the problems that can ensue from a divorce. One man with primary custody of his two young daughters paused, stared into space, and responded to my question regarding what single parenting was like: "It is just *real* hard."

Monetarily the burden of single parenting can be constricting. Unless the people are financially independent, the squeeze of the divorce is felt financially, socially, and in terms of time. Sitters are expensive, and yet it costs the parent a great deal not to allow himself or herself to socialize. Therefore in terms of both time and money it is a difficult situation.

Once the divorce is final the parents are in the third phase of getting on with life as unmarried persons and single parents. They may then involve a new person into the newly established network. This presents added problems. The situation becomes even more complicated because the single parent is juggling ways of creating alone time, family time, and now time for developing a new relationship. As a young man stated, "I can't be as spontaneous as some of my single friends." The freedom of single life is not present in single parenting. But while the task is exhausting, it can be rewarding and certainly is an invitation for creative and cooperative living.

STATUS OF RELATIONSHIP CHANGE

I see divorce as a growing apart. The two people no longer share the same interests and goals. If the divorce is part of the growth process mutually agreed on, then the situation tends to be less complicated. If the process of divorce brings with it insurmountable conflict and is destined to leave everyone involved feeling not OK, stress mounts and the chance is greater that the stress will produce illness, disease, and destruction.

If a single life-style does not emerge, the divorce never ends. If another marriage follows an incomplete divorce process, a rerun of the problems in the first relationship will occur. In order for a person to emerge successfully from the divorce process, he or she must live in an independent life-style for at least a year.

Before, during, or after the divorce filing, partners of a dying relationship begin to experience changes in their relationship as well as the changes involved in developing new relationships. One area in which to observe change is in sexual adjustment. I define sexuality as the desire for human contact and this includes the basic needs for affection, touch, tenderness, and love. I see sex and sexuality as a need for human touch and comfort, and it can be included in Maslow's hierarchy of human needs[19] (Fig. 3).

We are human sexual beings from conception to death. We need comfort even if only in the form of human touch. Many of us, however, are programmed not to be close to people and not to touch them. If we receive this message in childhood, we rework it and struggle with the fear of closeness through the divorce process. It is frequently very difficult to work through the fear of closeness and the problem of adjusting to a severance in a relationship. Our sexual value system dictates our rules for closeness. The problem in divorce is that many times the people in a divorce are faced with having to change their sexual value systems and learn how to be close.

The process of change involves three areas. The first area is being aware that one needs to change. The second is sharing the data with someone else, either in a therapeutic setting or outside of the therapeutic setting. The third is deciding on an action resulting from one's awareness.[20] The process of change may enhance growth. A prerequisite for growth is becoming aware of where one is and then moving toward change.

Basically the stages of a relationship change move from a "Don't be close" decision to a "Get close" decision (see Fig. 4, A). In between these two extremes there are various stages of relationship changes. Some

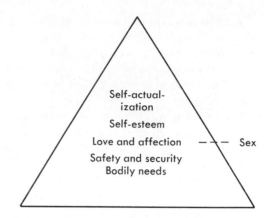

Fig. 3. Maslow's hierarchy of needs.

people never move from a "Don't be close" pattern; others get stuck somewhere in between. Because of the pain of a divorce few move on to developing closeness in a relationship where two people can be two total people sharing the relationship; dependency and fear in relationships after a divorce process prevail. Only when the parties become independent people, having licked their wounds, are they able to move on in the relationships. The process of the change to reentry into a relationship may look like Fig. 4, B.

The persons move from a position of "scare" to a position of independent risk taking and working to make their life work for them. They may never completely stop the scare and they move about despite the scare. This is a healthy adjustment and a desired outcome of the divorce process. The parties eventually develop a significant relationship and once again—or it may be for the first time—are able to develop a primary relationship and get close to another person.

If a person is raised to merge his identity in the marriage, however, a different or added process occurs. The person must reevaluate his value system and detach from the partner. From here the crisis of the separation and

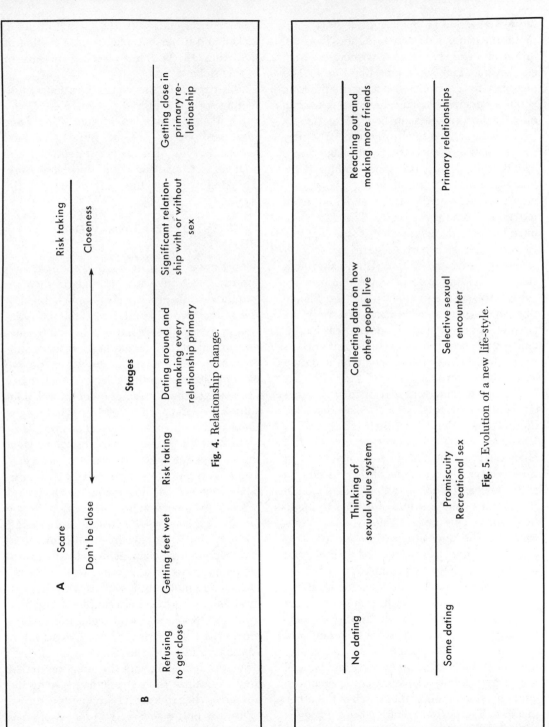

Fig. 4. Relationship change.

Fig. 5. Evolution of a new life-style.

individualization is open and, if it is complete, the panic in divorce is higher. The evolution of a life-style that is without internal conflict may look something like Fig. 5. The person may go from no dating to thinking about a personal sexual value system and go on to collecting data on how other people live, which may be totally different. The person may then reach out and make more friends and finally do some dating. After many months or years of dating, the person may become sexually active and may even move into some promiscuity. The next step, once the person decides that it is acceptable to get closer to a partner, is to do so with selected sexual encounters. The final growth stage is deciding to settle down to a primary relationship. At any point during the change the person may recycle back to a previous position. For example, if a person has a difficult sexual encounter after the beginning dating period, he may swing back into no dating and remain there.

The person may get stuck in an area, recycle, and decide to stay stuck. The thread is the message "Don't be close."

Another way of looking at relationship change is with the Karpman triangle.[16] Most divorced people fall in one of the positions of rescuer, persecuter, or victim. The person in the rescue position is into "I'm only trying to help you." This person usually does something for the opposite partner to help that person through the process of divorce, but actually does it to help himself feel better. This person is unable to separate from the partner. Again, this attachment is in direct proportion to how much self-identity the person has had in the marriage, not the length of the marriage. The person in the persecuter position is making the other party feel not OK at any opportunity. This is a one-upmanship game in which one partner catches the other in a flaw. The person initiating the game ends with the feeling of one-upmanship and the other person ends with the feeling of being kicked. Both persons play from a feeling of not being OK. Both feel insecure and unsure of themselves.

The person in the victim position is into feeling sorry for himself. "Poor me," "Why does it always happen to me?" and "See how hard I try?" are the games they find themselves in. The only way out of the triangle is to use the adult state and think. Thinking will get the partner out of the game.

INTERVENTION PROCESS IN PEOPLE HELPING

So far we have discussed love, marriage, the causes of divorce, the kinds of divorce, and the divorce process. As people helpers, it is essential for us to understand the intervention process. I intervene by inviting the clients to look at their situation as an opportunity to grow. By applying a growth model we explore the contributing factors each party has made to the deterioration of the relationship. These data are helpful in avoiding the same problems in a new relationship. After identifying the issues we then explore what the partner (or partners) want to change to avoid a rerun of the previous marital discord. Some people do not want to change. I respond by encouraging the person to see life, divorce, and grief on a continuum, and I teach cycling and recycling, and contracting and diagramming changes from family to single-parent roles. In addition, I work with various talking methods as well as with communication tools, which help couples to separate from an OK place. I also teach the divorce process as a life crisis, and I use crisis intervention. I identify the client's (or clients') strengths in dealing with the situation so that they will utilize their strengths in facing the new crisis. In a divorce situation it is essential to use the entire seven-step process of crisis theory.

Life crisis theory

In a life crisis a person is especially open to problem solving and new changes. The client is particularly susceptible to new input in making his life work and in finding new ways of problem solving.

Symptoms that are prevalent in a crisis are the recycling of past events, especially around previous losses, whether real, imagined, or anticipated. Clients also may experience a lack of self-confidence. Often they are upset and anxious; they may be crying, immobile, withdrawn, confused, angry, and scared. They may undergo behavior changes, for instance, sleep disturbances, changes in eating patterns, or general changes in their relations with people. These changes are frequently a part of the recycling.

Recycling is a part of the healing process.[19,21] The conflicts and tasks unresolved in earlier stages and phases are recycled when new tasks, conflicts, and losses appear. When conflicts remain unresolved, the human growth process is inhibited and the person stagnates, or remains fixed, at that particular stage of growth.

People frequently make early life decisions—as early as 6 months of age (or earlier if the person was severly emotionally abused). As their life progresses, early decisions no longer fit the stage of later development. Knowing where the client is in his recycling process is essential to effectively help him through his own process. Finding out what decisions were made and when they were made will help the client reexamine his life goals.

How do I find out? I ask the client! I may even draw a continuum and diagram the client's life crisis to help him help himself by seeing himself more clearly.

In addition to helping the client to identify his early life decisions, I teach him an adaptation of the problem solving process that was developed by Zahourek, Babcock, and myself.[19A] There are six steps through the process of problem solving:

1. Help the client identify the situation now. What are the stresses? List the things in the life stress scene.
2. Identify the client's feelings (anger, fear, and so forth).
3. Normalize when the stress is normal. People are not educated to normal human stress; teaching the client this can reduce his anxiety.
4. Teach the client to decide on a plan of action. I also help the clients to set goals for themselves, especially goals that would be helpful to them right now. Long-range goals may be included, but they need to focus on what is needed now.
5. Decide what the client can do now— what his priorities are and what he can do right now. I find out also what I as a clinician can do now.
6. Evaluate the client. I ask the client what is helpful to him or her. I ask what he needs but is not getting. I also ask what he needs in order to help himself. I take a look at what is not helpful to him, and I work with him to help to change what is not helpful. If I cannot help him to change what is not helpful, I refer the client to a place where he can get what he needs or to someone who is better able than I to help him.

Providing my intervention is helpful; the client and I review the above process and identify the new behavior. These new patterns are identified for the client, and he leaves the therapeutic process with a clear idea of what he can do to prevent the next crisis in a relationship.

Active listening

In addition to life crisis theory and the problem solving process, I also teach active listening.[20] In active listening the partner sets aside problem solving until he has heard everything the other partner has to say.

The process of active listening may be viewed as a five-step process: (1) listen quietly, (2) ask questions, (3) nod in response to the partner's communication, for example, "Un huh" (4) ask the other partner to clarify the issue and clarify for the partner what he heard the partner say, and (5) combine the above and offer suggestions—problem solve. The clarification and validation process includes both exact and approximate paraphrasing.

The first four steps of active listening come before problem solving can occur. Most partners err when, instead of listening, they begin problem solving in their heads and never hear what their partner said. A combining of all the above five steps, including problem solving, is active listening. The five-step process works into a delightful exercise for couples who are willing to practice the art and skill of active listening.

Stress

In addition to the skill of active listening, I also teach people who are going through a divorce to use the Social Readjustment Rating Scale.[22-24] This scale was introduced in 1967 by Holmes and Rahe. It lists 43 life events and assigns a value to each event. The life changes are added; for instance, if a person accumulates from 150 to 199 life crisis units, there is a 37% chance he will have a health-associated problem within 2 years. If the value is between 200 and 299 life crisis units, there is a chance that he will report a health change. If he has a score of 300, he has a 79% chance of illness or injury. The changes in health follow the life crisis in about a year.

As seen in the Social Readjustment Rating Scale, divorce is the second highest of the stresses leading to possible changes in health. Divorce is given a value of 73; death, a value of 100. If there are other changes in one's life, the chance of illness within a 2-year period of time is 37%. This means many things from pacing a life crisis to planning a divorce.

When I am working with a person in a life crisis, I help him to add up the amount of stresses that he is under. From this I can do preventive psychiatric counseling and teach coping behavior to help the client help himself to avoid possible physical manifestations of stress.

Other interventions

There are a number of other interventions that I use to help couples with their relationship or to help them sort out whether or not divorce should be their option: (1) identifying a contract between the partners (even if the contract is unspoken); (2) identifying rules and norms established along the way—rules and norms that had not been clearly defined or talked about by the couple; (3) teaching the partners skills in active listening;(4) observing a couple as they talk with each other and helping to point out the pitfalls of dysfunctional communication; (5) if the couple is in the growing process, giving them permission for the process to be fun; (6) if the couple is separating, working toward the enhancement of an OK separation; (7) if the couple fears the growing and changing relationship, referring them to therapy to facilitate individualization; and (8) teaching them to use the Karpman triangle.

I find that it is helpful for a couple going through a divorce to see their lives on the continua of relationship change, grief process, and anger racket. I use the Karpman triangle to help them visualize their life positions. If I visualize where a couple is, I can help them to see where they are and what their options are for change and growth. It is an exciting way to view the divorce process and a helpful tool in therapeutic practice.

Another way of helping people through a

divorce process is to contract with them for a separation and life change pattern. I contract with them for individual or couple therapy[24] by asking them (1) What are the problems? (2) What do you want to change? (3) How will you know when it is changed? (4) What are you willing to do now? and (5) What do you want from me? The contract can be limited to one partner in a relationship. He or she can do self-contracting using the above formula and moving through the process. This is helpful especially when there is an unwilling partner.

Another tool in therapy is to work with clients in identifying the ways in which they have coped previously with their losses. If the mechanism is helpful to them, I help them plug in that mechanism to cope with the grief of the divorce process.

In my practice, I use the intervention process analysis identified by Risley[26] as it applies to my clients who are going through a divorce. I identify (1) my needs, (2) my feelings, (3) my intervention on behalf of myself, (4) the client's needs, (5) the client's feelings, and finally (6) the intervention on behalf of the client. This six-step process is a guideline to my therapeutic intervention.

The use of a continuum in viewing both myself and my client is another helpful tool in decision making. I see life as a continuum. It has a beginning, a middle, and an end. The stages and phases of growth and development can be plotted on a continuum flow. Viewing a person in his growth stages is one of the guidelines for my therapeutic practice. With this, the client sees where he is in relation to where he needs or wants to be. I see an overview of the possible areas for change and use the continuum from which to view the change. The continuum then becomes a guideline for therapeutic intervention. An example of this is a 45-year-old woman who is divorced, living alone, and having problems coping with the independent unmarried state; she seeks therapy to stop crying and to become independent. Her continuum may look like Fig. 6. In looking at the continuum with her, I can see her phases of life change, where she has come from, where she has recycled to, what developmental tasks she has not completed, and where she needs to

Divorce continuum

Married	First child	First thought of divorce	Second child	Children have left	Separated	Final divorce
1953	1954	1955	1956	1974	1977	1978

Life continuum

Born	School	Death of mother	Married	Child	Child	Separated
1933	1939	1943	1953	1954	1956	1977

Grief continuum

1943 ---

Death of mother   1977 divorce

| Denial | Anger | Bargaining | Depression | Acceptance |

Fig. 6

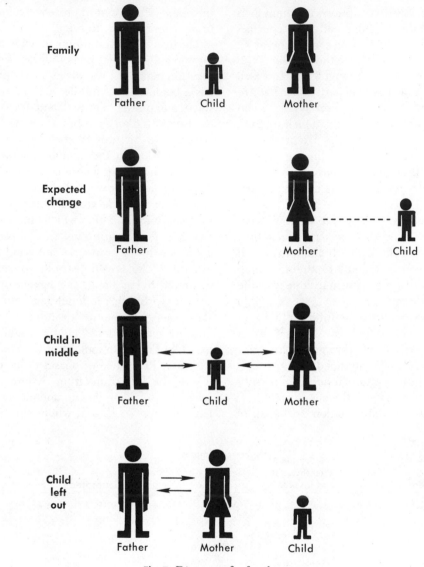

Fig. 7. Diagram of a family system.

go from here. Scanning the continuum will be a helpful tool for her to make independent commitments for change.

Another prevention tool I use in working with clients in a stressful situation is an adaptation from Zahourek's family stress model.[25] These stress models include the diagramming of family systems, which is the part that I use. I have the family members draw themselves as they are now and then with their anticipated changes (Fig. 7). The family members may visualize themselves differently as separate entities than they do within the family unit, for example, a father, mother, and child.

The child may be in the center of the family with the communication in, around, and through the child. The same family may visualize an expected change as the mother and child existing without the father. In actuality the change may lead to a situation in which the child is caught directly in the middle and the communication takes place only through and with the child. Another example of this would be if the child were left out of the communication in the relationship.

Sometimes when the couple becomes aware of the possibility of placing a child in a victim position, it is enough impetus for them to take a different course of action. It may open paths for more effective communication between these partners.

There are many other diagrams and possible options using family stress models, and it is useful to help the family or couple in visualizing how they would like to continue parenting roles once the marital relationship is severed. This diagramming may be most valuable, and frequently offers direct input on the dysfunction in the development of the marital discord. Children are frequently aware of the problems in a marital relationship even if they have never been directly involved by the couple in their talking. The child's input into the family change may be valuable, particularly at the time when the couple definitely has decided to divorce and the problem-solving process of a single unit is underway. Much before this time it is too premature and too stressful for the child.

In divorce the couple's marital status ceases but their parenting roles will continue. This is why it is so essential in counseling to work out the most OK process, the least anger-provoking agreement in the most stimulating growth environment. If they do not, the children will most surely become victims of the marital cessation and their life scars will be deep. Parents should continue to be parents; the children still need to be taken care of, and they should not be caught in the middle.

One of the most essential tools in people helping is teaching the divorce process and teaching what is normal. Most people are unfamiliar with the process; usually their acquaintance with the divorce process is only with the person who has been in an extreme anger situation. This is certainly not the only way to separate. Facilitating the growth model is the most effective way a therapist can help people.

SUMMARY

Divorce is a life crisis. It can be a creative time of change and a growing process for those involved; or it can be a destructive, marring experience that leaves life-long scars. The degree to which the anger is unresolved is related directly to the lethality of the divorce. The more unresolved the anger is, the more negative the divorce process is. The divorce process has a beginning, a middle, and an end. Divorce seldom ends with the final hearing and signing of the papers.

As people helpers we can help people to help themselves through the process of divorce by first learning about the process and then by knowing the options for intervention.

There is life after a divorce and the coping problems are related to family structuring, finances, and how OK the divorce process is. The more OK the divorce is, the more anger is resolved, and the less trauma there is for the children.

REFERENCES

1. Statistical abstract of United States: 98th annual edition, Washington, D.C., 1977, U.S. Department of Commerce, Bureau of Census;
2. Heller, P. J., and Heller, M.: 3 out of 4 marriages this year will end in divorce: Denver is No. 1. What is being done? Denver, vol. 5, 1977.
3. Satir, V.: Conjoint family therapy, ed. 2, Calif. 1967, Science & Behavior Books, Inc.

4. Bevis, E. O.: Curriculum building in nursing: a process, ed. 2, St. Louis, 1978, The C. V. Mosby Co.

5. Aguilera, D. C. and Messick, J. M.: Crisis intervention, ed. 3, St. Louis, 1978, The C. V. Mosby Co.

6. Kübler-Ross, E.: On death and dying; New York, 1975, Macmillan Publishing Co., Inc.

7. Zahourek, R. and Jensen, J.: The loss of the newborn: nursing implications, Feb. 12, 1971, unpublished.

8. Zahourek, R. and Jensen, J.: Grieving and the loss of the newborn; Am. J. Nurs. **73:**836-839, May 1973.

9. Thaler, O. F.: Grief and depression, Nurs. Forum **5:**9-22, 1966.

10. Ujhely, G. B.: Grief and depression: implications for prevention and therapeutic nursing care, Nurs. Forum **5:**24-35, 1966.

11. Engel, C.: Psychological development in health and disease; Philadelphia, 1962, W. B. Saunders Co.

12. Lindeman, E.: Symptomatology and management of acute grief; Am. J. Psychiatry **101:**141-148, September 1944.

13. Engel, G. L.: Grief and grieving; Am. J. Nurs. **64:** 93-98, September 1964.

14. The world almanac and book of facts, 1975, New York, 1974, Newspaper Enterprise Association, Inc.

15. Krantzler, M.: Creative divorce, New York, 1974, M. Evans & Co., Inc.

15A. Goldberger, D.: Notes from workshop with Rev. Jim Smoke of California, Denver, Pastoral counselor.

16. Karpman, S. B.: Fairy tales & script drama analysis, Transactional Analysis Bulletin **7**(26): 39, April 1968.

17. James, M., and Jongeward, D.: Born to win; Reading, Mass., 1971, Addison-Wesley Pub. Co.

18. Holmes, M., and Keepers, T.: Transactional analysis workshop, Denver, 1970, unpublished.

19. Babcock, D., and Keepers T.: Raising kids O.K., New York, 1976, Grove Press, Inc.

19A. Zahourek, R., Babcock, D., and Meagher, M.: Notes from Workshops on Problem-Solving, Life Crises, and Grief, Denver, 1970-1975.

20. Dodson, L. S.: Family therapy workshop, Denver, 1969.

21. Sheehy, G.: Passages, New York, 1976, E. P. Dutton & Co., Inc.

22. Holmes, T. H., and Rahe, R. H.: The social readjustment scale, J. Psychosom. Res. **11**(2):3-8, 1967.

23. Dudley D., and Welke, E.: Change: it could kill you, Denver Post, Oct. 23, 1977. How to survive being alive, New York, 1977, Doubleday & Co., Inc.

24. Attwell, T.: Self-awareness, self-responsibility and self-esteem: a treatment plan, Transactional Analysis Journal, **4**(2): 25, April 1974.

25. Zahourek, R.: Psychological aspects of the critically ill and their families, Vail, Colo., 1976, unpublished.

26. Risley, J.: Nursing intervention in depression, Perspect. Psychiatr. Care **5**(2):65-67, 1967.

7

Child abuse patterns in the family unit

Sharon L. Cross

Although abusive parenting behavior can be traced throughout history, it was not until 1961 that the term the "battered child syndrome" was first used by Dr. Henry Kempe to describe the plight of children throughout this country. Because of the frequency of its occurrence in communities and the desired potential to prevent the recurrence of abusive parenting, the problem of child abuse and neglect clearly becomes one of the responsibilities of community health nurses.

In an attempt to analyze more specifically the nature of the problem as well as the nurse's role in prevention and intervention, an epidemiologic model will be used. Thus the occurrence of the problem, the agent, the host, the suseptibility, and the nursing intervention to minimize negative effects will be discussed and explored.

OCCURRENCE OF CHILD ABUSE AND NEGLECT

According to 1975 statistics, there were 550,000 cases of suspected child abuse and neglect reported in the United States. The incidence of child abuse is thought to be approximately 500 new cases per million population per year. However, when neglect is also reported, it is expected that this figure may double.

In recent years all 50 states have mandated the reporting of suspected families by health professionals including nurses and a variety of other community individuals. Although these laws have assisted in increasing our awareness of the widespread nature of the problem, several factors continue to limit our knowledge of the problem's actual occurrence in the population.

One of the most perplexing factors that makes identifcation difficult relates to the complexity of analyzing parenting behaviors and determining to what degree abusive and neglectful behavior influences both the physical and psychosocial development of a child. The physically injured child or the abandoned or malnourished child is more easily detected. The challenge that remains is the recognition of those families in which the more abstract forms of abuse occur, such as verbal battery and parental rejection. Only when we are able to define the minimal nurturing a child needs to develop physically and psychosocially will we be more able to describe fully the occurrence of the problem in the population.

Another limiting factor in problem identification is the potentially undetected abuse and neglect that occur in middle-income and upper-income families. Some experts believe that identification occurs more readily in lower-income families because they have greater contact with professionals in public agencies. Additionally, the number of cases of sexual abuse identified and reported is believed to be far below the actual incidence in the population. The very nature of incest and its cultural taboos often lead to family secrecy and denial. Because of the dynamics present in incestuous families, the child-victim frequently assumes responsibility for maintaining family congruency and blame for the sexual encounters and thus does not report the incident. Young children also may believe that their sexual contacts are representative of all children's experience, even when they are aware of being the only involved child in the family. As they move into adolescence, they may then begin to recognize the differences in their family and again feel guilty and peculiar. These feelings inhibit their reporting of sexual abuse to helping professionals. As a result of these factors, combined with the problem community professionals may have in perceiving this kind of abuse, detection becomes considerably more difficult than when a child has a visible injury. Although our awareness of the problem has increased dramatically in recent years, the actual numbers of affected families are unknown.

THE AGENT

Research on abusive parents has contributed significantly to our ability to describe and identify the parental agent. Studies indicate that parents who abuse their children were themselves frequently abused by their care givers. As children they experienced a "lack of empathetic mothering." They frequently are found disciplining their children or responding to them in the same manner that their parents dealt with them. Although replicating past parenting behavior is a common finding in most parent-child relationships, it becomes a significant problem for the children of these individuals. If as children these parents were repeatedly told that they were mean, bad, ugly, or dumb, they frequently will use the same words to describe their children. Because these parents have not experienced alternative, positive parenting behaviors, they are unable to behave more positively toward their own children.

Another indicator of a high-risk potential for abusive behavior is based on the parents' inadequate self-concept. As a result of their own childhood, these individuals view themselves as negative persons who have no control over their lives, who set unrealistic goals for themselves, and who as a result are consistently negatively reinforced by failure. Because of their inability to define their own self-worth, they cannot identify their child's worth, and the cycle of personal degradation continues.

Inappropriate expectations of their children's behavior is another commonly found characteristic of abusive parents. A common example is the mother who describes looking forward to the delivery of her baby so that she will have someone to love her. Clearly this expectation is one that an infant physically and psychologically cannot accomplish. As a result of this inappropriate expectation, the mother experiences rejection, which further reinforces her belief that she is unloveable.

Another commonly reported example is the parent who allows iron cords or coffeepot cords to be within the reach of a toddler. Often the parent allows the child to pull on the cord to teach him through self-injury not to pull on electrical cords. Such an experience not only places the child in significant danger but it also places the child in a position of personal failure followed by parental reprimands and rejection, which fosters the development of a poor self-concept in the child.

Parents who use violence to deal with their

frustrations and discouragements are also at high risk for potential abuse. Women who are abused by their husbands or boyfriends frequently were physically and sexually abused as children. Some interpret the violent behavior as an expression of someone's caring for them. They then demonstrate similar behavior toward their children. Striking numbers of previously abused adults select partners with similar life experiences, thus limiting their experiential behavior alternatives in dealing with their children while continuing to experience self-rejection.

Social isolation is another factor that describes abusive or neglectful parents. On history taking one finds that these parents are unable to name someone on whom they could call if they needed help. Often these families move frequently, perhaps twice within a month or several times in a year. These moves contribute to the disruption of their lives, resulting in inconsistent relationships with neighbors or concerned professionals.

Despite parents' abusive behavior, studies indicate that no more than 10% of them are mentally ill. Instead, these abusive agents are products of their own childhood and need a great deal of help in learning alternative parenting behaviors. They are individuals who want to, and in their own way do, love their children.

THE HOST

To describe the host is to define the child and to recognize that it is the interaction between the parent and the child that makes for an abusive incident. A variety of studies have indicated that children with congenital anomalies are at risk for abuse because of the difficulty parents may have in forming an attachment to this child and his special needs and care requirements. These studies have also begun to explain why one child within a family may be at greater risk for abuse than another. The relationship of the parents and the prenatal, labor and delivery, and postpartum experiences are all significant factors contributing to the parent-child attachment process. If parents perceive these experiences negatively, the potential risk to the child increases. Similarly an infant who cries frequently or who is difficult to quiet may be perceived by the parent as rejecting the parent. Such an interpretation appears reasonable to a parent who has consistently experienced unsuccessful relationships. Also, an infant cry, which is frustrating to many parents, becomes more frustrating when there is no one else with whom they can leave the child. Similarly, extremely active children have been identified as at risk for abuse. The combination of frustrating child behavior, coupled with limited alternatives for dealing with the child, leads to abusive parental acts.

SUSCEPTIBILITY OF FAMILIES TO ABUSIVE BEHAVIOR

The susceptibility of families to abusive behavior intensifies when an event occurs that the parents interpret as a crisis. Because it is the parents' response to an event that makes it a crisis for them, the type of event that precipitates a crisis or abusive response is limitless. For some families it may be a financial concern; for others it may be the disappointment of unfilled holiday expectations coupled with a child's increased excitement around the holiday. Another example of a potential high-risk situation is the parents' having a flat tire on the way to a clinic appointment combined with a sick child who has a high fever and a parent who has no one with whom he can share his frustrations and feelings.

The agent and the host coupled with a crisis event present a complex set of factors that, when they occur together, create an abusive situation. Increasingly it is believed that any time the variables combine, anyone who has contact with a child is susceptible to abusive behavior.

COMMUNITY HEALTH NURSING INTERVENTION TO MINIMIZE NEGATIVE EFFECTS OF CHILD ABUSE

The purpose of nursing intervention in child abuse and neglect situations is to help parents to replace their negative personal and parenting behaviors with methods that foster healthy physical and psychosocial development in their children. In dealing with families and aggregates of families in the community, the role of the nurse includes (1) case identification and reporting, (2) assurance of follow-through of the medical plan after physical injury or nutritional deprivation, (3) assessment of the physical and psychosocial development of the parent and child, (4) instruction of parents regarding normal growth and development of children, (5) provision of alternative methods of child rearing, and (6) coordination of nursing intervention with the actions of other involved professionals. These particular roles have been selected because they effectively interface parent and child needs with the knowledge and skill of community health nurses. It is this crucial determination of family need and nursing ability that must be made in each case to ensure that nursing intervention will be beneficial in a specific family situation.

Although specific community health nursing interventions will be addressed, it is also essential to consider the process that nurses use to accomplish effective outcomes with families. Thus it is crucial that public health nurses understand the factors that make parents and children respond as they do. It is only when nurses understand abusive behavior that they can begin to formulate a plan in collaboration with the client. When one recognizes that these parents' experiences and views of themselves inhibit their ability to trust others, then one can purposefully

address this problem in the nursing plan and establish a long-term objective that deals with encouraging client trust. Several behaviors that have been shown to encourage client-nurse trust include (1) following through on all things agreed to with the client, (2) consistent visiting even when the parent appears angry with the nurse, (3) contacting a social worker or physician by telephoning directly from the family's home, (4) sharing written reports directly with the family, and (5) being certain to explain when and why a child abuse report is filed. Again, because the past experience of these parents may have altered their perceptions of why a nurse is suggesting something, it is important to explain clearly why a recommendation is being made and purposely allow the parent an opportunity to question further. The nurse also needs to remember that these families have had numerous experiences that have made them untrusting, and that it may take a long time before any trust with the nurse can be established. The development of trust, however, will be the cornerstone of the nurse's ability to work effectively with these parents.

Another effective method of intervention with these families is that of establishing a mutually defined contract. Until the parent begins to trust the nurse, it may be difficult to develop a functionally effective agreement. In this process one can use either a written or verbal agreement depending on the learning style of the parent. Through this process both the parent and the nurse define specific problems that they want to address. This first step affords the client an opportunity for problem identification while also allowing the nurse to share her professional assessment of the family's needs. It also provides the nurse with the opportunity to define specifically which problems she can help the family with and which ones would benefit from other professional intervention; then nurse and family can proceed to define the problems they will work on and discuss what alternatives are available to resolve them. This step is followed by identifying what actions the parent will take and what responsibility the nurse will have. A time can be set for mutually evaluating the outcomes of the contract. After the evaluation process the contract can be renegotiated, continued, or terminated. The benefits of using contracting include problem clarification, clarity and honesty between parents and nurse, mutual rather than nurse responsibility, and application of the problem-solving process, which families can learn to use in other situations.

The third process to be considered by community health nurses is that of being as concrete as possible in teaching and counseling. Although role modeling can be an effective teaching method, its impact is enhanced when the community health nurse verbalizes to the parent what she is doing and why. In this way the nurse and the parent can better understand, recall, and apply the learning that has occurred. Because of their experience and perceptions, these parents often do not understand the multiple behaviors that combine to nurture a child effectively. To clarify these behaviors and allow the parent to use them with the child, the nurse might be very directive with the parent by setting limits on the parent's behavior. At another time she might listen to the parent and demonstrate concern for his feelings. After each behavior, the nurse might then describe what parental role she was assuming and then have the parent demonstrate a similar response to the child. In some situations it may also be helpful to use pictures that depict the accompanying appropriate nonverbal behavior. Such methods assist the nurse to make abstract behaviors concrete, thus enabling the parent to replicate them.

Because of the complexity of the problem of child abuse and neglect, there are no simplistic formulas or methods for accomplishing effective nursing intervention. There are, however, activities that are the responsibility of the community health nurse working with abusive families.

When taking a history of a family, the nurse should be certain to include questions that explore (1) the parents' view of discipline, (2) their view of their own childhood and how they would like that of their children to be similar or dissimilar, (3) their support systems, (4) their perception of themselves compared to how they see others, (5) their description of their child and his or her behavior, and (6) their expectations of their child's behavior. Dependent on the parent's responses and the parent-child interaction, the nurse may make a report to the local child protection agency. It is absolutely essential, however, that the nurse inform the family of the report. In so doing, the nurse may say, "It doesn't appear to me that the injury could have happened in the way you described. I'm interested in helping you; I know that you love your child and that you don't want to hurt him." When this information is shared, one typically finds that the parents deal more effectively with their anger and are able to use social service help faster. Any time a nurse observes a child's injury, it is important to include a description of an injury including the location, size, number of marks, and estimated duration of the injury. Any time a child has been abused it is important to include in the parent-nurse contract an opportunity to inspect the child. When completing a physical assessment, the nurse should also check the child in less visible areas such as the soles of the feet, between the toes, and the fingers and scalp.

If the nurse is intervening for follow-up of a medical plan, it is important that the parents get specific, consistent information from the public health nurse and that they fully understand what is expected of them in caring for the recovering child. In an infant with failure to thrive or low weight gain, the nurse should specifically observe the parents' feeding or food preparation technique. In so doing, the nurse is better able to detect problem areas and will then be prepared to use the most effective method of intervention. In such a case it is necessary for the nurse to graph regular weight and head circumference measurements. It is also important to remember the parents' needs and not demonstrate concern solely for the child.

Through the use of tools such as the Denver Developmental Screening Test, the Draw-A-Man Test, and the Piaget experiments, the nurse can assess the child's physical and psychosocial development. Most parents find these screening mechanisms interesting. Although the screenings were not developed as teaching mechanisms, they do effectively demonstrate realistic expectations for children of specific ages. In this way parents are helped to gain information about normal growth and development. Again, the nurse can be helpful in drawing the parents' attention to a child's specific behavior. As noted earlier, these parents may not recognize or understand why a child is behaving in a specific way. For example, the parent who becomes angry when an infant spits out cereal needs to understand the child's tongue thrust and that oral exploration is normal behavior and not a rejection of the parent. A child's "no" response needs to be recognized as normal infant behavior and not rebellion. Often parents can gain more realistic expectations of their children if nurses can expose them to the behavior of children of similar ages to those of their own. In this way groups for parents can be extremely beneficial.

Once parents begin to identify the problems inherent in their parent-child relationships and begin to trust helping professionals, their involvement in groups may be an important consideration for the intervention plan. Whether the group is a local chapter of Parents Anonymous or another similarly directed group, the effective utilization of the group process can assist parents to (1) gain support from others by recognizing the similarity of their problems, (2) develop more effective personal interaction skills, (3) perceive themselves and their experiences more realistically, (4) define alternative solutions to problems that previously had been outside of the parents' own experience, and (5) enlarge their personal support system.

It is crucial that teaching these parents about children be done in a manner that recognizes the parents' ability and knowledge, no matter how limited. After the parents' input is gained, the nurse can expand on the information that the parents have shared while positively reinforcing the parents' contribution. Because of their lack of experience with "empathetic mothering," these parents initially may not be able to identify their child's needs or feelings. Thus the nurse may first need to have the parents express how they would feel in a particular situation. After the parents have verbalized their feelings, the nurse will need to help them recognize that this may be how their child feels also. In some cases the nurse may need to tell the parent specifically what to do; for example, "Hold the baby closely." "Kiss the baby." "Ask John what he did in school." "Tell Beth why her picture is good." Again, after the parents follow through, the nurse has an opportunity to reinforce the parents' positive attempts while simultaneously providing the parents with a concrete alternative to their past behavior. Another apparently effective method of reinforcing parental behavior while improving parents' self-concept, is to have them define those positives that they have demonstrated during the nursing visit, as well as during the past day or week.

For these parents and their children, it is important that the community health nurse use creativity in dealing with their complex problems. Similarly it is critical that the nurse clearly delineates her biases in working in abusive situations, for these biases may be detrimental to the family. Only when the nurse is able to recognize and deal effectively with her fears, anger, and frustration will she be able to intervene in a manner conducive to an abusive family's positive development. Similarly, the community health nurse must benefit from effective supervision in case management. It is unreasonable for the nurse to deal with these families, whose care is long term and whose progress is slow, without the support of effective nursing supervision in addition to collaboration with other professionals.

Finally, if community health nursing intervention is to be truly significant in altering abusive parenting practices in this country, we must attack the problem from two additional perspectives. The first to be explored is that of working collaboratively with other community professionals to develop mechanisms that will break the cycle of dysfunction-al parenting and child abuse and to promote positive parenting. The second area of need is that of objectively evaluating community health nursing intervention through research. Only as community health nurses continue to explore, experiment, examine, and evaluate and are professionally and empathetically involved with abusive families will we be able to improve the staggering experiences of many parents and children throughout this country.

SUGGESTED READINGS

Helfer, R. E., and Kempe, C. H.: The battered child, ed. 2, Chicago, 1974, The University of Chicago Press.

Helfer, R. E., and Kempe, C. H.: Child abuse and neglect: the family and the community, Cambridge, Mass., 1976, Ballinger Publishing Co.

Josten. L.: Out-of-hospital care for a pervasive family problem: child abuse, Am. J. Maternal Child Nurs. 3:111, March/April, 1978.

Justice, R., and Justice, B.: The abusing family, New York, 1976, Human Sciences Press.

Schmitt, B. D., ed.: The child protection team handbook, New York, 1978, Garland STPM Press.

8

Fertility and family planning in the United States
progress, programs, and challenges

Michael C. Chulada

Significant changes in the fertility of Americans have taken place in recent years. Although many factors have influenced the fertility aspirations of our population, one factor has enabled people to meet the fertility goals that they have set for themselves—the availability of family planning methods and services. Many people, particularly those who are young or poor, are provided with the means to realize their goals through a nationwide network of publicly subsidized family planning programs. This chapter provides a brief overview of the progress made in recent years, the part that family planning programs have played in that progress, and the challenges that face these programs as they attempt to address the remaining family planning needs of Americans.

CHANGING FERTILITY PATTERNS

Dramatic reductions in the fertility of Americans have taken place during the past two decades. Beginning in 1958, after 10 years of the baby boom and relatively high birth rates, a steady downward trend in American birth rates began. As a result, in the 20-year period from 1958 to 1977, our crude birth rate (births per thousand population) plummeted from 24.6 to 15.3, a drop of almost 40%.[1,2] Had the birth rate remained the same as in 1958, Americans would have experienced over 2 million more births than they actually did in 1977.

Much of this decline has been attributed to a reduction in unwanted and mistimed births among married couples. In the mid-1960s, 1 in 5 marital births was termed unwanted by the parents at the time of conception. By 1973 this rate had dropped almost 60% to 1 in 12.[3]

Although these shifts in fertility patterns are dramatic in and of themselves, it is important to note that during this period the reduction in birth rates and rates of unwanted fertility was most pronounced in groups that previously had the highest fertility rates—the poor, ethnic minorities, and residents of rural areas.[4] Differentials in unwanted fertility still exist between income and racial groups, but these differentials have been reduced significantly in the recent past.

The major subgroup of the population that has not shared in this significant fertility decline is females 17 years old and younger. While other age groups experienced birth rate decreases of from 25% to 40% during the

1970s, females aged 10 to 14 experienced no decrease, and those 15 to 17 experienced only a 10.8% decrease.[5] The consequences of this are serious for both adolescents and society as a whole.

CAUSES OF FERTILITY DECLINE

Certainly no single factor can account for the dramatic reduction in fertility that we have witnessed in recent years. A variety of social, personal, legal, economic, and medical factors have all had an impact. Those most frequently mentioned are the changing roles and aspirations of women, recent economic trends including a steady increase in the cost of living, concern about environmental issues and overpopulation, the desire for upward mobility in an increasing segment of the population, and the removal of legal and cultural barriers to the practice of family planning.

These factors and without doubt many others have led to significant changes in the birth desires and expectations of Americans. According to the U.S. Bureau of the Census, the average number of children anticipated by married women aged 18 to 39 fell from 3.1 in 1967 to 2.4 in 1976. Furthermore, the younger the woman, the lower her birth expectations were. Those women aged 18 to 24 expected an average of 2.1 children and those 35 to 39 expected an average of 2.9.[6] Opinion polls have also reflected trends toward smaller family expectations. In 1968 41% of the respondents in a national survey indicated that four or more children constituted their ideal family size. By 1977 only 13% considered four or more children as ideal. The 1977 poll also reported that 72% of the respondents considered two or three children ideal; 2% felt that one child was ideal; and 1% said they wanted no children; while 11% had no opinion on the matter.[7]

What does this mean for future fertility? While these data reflect changing attitudes about childbearing in our culture, they can be used only as crude predictors. Some demographers think that our low fertility rates are simply a result of changes in the timing and spacing of births. They predict increases in fertility rates in the future. Others disagree and predict a leveling off at or below current rates. It is important to note that data gathered in the 1970 and 1975 national fertility studies indicated that the actual fertility of Americans was 16% lower than their expected fertility.[8] If this trend continues we may be entering a period in which the average American family has only two children.

THE CONTRACEPTIVE REVOLUTION

The significant reduction in fertility in the recent past makes it apparent that childbearing is under a greater degree of voluntary control today than ever before. We have witnessed a number of important changes in the fertility control practices of Americans in the past decade; some have termed these changes the "contraceptive revolution."

In 1976 about 90% of all married couples at risk of an unintended pregnancy were using either sterilization or a temporary method of contraception to prevent pregnancy. This compares with approximately 70% a decade ago.[3] During this same period the percentage of married couples choosing the most effective contraceptive methods (sterilization, pill, and IUD) almost doubled, and the percentage using the least effective methods (douche, withdrawal, and rhythm) declined by over one half. Table 2 details the changes in contraceptive choices of married couples from 1965 to 1976.[9,10] These changes truly represent a revolution in contraceptive practices among married couples, and they closely parallel the dramatic declines in both general fertility and unwanted fertility during the period.

Perhaps the most significant change in the past decade has been an increase in reliance

Table 2. Percentage of distribution of married women aged 15 to 44 using contraception, by current method used and percentage of change, United States 1965 and 1976*

Current method used	1965(%)†	1976(%)†	Percentage point change, 1965-1976
Wife sterilized‡	7.0	14.1	7.1
Husband sterilized*‡	5.1	14.3	9.2
Oral contraceptive (pill)	23.9	32.8	8.9
Intrauterine device (IUD)	1.2	9.0	7.8
Diaphragm	9.9	4.3	−5.6
Condom	21.9	10.6	−11.3
Foam	3.3	4.4	1.1
Rhythm	10.9	5.0	−5.9
Withdrawal	4.0	2.9	−1.1
Douche	5.2	1.0	−4.2
Other	7.5	1.3	−5.2

*Data from Westoff, C. F., and Jones, E. F.: Contraception and sterilization in the United States, 1965-1975, Family Planning Perspectives 9:154, July/August 1977; U.S. Public Health Service: Advance data: contraceptive utilization in the United States, 1973 and 1976, No. 36, Washington, D.C., 1978, U.S. Government Printing Office.
†Percentages may not total 100 because of rounding.
‡Includes only those people sterilized for contraceptive purposes.

on surgical sterilization for contraceptive purposes. The use of sterilization more than doubled among married women and nearly tripled among married men between 1965 and 1976. For the first time more men than women have been turning to sterilization. It is by far the most popular contraceptive method for couples who have all the children they want. The percentage of these couples choosing sterilization (43%) is almost double the percentage using the pill (24%), the second most frequently used method.[10]

Analysis of available data for 1973 and 1976, reflected in Table 3, points out some of the more recent trends and racial differentials that exist in contraceptive choices. Analysis of these data shows the following:

1. Although rates of use for the pill and IUD continued to rise between 1965 and 1973, a slight downturn occurred between 1973 and 1976. Approximately 4% fewer couples were using these methods in 1976 than were in 1973. Since approximately 60% of the couples used either these methods or sterilization in both 1973 and 1976, this change may be primarily the result of a shift to sterilization among couples previously using the pill or IUD.

2. A slight upturn in the use of rhythm, diaphragm, and douche reversed the trend toward decreased reliance on less effective methods. Approximately 3% more couples employed these methods in 1976 than did in 1973.

3. A significant decrease, almost 11%, took place in the percentage of black couples using the most effective methods (sterilization, pill, and IUD).

The shifts in contraceptive practices between 1973 and 1976 may be partly attributable to increased publicity about the potential risks and side effects associated with use of the pill and the IUD. Whatever the reasons, the increase in use of the least effective methods by all couples using contraception and the decrease in use of the most effective methods by black couples in particular are

Table 3. Percentage of currently married couples who use contraception, by method of contraception, according to race, United States, 1973 and 1976*

Method of contraception	All couples (%)†*		White (%)†		Black (%)†		Hispanic origin (%)†	
	1976	1973	1976	1973	1976	1973	1976	1973
Contraceptive sterilization§								
Female	14.1	12.4	13.9	11.6	18.9	22.7	11.8	16.3
Male	14.3	11.2	15.2	11.9	3.3	1.7	7.1	7.6
Contraceptive method								
Oral contraceptives	32.8	36.1	32.6	35.6	37.7	43.9	34.9	35.0
Intrauterine device	9.0	9.6	8.8	9.3	10.5	12.7	17.5	13.3
Diaphragm	4.3	3.4	4.3	3.5	3.1	2.0	4.0	2.7
Condom	10.6	13.5	10.7	14.0	7.7	5.3	10.3	10.7
Foam	4.4	5.0	4.2	5.0	6.5	5.0	5.9	2.7
Rhythm	5.0	4.0	5.1	4.1	2.4	1.2	5.2	3.2
Withdrawal	2.9	2.2	2.9	2.3	3.1	.7	1.8	3.4
Douche	1.0	.9	.7	.7	4.6	3.0	.2	.9
Other	1.3	1.9	1.3	1.8	2.1	1.7	.8	4.1

*Data from U.S. Public Health Service: Advance data: contraceptive utilization in the United States, 1973 and 1976, No. 36, Washington, D.C., 1978, U.S. Government Printing Office.
†Percentages may not total 100 due to rounding.
‡Includes all races.
§Includes only those couples sterilized for *contraceptive* purposes.

significant. It is likely that we will see the results when data regarding contraceptive failure and unwanted fertility become available for the period beginning in 1976.

Contraceptive failure

Although the percentage of people at risk of unintended pregnancy who are using contraception has steadily increased, contraceptive failure is a continuing problem. In the 3-year period from 1970 to 1973, 3.7% of married couples who wanted no more children at any future time experienced a failure within the first year of contraceptive use. Of those couples attempting to delay pregnancy to some future time, 7.3% experienced a contraceptive failure.[11] While these rates of contraceptive failure reflect a high degree of effectiveness for the population as a whole, they

certainly indicate that there is much room for improvement. Table 4 depicts theoretical and actual effectiveness rates of contraceptive methods. The theoretical rates refer to the number of failures that can be expected when a method is used correctly and consistently. The actual rates refer to the actual number of failures experienced by users of the method and takes into consideration human error. First-year failure rates for methods other than sterilization range from 4% for the pill to 40% for douching. These rates clearly point out the inadequacy of currently available methods.[12]

As important as rates of contraceptive failure are, the rates of failure to use contraceptives are even more serious. In 1976 10% of married couples who were at risk of an unintended pregnancy were not using contracep-

Table 4. Theoretical and actual contraceptive failures during first year of use per 100 women who want no more children*

Method	Theoretical failures	Actual failures
Female sterilization	0.04	0.04
Male sterilization	0.15	0.15
Oral contraceptive (pill)	0.34	4
Intrauterine device (IUD)	1-3	5
Diaphragm	3	17
Condom	3	10
Foam	3	22
Rhythm	13	21
Withdrawal	9	20-25
Douche	?	40

*Data from R. A. Hatcher et al.: Contraceptive technology, 1978-1979, New York, 1978, Irvington Publishers, Inc.

tion.[9] The magnitude of this problem becomes evident when one realizes that 90% of these couples will experience a pregnancy within 1 year. It is not surprising that more than two thirds of women seeking abortions in the United States have not used contraception to prevent pregnancy. Clearly the rates for both unintended pregnancy and abortion could be lowered considerably if a greater percentage of married couples used contraception.

Analysis of existing data raises the following concerns about contraceptives and contraceptive practices:

1. A significant proportion of married couples who do not wish pregnancies do not use contraception.
2. The effectiveness rates for all methods, with the exception of sterilization, leave much to be desired.
3. There are significant differences between contraceptive effectiveness rates for couples wishing to prevent and those desiring to delay pregnancy and between the theoretical and actual effectiveness rates for each method of contraception. This indicates that human factors such as inconsistent or improper use have an important effect on the ability of people to prevent an unintended pregnancy.
4. In 1976, of every 100 couples who did not wish a pregnancy, approximately 9 experienced pregnancies because they failed to use contraceptives, and 5 because of failures in the contraceptives they were using.

These data point strongly to the need for contraceptives that are more effective as well as to the need for more effective use of the contraceptives that are available. The latter presents a challenge to those in family planning programs; the former, to those working in contraceptive research.

Contraceptive technology

The array of contraceptives available today represents significant advances over what was available to Americans just 20 years ago, but much progress remains to be made in the area of contraceptive technology. The most effective temporary methods, the pill and the IUD, carry with them a number of risks and side effects. Because of this a significant percentage of people cannot or will not use them. Sterilization is highly effective and relatively safe, but until reversibility can be guaranteed it will be appropriate only for people who have completed their families. Barrier methods such as condoms, spermicides, and diaphragms are free from serious side effects but are more subject to human error in their use. Natural family planning methods are of limited effectiveness for many people.

Many people find none of the available methods adequate. Nevertheless, for people who choose to be sexually active these methods represent their only means of preventing pregnancy. If one envisions the ideal contraceptive, the shortcomings of current methods become readily apparent. The ideal contraceptive would be 100% effective and have no side effects; it would be coitus-independent and provide continuous protection, it would be reversible and have no effects on future fertility, it would be highly acceptable, easy to get, and affordable to everyone; and it would be easy to use, with no possibility of human error.

The probability that a method will be developed that can meet all of these criteria is remote. It is clear that contraceptive researchers will have to develop a number of different methods that people can match to their individual needs and life-styles. A recent Ford Foundation report details both the promise and the problems in the area of contraceptive research today. The report, which draws on the expertise of 160 experts from 26 countries, points out that more than 200 promising research leads have been identified including once-a-month contraceptives, vaccines to prevent pregnancy, a male pill to suppress sperm formation, and agents that prevent implantation of fertilized eggs.[13] The report also states that the development of improved methods may be significantly delayed by a low-level of funding. In 1976 actual funding for contraceptive research was less than 30% of the level needed to ade-

quately pursue the existing scientific leads. Given that it takes between 10 and 20 years to develop, test, gain approval for, and market a truly new contraceptive, it is likely that we will have to rely on our current imperfect methods for some time to come.[14] Most important, if we expect to see any significant advances by the turn of the century, a drastic increase in funding is needed now.

FAMILY PLANNING PROCESS
What is family planning?

Family planning is a process through which people establish their fertility goals and then take specific steps to assure that those goals are met. From a logical and systematic point of view the process of family planning includes at least four general steps: (1) gathering information about needs, desires, goals, abilities, and resources; (2) analyzing that information and determining how having children will influence one's life and life goals; (3) deciding if and when one will have children including how many children to have and when to have them; and (4) implementing a plan of action that is designed to assure that the established goals are reached.

It is rare, however, for family planning decisions to be based solely on criteria and processes that are so logical. To assume that the decision to have or not to have children is mostly a rational one is to dismiss the importance of a myriad of psychological, emotional, cultural, and social factors that operate on human beings. Each step of the process is influenced by who we are, where we are, where we have been, and where we perceive we are going.

Health and economic benefits of family planning

Children are valuable. Most fundamentally they provide for the continuation of the human species. If births were to cease mankind would become extinct within the span of a lifetime. But this reason for wanting children is usually not uppermost in the minds of parents. To them children are valued as sources of joy and happiness, companionship, and pride. It is safe to state that most people want and have children. It is also true that if the only limiting factor to childbearing were biological ability to have children, there would be a lot more children in the world today. Most people practice family planning at some time in their lives. Those who conscientiously plan their families tend to have fewer children, to space their births at intervals most advantageous to both themselves and their children, and to experience fewer unwanted pregnancies and births. This results in significant health and economic benefits to the families.

We can best determine the health benefits of having smaller, well-spaced families by analyzing the differences in health status between smaller, well-spaced families and larger, poorly spaced families. Seigal and Morris, in an evaluation of the health rationale for family planning, found that increased family size and short birth intervals were associated with higher rates of prematurity; increased maternal, infant, and fetal deaths; poorer growth in child height and weight; lower IQ scores among the children; a greater chance of child abuse; increased evidence of infectious diseases in both parents and children; and a higher prevalence of certain diseases such as rheumatoid arthritis, peptic ulcers, and diabetes in either the mother or the father.[15]

Significant evidence exists to show that the age of the mother at time of childbearing also affects family health. In general the safest time to experience pregnancy and childbirth is during the 20s and early 30s. The further a woman is from this age group the more likely it is that she or her baby will suffer.[16]

The risk of having a baby with congenital defects is significantly higher for women in the extremes of the childbearing years. Babies born to mothers under 15 years of age are three times more likely to have congenital defects than those born to mothers in their 20s. Those born to mothers over 35 are twice as likely to have congenital defects.[17] Perhaps the most clear-cut example of the relationship between maternal age and congenital abnormalities is Down's syndrome (mongolism). In mothers less than 30 years of age the risk of having a baby with Down's syndrome is 1 per 1,000 live births; at age 40 it is 1 in 100; and in women 45 or older it is 1 in 45.[18]

Maternal and infant mortality are also affected by the age of the mother. Women under 14 have maternal mortality rates 60% higher than mothers in their 20s, while those in their 30s have rates 100% higher.[16] In addition, rates for toxemia, anemia, miscarriage, and premature births are all associated with maternal age.[18,19]

It is clear that the health status of mothers and their children can be enhanced when pregnancy and childbirth take place during the prime childbearing years (the 20s and early 30s), when families are kept relatively small, and when the interval between pregnancies is of sufficient length.

When planning their families people typically pay more attention to economic considerations than they do to health considerations. It is important to note, however, that people greatly underestimate the cost of having children and thus often make their childbearing decisions based on inaccurate perceptions of the economics involved.

The research of Espenshade,[20] a Florida State University economist, clearly points out the importance of looking at economic considerations when planning a family. When analyzing the economic implications of having children, one must consider both the direct costs such as food, shelter, clothing, medical care, and education as well as the indirect costs that result from lost opportunities for the parents in their ability to generate and invest income.

Espenshade found that in 1976 the cost of bearing a child, raising it to age 18, and financing a public college education ranged from about $77,000 to $107,000. This cost had increased over 60% between 1968 and 1977. The largest cost of rearing a child is direct maintenance, which includes food, shelter, clothing, and medical care. He estimated that in 1977 the cost of direct maintenance for a first child, from birth to age 18, ranged from about $33,000 for a farm family consuming inexpensive food to about $54,000 for an urban family consuming moderately priced food. A middle-income family now spends more than 30% of its annual income to raise a first child. The cost of raising an additional child to age 18, not including college costs, is about one half that of a first child.

Influences on family planning decisions

Pohlman, in his book, *Psychology of Birth Planning*, addresses motivations for childbearing.[21] After concluding from his research that most people want children, he attempts to answer the question why. Most parents, when asked this question, would probably not recite the list of reasons that Pohlman puts forward in his book. Nevertheless, many of these reasons, consciously or subconsciously, influence the decision to have a child. Pohlman suggests that the following are typical reasons for childbearing: a basic liking of children; an innate or socially learned desire for children; a need to help or to be responsible for others; a need to prove potency, sexual maturity, and the ability to reproduce; a sense of immortality because a part of the parent lives on in the child; a desire to strengthen marital relationships; a desire for existing children to have siblings; the wish to have a child of the opposite sex once a boy or girl has been born; a belief that motherhood is a socially acceptable role for women, one that validates their existence and makes their lives complete; and a need to fulfill religious influences, which equate childbearing with goodness, theology, and so forth.

Needless to say, this is not a complete list of possible psychological and emotional factors that affect people's childbearing decisions. Nor can it be said that any, or all, of these factors will affect the family planning decisions of a specific individual or couple. It is important to recognize, however, that childbearing decisions that people make, though they may not appear logical or rational, often have a psychological or emotional justification.

A variety of social factors also influence decisions about childbearing. Perhaps the primary social factor in the recent past has been the increased attention paid to the status and roles of women in our society. There is little doubt that childbearing and child rearing historically have had the effect of reducing educational, personal, and economic opportunities for women. Conversely, the control of fertility has had the effect of increasing these opportunities. Women with few children typically have had more opportunities outside of the home than those with several children. As the traditional role of women continues to be questioned, the automatic social response of marriage, childbearing, and homemaking by women is becoming less the norm. In fact between 1960 and 1976 the proportion of women in their prime childbearing years (20 to 34) who were working increased from 40% to 60%.[22] It is important to note that during this same period both fertility expectations and actual fertility levels decreased significantly.

Another important social influence on many people has been an increasing concern about the size of our population and its effects on the quality of life. Recent energy shortages, rising pollution levels, and increased competition for limited recreational and other resources have heightened awareness of the relationship between the quantity of life and the quality of life. The response of people most influenced by this social condition has been a careful assessment of their fertility goals and how those goals will affect society as a whole.

Sociologist Janet Griffith has studied the effects of social pressure on family planning decisions. She found that there is considerable pressure on couples to conform to generally accepted family size norms. According to her research, two children are widely accepted as the bottom limit of this norm, and four children as the upper limit. People who consider varying from the norm are subject to considerable family, peer, and social pressure to conform.[23]

FAMILY PLANNING PROGRAMS

We have discussed the significant changes that have occurred in the fertility and fertility goals of Americans in the recent past. A variety of factors have affected these fertility goals, but one factor has enabled people to meet them—the availability of family planning methods and services. The advent of the oral contraceptive, refinement of intrauterine devices, and improved technology in surgical sterilization have all made major contributions.

Many people need only seek contraceptive services from their private physicians. For low-income people with limited resources, however, this is not the case. Organized family planning services with extensive financial support from the federal government have been uniquely successful in providing low-income people with the means to reach fertility goals. Between 1970 and 1975 alone federally assisted programs helped low-income and marginal-income people to avert 1,098,000 unintended births, and higher-income teenagers to avert an additional 266,000 unintended births.[24]

In 1976 an estimated 4.1 million women received subsidized family planning services from a network of 2523 organized family planning programs in the United States. This network was comprised predominantly of health departments, hospitals, and affiliates of the Planned Parenthood Federation of America.[25] The Department of Health, Education, and Welfare estimates that in 1976 the federal government supported these programs at a level of 384 million dollars.[26] Although the accuracy of this estimate has been questioned, it is clear that the federal government is providing extensive financial support to the nation's family planning programs.

Historical perspective

The first family planning clinic in the United States was opened in the slums of Brooklyn in 1916 by Margaret Sanger, a public health nurse. Working with the poor, she regularly witnessed the hardships and sorrow that resulted from unchecked and unintended childbearing, and the deaths associated with self-induced and back-alley abortions. The shocking death of one of her impoverished patients, which resulted from her second self-induced abortion, provided the impetus for Sanger's decision to open a clinic. This led to her immediate arrest, the first of many. It was not until 1923 that a clinic was able to remain open.

In 1921, despite legal and public harassment, the nation's first official family planning organization was formed. Termed the American Birth Control League, its dual purpose was to "disseminate knowledge concerning contraception and to promote the distribution of contraceptive devices." By the end of the 1930s local voluntary groups were providing birth control services in most large and medium-sized cities. These voluntary groups eventually joined efforts and formed the Planned Parenthood Federation of America.

The public sector became involved in 1935 when Mississippi became the first state to provide birth control services through its public health departments. Several other states had followed suit by the mid 1940s. For the next two decades, growth in the family planning movement was relatively limited. This trend was reversed in the 1960s when a significant expansion phase began.

The federal government becomes involved

With Congressional passage of the Economic Opportunity Act, the federal government became involved in the funding of family planning services. The first federal grant to a specific family planning program was awarded in 1965 to a Planned Parenthood affiliate in Texas. By 1967 grants from this act totalled just over 4 million dollars.[27] From 1968 to the present, federal support of family planning services has perhaps been the single largest determinant of family planning policy in America. It is estimated that between 1971 and 1976 annual federal support of family planning services increased from 129 million to 384 million dollars.[26] During that same period the number of patients being served annually in these federally assisted programs increased from 1,889,000 to 4,083,000.[25]

Congressional impetus for the financing of family planning services has stemmed from three general priorities:(1) a recognition that all persons should be able to determine the number and spacing of their children, (2) an interest in improving the health and welfare of women and children, and (3) an effort to reduce poverty and dependence. Few people would quarrel with these priorities. Some may raise the question, however, of whether the federal government should be spending even limited tax dollars to subsidize family planning programs, regardless of the possible benefits to individuals who utilize these programs. After all, there are a number of other health and social service programs that need funds.

Jaffe and Cutright studied the short-term benefits and costs of family planning pro-grams from 1969 to 1975 in an attempt to determine the financial justification for these programs. The results of their analysis were significant. By helping their patients avert unwanted and mistimed births, family planning programs saved the federal government 1.1 billion dollars during the period from 1969 to 1975. During this same period the federal expenditures for family planning services totalled 584 million dollars. One dollar invested in family planning services in 1 year saved the federal government $1.80 in the next year alone. The bulk of these savings came from reductions in expenditures for public assistance and medical care associated with pregnancies, which would have been required had those births not been averted.[24]

It is unlikely that many, if any, publicly funded programs in the United States could provide this level of return on investment within 1 year. The long-term savings are even more impressive, however. It has been estimated that, over the long term, family planning programs save the public 26 dollars for every dollar spent. Thus the cost effectiveness of family planning programs, plus the benefits to individuals and society that result from the prevention of unwanted and mistimed births, tend to support continued government funding of family planning services.

Family planning network

In 1976 the nation's network of family planning programs was comprised of 3112 agencies, of which 2523 were direct service providers. Table 5 details who these providers were and how many patients they served. The primary providers of subsidized family planning services in the United States are health departments and affiliates of the Planned Parenthood Federation of America. Between them, they serve two thirds of the patients seen in publicly subsidized programs.

Table 5. Direct providers of family planning services in the United States by type of agency, distribution, and case load, 1976*

		Type of agency			
	Total	**Health departments**	**Planned parenthood affiliates**	**Hospitals**	**All others†**
Number of agencies	2,523	1,476	180	339	528
Percentage of total agencies	100	58.5	7.1	13.4	20.9
Total patients served (in thousands)	4,083,000	1,723,000	1,108,000	563,000	689,000
Average patients served per agency	1,618	1,167	6,156	1,661	1,305
Percentage of total patients served	100	42.2	17.1	13.8	16.9

*Data from Alan Guttmacher Institute: Data and analyses for 1977 revision of DHEW five year plan for family planning services, Contract No. 105-74-193, New York, 1977, The Institute.
†Includes community action agencies, neighborhood and community health centers, free clinics, university health services, and various other public and private, nonprofit organizations.

The typical patient in American family planning programs in 1976 was of low income (78% were below 150% of the poverty level, $8250 annual income for a family of four); she was young (28% were below age 20; and 57%, between 20 and 30); had one or no children (51% had no children; 22%, one child); and left the clinic with a more effective contraceptive method than she previously used. (Prior to clinic attendance, 31% of patients used no method, and 18% used the least effective methods; after clinic attendance, 76% of patients used the most effective methods.[28])

Perhaps the most important of these patient characteristics are age, income, and contraceptive behavior. Family planning programs exist primarily to assist people who are at risk of unintended pregnancy, but who have limited access to services in the private sector. Two of the major subgroups of the population that fall into this category, for a variety of social and economic reasons, are low-income persons and teenagers. It is obvious that family planning programs are serving many of these people.

Services provided by family planning programs

The major objective of family planning programs is to help people realize their fertility goals. Historically the primary activity of these programs has been the provision of contraceptive services. It is important to note that these programs typically have provided a number of important ancillary services as well.

Contact with the health delivery system is extremely limited for many low-income and younger people. Often family planning programs serve as a primary health care provider to these people. Routine health screening procedures such as pelvic and breast examinations, pap smears, VD screening, and blood and urinalysis as well as treatment for minor gynecological problems are provided as an integral part of family planning services. These programs also serve as an important source of referral to other medical providers.

Education and counseling services are also important aspects of family planning programs. Typically clinics provide education about family planning, sexuality, and health to both their patients and the community. Counseling for most family planning-related problems is usually provided directly or by referral to other agencies.

As family planning programs have become more stable and sophisticated, many have begun expanding the scope of their medical services. It is not surprising to find programs that are providing male and female sterilization, infertility services, abortion, prenatal care and delivery, and a variety of other gynecological and health services. Some of this expansion has been in response to direction set by the federal government, but more often than not it has been in response to community needs that have been perceived as not being met. American family planning programs have established a solid base for the provision of family planning and other health services. The accomplishments during the past decade have been impressive. It remains for these programs to maintain, and build on, that base.

FAMILY PLANNING AND THE FUTURE
Needs that remain

Although significant progress has been made in the family planning field, the job is far from done. It is clear that millions of people are still unable to regulate their fertility in accordance with their needs and desires. The following statistics, based on the most recent data available, show the magnitude of the problems that must be addressed:

1. One of every 11 marital births is termed unwanted at the time of conception.
2. One of every 7 births occurs out of wedlock. One in 10 adolescents become pregnant each year and two thirds of their pregnancies are conceived out of wedlock. In 1976 this resulted in 1 million pregnancies in adolescents 15 to 19 years old and 30,000 in those 14 years old and younger.

3. In 1976 1.1 million abortions were performed, and over two thirds of the women seeking those abortions had not used a method of contraception to prevent an unintended pregnancy.
4. Nearly 1 million couples are infertile and cannot have the children they want.
5. Each year 250,000 babies are born with congenital defects.

Each of these remaining needs will require significant effort on the part of our entire health delivery system. A large proportion of the people who make up these statistics could be categorized as the hard to reach: the poor, the rural, and the young. This will place a significant part of the responsibility for meeting their needs on the nation's family planning programs. Their record to date is excellent, but much remains to be done.

Challenges that remain

While attempting to address the remaining family planning needs of Americans, family planning programs will be faced with many challenges. Most important among those challenges are the following.

The need to significantly expand the existing family planning network. This expansion must include increases in both the number of family planning sites and the number of patients served at each site. Much of this expansion could be accomplished if health departments could expand their case loads. If the average case load of health departments were equal to those of all other family planning programs, they would serve an additional 1.6 million people per year. The addition of a greater number of hospitals as service sites could also have a major impact. The total of 339 hospitals currently providing services represents an extremely small proportion of all U.S. hospitals.

The need to expand the scope of family planning programs. Significant gaps exist in the availability of reproductive health services in many communities where family planning programs are located. Current programs could do much to fill these gaps by adding services in areas such as infertility, sterilization, prenatal care, abortion, and other related problem areas.

The need for more trained medical and paramedical personnel. Organized family planning programs were among the first health programs to address a rapid increase in demand for services in the face of a severe physician shortage. Nurse practitioners, midwives, and other nonphysician clinicians have provided a vital solution to the personnel shortages facing these programs. They have been well accepted and have performed admirably, but there simply are not enough of them to meet the need. Training programs are expensive and oversubscribed. Family planners will have to work toward the expansion of training programs to help alleviate the problem.

The need to address further the process of family planning. Family planning programs have been primarily involved in the provision of contraceptive methods to their patients. They need to begin addressing motivations for childbearing and factors that influence people's family planning decisions. Educational and counseling services should be geared toward the provision of well-balanced, accurate information and toward helping people as they go through the family planning decision making process. Clearly people must make their own decisions, but those decisions should be based, to the extent possible, on fact and reality.

The need for better contraceptive methods. As discussed in the sections regarding contraceptive failure and technology, the current methods leave much to be desired. Family planning programs must serve as advocates for the general public by working to convince the private and governmental sectors that what we have is inadequate, and that much more emphasis on funding for contraceptive research is required.

The need for increased public information and outreach programs. As mentioned earlier, a large percentage of the people still needing services are difficult to reach. It is unrealistic to expect that most of these people will seek out family planning programs. Instead, the programs must develop innovative ways of reaching out to them with information about the benefits of family planning as well as the availability of services.

The need to remove existing legal barriers. A number of critical questions need to be answered by our legal and judicial systems. The right of minors to consent for medical services, the right of poor people to have access to safe, legal abortion services, and the right of all people to have the information needed to make intelligent family planning decisions are primary among these unanswered questions. Family planning programs must actively seek answers to these questions.

The need to defend family planning programs against increasing opposition. Every American President since Dwight D. Eisenhower has referred to family planning as a basic human right, and an overwhelming majority of Americans support the activities of family planning programs. Nevertheless, a small but vocal minority is actively involved in attempts to undermine family planning efforts. These people are typically opposed to the policies or activities of programs in the areas of services to minors, abortion, and sex education. Family planners will have to do a better job of publicly articulating their purposes and goals, their positions on these controversial issues, and the reasons for those goals and positions. Unless this is done in a positive manner and on a continuing basis, it is possible that this vocal minority will exert strong influence against family planning programs.

The need for better management and coordination of programs. As is often the case in health and social service programs, many family planning programs are managed by people with little or no management experience or training. Former nurses, educators, social workers, and other professionals with limited management experience or education often find themselves directing large and complex programs. Much attention needs to be paid to upgrading their knowledge and skill levels. There is also a need for more effective and efficient interagency coordination among family planning programs. Better coordination among the programs themselves could make it possible to reduce the amount of funds being spent for administrative costs by third-party coordinators such as umbrella agencies and area family planning councils. This could result in the reallocation of these vitally needed funds to direct service providers.

The need for increased funds. The ability of programs to meet the remaining needs and face the challenges ahead will to a great extent depend on the availability of additional financial resources. Although federal funds are increasingly being made available, it is unlikely that these funds alone will be adequate. There is a need to increase funds from state and local sources, from insurance companies and other third-party sources, from patients, and from the general public. Family planning programs have been proved to be among the most cost-effective of health programs. In these days of budget deficits and taxpayer revolt, it is important that this fact be stressed when additional funds are being sought.

CONCLUSION

This chapter represents a modest attempt to review family planning in the United States. Entire books have been written about many of the issues that have been mentioned here only briefly. The recent attention of the media and professional journals to issues such as adolescent pregnancy and abortion has been extensive, and it is rare not to find several references to fertility or family planning at most any magazine rack. The fact that the first major television coverage of family planning occurred only 16 years ago points out the recency of the progress that has been made in the field.

People have children; they always have had and always will. The important change that has occurred in recent years is the increasing number of people who are seriously considering their childbearing decisions and goals and are having children at times most appropriate in their lives. The availability of publicly subsidized family planning programs has helped countless people who for a variety of reasons have been unable to reach their fertility goals. This has been and will continue to be vitally important to parents, their children, and ultimately to society as a whole.

REFERENCES

1. U.S. Public Health Service: Vital statistics rates in the United States: 1940-1960, PHS Publication No. 1677, Washington D.C., 1968, U.S. Government Printing Office; also
2. U.S. Public Health Service: Monthly vital statistics report: births, marriages, divorces, and deaths for 1977, PHS Publication No. 78-1120, Washington, D.C., March 13, 1978, U.S. Government Printing Office.
3. Ad Hoc Committee for a Position Paper on the Status of Family Planning in the United States Today: Planned births, the future of the family, and the quality of American life: towards a comprehensive national policy and program, New York, June 1977, Alan Guttmacher Institute.
4. Sweet, J. A.: Differentials in the rate of fertility decline: 1960-1970, Fam. Plan. Perspec., **6:**103, Spring 1974.
5. U.S. Public Health Service: Monthly vital statistics report: final natality statistics, 1976, PHS Publication No. 78-1120, Washington, D.C., March 29, 1978, U.S. Government Printing Office.
6. U.S. Bureau of the Census: Prospects for American

fertility: June 1976, Current Population Reports, Series P-20, No. 300, Washington, D.C., 1976, U.S. Government Printing Office.

7. Gallup, G.: Big families out of style in U.S. and Europe, news release, Princeton, N.J., March 24, 1977, The Gallup Poll.

8. Westoff, C. F.: The predictive validity of reproductive intentions, paper presented at the annual meeting of the Population Association of America, St. Louis, April 21-23, 1977.

9. U.S. Public Health Service: Advance data: contraceptive utilization in the United States, 1973 and 1976, No. 36, Washington, D.C., August 18, 1978, U.S. Government Printing Office.

10. Westoff, C. F., and Jones, E. F.: Contraception and sterilization in the United States, 1965-1975, Fam. Plan. Perspec. 9:154, July/August, 1977.

11. U.S. Public Health Service: Advance data, contraceptive efficacy among married women 15-44 years of age in the United States, 1970-1973, No. 26, Washington, D.C., April 6, 1978, U.S. Government Printing Office.

12. Hatcher, R. A., et. al.: Contraceptive technology, 1978-1979, New York, 1978, Irvington Publishers, Inc.

13. Greep, R. O., et al.: Reproduction and human welfare: a challenge to research, Cambridge, Mass., 1976, The MIT Press.

14. Southern, E. M.: The industrial challenge in reproductive drug development. In Providing contraceptive technology, Washington D.C., Summer 1977, The Draper Fund for the Population Crisis Committee.

15. Seigal, E., and Morris, N. M.: Family planning: its health rationale, Am. J. Obstet. Gynecol. 118:995, 1974.

16. Beasley, J.: Benefits of family planning to family health, In McCalister, C. V., et al. : Readings in family planning, St. Louis, 1973, The C. V. Mosby Co.

17. Parsons, L., and Sommers, S.: Gynecology, Philadelphia, 1963, W. B. Saunders Co.

18. Guttmacher, A. F.: Pregnancy, birth, and family planning, New York, 1973, The New American Library, Inc.

19. Alan Guttmacher Institute: Eleven million teenagers, what can be done about the epidemic of adolescent pregnancies in the United States, New York, 1976, The Institute.

20. Espenshade, T. J.: The value and cost of children, Population bulletin, 32(1), 1977.

21. Pohlman, E.: Psychology of birth planning, Cambridge, Mass., 1969, Schenkman Publishing Co., Inc.

22. U.S. Bureau of Labor Statistics: New labor force projections to 1990, Special Labor Force Reports, No. 197, Washington, D.C., 1976, U.S. Government Printing Office.

23. Griffith. J.: Social pressure on family size intentions, Fam. Plan. Perspec. 5:273-242, Fall, 1973.

24. Jaffe, F. S., and Cutright, P.: Short term benefits of U.S. family planning programs: 1970-1975, Fam. Plan. Perspec. 9:77-80, March/April, 1977.

25. Torres, A.: Organized family planning services in the United States: 1968-1976, Fam. Plan. Perspect. 10:84, March/April, 1978.

26. Dryfoos, J. G., and Doring-Bradley, B.: The hundred million dollar misunderstanding, Fam. Plan. Perspec. 10:144, May/June, 1978.

27. Metropoliton Executive Director's Council of the Planned Parenthood Federation of America: Toward continued strengthening of the Planned Parenthood Federation of America, unpublished discussion paper, May 1975.

28. Alan Guttmacher Institute: Data and analyses for 1977 revision of DHEW five year plan for family planning services, HSA Contract No. 105-74-193. New York, 1977, The Institute.

PART THREE

Health services for today's population

☐ In Part Three the reader is offered a wealth of material on health services that are available to people in a variety of community settings. Eight chapters describing various areas of health service delivery are included; each addresses a specific subject that will aid the health care professional in dealing with current health problems. The contributors to this section offer innovative concepts and approaches along with updated references, all of which afford the reader an opportunity to expand knowledge and horizons.

In Chapter 9 Bible has clearly outlined essential guidelines for the creation and operation of community health care systems in rural areas. He describes the personnel needed for the operation of such rural community health care systems and underlines the importance of the community's involvement in the planning of such systems. Bible points out that "Health is but one aspect of the quality of life which includes all of the socioeconomic, ecological, and educational factors that make for a satisfactory living situation."

The role of the community health nurse and her contribution to the health of the adolescent in today's changing social structure is addressed by Rosenberg in Chapter 10. The author presents the historical development of adolescence in our society as well as the health needs of this age group, and includes some models of health care delivery that attempt to meet the adolescent's needs.

Rosenberg emphasizes the need for greater commitment to preventive health care for the adolescent, utilizing the primary health care model.

Chapter 11, contributed by an interdisciplinary team consisting of a physician, a nurse, and a social worker, outlines the work of the Rape Treatment Center at Jackson Memorial Hospital, Miami, Florida, which is devoted to the health care of the victim of sexual assault. The material describing this unique center (developed as a result of the feminist movement) offers the health care professional a variety of ideas and information that should contribute to the establishment of similar centers in other communities throughout the nation.

Wortman and Curran, two perceptive social workers, present in Chapter 12 a diagnostic framework for understanding victims of sexual assault. Three types of relations that are found between the family and the victim affect the victim's ability to resolve crisis and determine the type of intervention that would be most helpful. The three relationships dealt with are (1) the family is negative to the sexual assault victim; (2) the family is positive and supportive of the victim; and (3) the victim has little support and few significant others to whom to turn. Close study of this material will assist the community health nurse in working with these victims and their families.

Home health care services for the family

with an elderly parent are discussed by Scheel in Chapter 13. The author answers many questions concerning the care of the elderly parent and gives an example of how home health care services can operate in communities through the community health nurse's creative use of available facilities and through contacts with specialists in other disciplines for part-time assistance.

Occupational health nursing focuses on people in their work environment. In Chapter 14, Hornyack has described the role of the occupational health nurse and the necessity for the nurse to work in a cooperative and coordinated relationship with other health care professionals. The writer stresses the need and importance of up-to-date knowledge in solving today's industrial health problems.

The viability of the school health nurse will depend on the nurse's ability and willingness to build effective team relationships, expand her educational base, and interpret her role as nurse, as pointed out by Wold in Chapter 15. She describes three topics of importance: (1) the historical development of the school nurse role in this country, (2) problems that plague the school nurse, and (3) future needs and prospects for survival and expansion of the school nurse's role.

Many physicians and nurses are uncomfortable with the dying patient, rejecting them through behavioral cues and physical isolation. Chapter 16, contributed by Ufema, a nurse thanatologist, is a sensitive, perceptive, and highly personal statement about the author's caring for and sharing of her humanness with dying patients. May her message modify our socially conditioned fears of death and help us work lovingly with dying patients.

9

Guidelines for creation and operation of community health care systems in rural areas

Bond L. Bible

Organization for health services and for health manpower distribution are the two most basic health care problems for the rural areas of the nation. Solving either of these problems would aid in resolving the other. Community organization for the provision of group practice can make recruitment and retention of physicians, nurses, and other health manpower easier to accomplish. Adequate manpower enables the task of organization to go further than it otherwise could. Group practice for physicians seems to hold the greatest promise in recruitment of physicians for rural areas.

In comparison with urban areas, rural communities differ widely in their characteristics, but generally in rural areas the physician and nurse shortage is more acute, persons must travel longer distances to obtain health care, emergency services are more deficient, work-related injury rates are higher, the rural poverty rate is higher, and a comprehensive approach to health care delivery often is not present.[1]

In 1975 the physician population ratio ranged from a low of 495 persons per physician in urban counties of 5 million or more inhabitants to a high of 2950 persons per physician in rural counties of less than 10,000 inhabitants. This is almost six times as many people per physician in rural counties as in urban.

These extreme differences do not mean that people in rural counties are without care, but it does have two important implications: first, rural people may have to travel longer distances to find health care; and second, it may be difficult to get appointments with physicians because they already have a greater patient load than they can handle.

Physicians often express concerns regarding rural practice, such as longer hours, lack of peer support and stimulation, limited access to continuing medical education, less availability for group practice, lack of management assistance, negative reaction of spouse to rural location, and limited cultural, social, and educational opportunities.

This chapter will examine ways in which rural communities can help to develop comprehensive health care delivery services for the people and thus overcome some of the rural health problems.

RURAL HEALTH CARE SYSTEMS

To meet the health needs of everyone in the rural community it is necessary to make arrangements to take care of the varying needs of the people. This is generally referred to as a health care system. Specifically, a rural health care system is a formal arrangement in which a variety of health care resources are linked together to provide for the delivery of the complete range of the health services deemed appropriate for a designated geographic area or for a given population.

Rural communities must consider four basic issues before building a health system:

1. Are there enough people to require the services of one or preferably two physicians?
2. Is the community able financially to support a variety of health care personnel and facilities?
3. Where does the population currently obtain health care?
4. Are major health resources available and accessible in the larger region for required backup services?

Initial planning by rural communities is basic to the development of rural health systems. Planning must involve all segments of the community, provider and consumer alike, with the support and involvement of the health systems agency that is responsible for planning for the community concerned. It must also be tailored to the geography and the potential resources of the locality.

It is generally recognized that primary health care can be provided on an ambulatory, or walk-in, basis within reasonable distance of the people being served. For patients in need of specialty care and hospitalization, primary ambulatory care should be linked to secondary levels of care. A complete health system must provide access also to a tertiary care facility where highly developed diagnostic skills are available and unusual procedures such as heart surgery or organ transplants can be performed.

No one rural community will have all of the

health care needed by its population. However, each community can have access to basic primary care and be linked through formal arrangement to higher levels of care in the same or another community, on the state level, or in another state.

Many small communities that once had their "own" physician will never again have one. For some rural areas solutions completely different from the traditional "physician in residence" must be sought. For some communities emphasis may be needed on expanded transportation and communication capabilities, part-time use of physicians and greater reliance on nurse practitioners and physician's assistants, improved biomonitoring technology, use of new physician-support occupations, better understanding and use of individual health practices, and development of emergency care and self-help methods to ensure rural health coverage.

CREATION OF SYSTEM THROUGH ORGANIZED EFFORT

Although the readiness of a community to plan for its health services and to carry out these plans are dependent on many factors, a seemingly important factor is the presence of an organizational structure. The organization of a community health board (often called a council or committee) is essential to secure effective participation and action. The board then can do the following:

1. Assess the community health problems
2. Seek information from the regional or state health systems agencies
3. Establish local priority projects
4. Facilitate communication among government, private, and program agencies
5. Act in a fund-raising or grant-seeking capacity
6. Negotiate with neighboring areas having similar needs or problems

A health board must have broad-based community support. At first a community may be able to utilize an existing organizational structure such as a health subcommittee. But eventually the board should be a self-standing body with consumer support. Since the decision-making process of each community operates on a unique power structure, it simply is not possible to establish absolute guidelines that apply to every community or every situation. The suggestions that follow should be adapted to the special needs of individual communities.

The composition of the board will generally change and expand as it begins its work. It is necessary to begin with a strong, diverse leadership. Both providers and consumers must become involved along with, possibly, representatives from the health professions, service clubs, farm and youth organizations, religious groups, women's organizations, local and area extension staff, and educational leaders including schools, colleges, and universities.

An effective method of creating an awareness of a health care problem is to provide additional documentation to support the initial perception of the problem. Such information will help to legitimize the new organization's efforts and to develop added support for what needs to be done. It is necessary to identify and contact not only influential citizens in the community but also those who will be affected by the services of the program. Such possible health field sources can be categorized under health service providers and educational institutions, influential community groups and individuals, and consumers of health services.

An educational process is necessary to enable the board to understand more clearly the problem it faces and to help convince the community of the validity of its conclusions about health care services. The U.S. Department of Health, Education, and Welfare

Bureau of Community Health Services offers information on existing federally funded health programs such as the National Health Service Corps, Rural Health Initiative, Health in Underserved Rural Areas, Maternal and Child Health Services, and Emergency Medical Services Systems Program. The U.S. Department of Agriculture's Farmers Home and Rural Development Service as well as the Cooperative Extension Service can also provide information.

There is no "right" way to organize a board; however, certain principles are recommended:

1. A formal structure should be set up with officers and staff, if possible. The chairperson, elected by the board membership, will preside over the meetings, assist the staff in the preparation of an agenda for meetings, and represent the board on official business or designate a substitute.
2. The board should have a stable membership since effective planning is a permanent process.
3. Although a constitution and bylaws may be adequate for most groups, incorporation is useful for handling both private and public funds.
4. The size of the board membership as well as its length of tenure and method of member selection should be determined by the board in the development of its constitution.
5. The board should supervise and coordinate health planning activities and make decisions based on recommendations and alternative courses of action; the board should also determine general program policies.
6. Medical and nursing societies as well as other established health care service organizations or agencies should be represented on the board.
7. Ideally the board should serve an area

large enough to support a part-time or full-time staff.

8. Board members should be able to stimulate the implementation of planning by influencing necessary political action and financing.

9. Board members selected for their leadership abilities should be expected to act as "community trustees" rather than in their organizational interest.

10. The board should focus on the total spectrum of health activities and maintain effective liaison with other organizations and agencies that have mutual concerns.

11. The number of board subcommittees can be determined by the scope of the program; for example, standing committees might include health manpower, financing, health care delivery, health education, and health care organization.

Determining the boundaries of the community health system area is one of the board's first tasks. Close communication should be maintained with the health systems agency in the area. This may mean redefining "community," and perhaps enlarging the board at some future time. Careful consideration should be given to the retail economic trade area. This usually means at least two or more communities already linked by common business, social interests, and transportation systems. An entire county or several counties may be included in the service area in sparsely populated rural sections. The county cooperative extension agent can assist with the demographic survey.

Today, planning for health services, especially in rural areas, means thinking in terms of time rather than distance. At least 50% of the service area population should reside within 30 to 40 minutes' driving time from the nearest health center and hospital. If greater distances are involved arrangements need to be made for satellite clinics.

Health planning for rural communities should involve area-wide or regional cooperation. Because of modern transportation and communication services, physicians are not needed in every town, village, and township. Several communities within a trading or service area can plan together to develop health care systems on an area basis, to attract needed health manpower, and to provide home, clinic, and hospital care. Health and medical resources can be consolidated in much the same way that educational services have been—providing the health service area is carefully chosen. There are some factors to consider:

1. Is there a sufficient population base at various age levels to warrant one or more physicians and the necessary nursing personnel?

2. Is the community capable of providing adequate financial resources to support personnel and facilities?

3. Where must people travel for health care at present?

4. Are there readily accessible, major health centers available in the larger community area?

The information needed to determine the size and scope of the health services needed to cover the entire population includes demographic, socioeconomic, and geographic data, health status indicators, medical provider profiles, and data on health department, hospitals, long-term institutions, and mental health programs. The health care providers located in a service area have an important responsibility in assessing health needs as well as in helping to determine the health service area.

One goal of the board is to design a primary health care program that will meet the health needs of the community. Consideration must be given to the services to be provided, who will provide the services, delivery methods for the services, how to finance the services, and the nature of securing continued community involvement.

It is important to note that the process undertaken to achieve the program goal will involve long discussion as well as the preparation and revision of several program drafts by the board. At times the preferred program solution will be tempered by the practical consideration of what the community can afford. There is a need to have extensive community support in all phases of community effort, which implies the inclusion of many viewpoints and the weighing of various approaches to develop the best solution and program of action.

A review of various approaches should produce a tentative list of all the services the community would like to include in a primary care program. Further review may determine that some services cannot be provided within the limits of available resources and careful planning; for example, a service package may include 24-hour physician and nursing services, family planning services, transportation for the elderly, basic laboratory and X-ray services, and health education and other preventive services. In addition, an important task will be to determine the kind of program that can deliver the service package and still be financially feasible. It must be decided whether or not a primary care center is sufficient or if a satellite arrangement connected to the primary care center is necessary. In some cases a mobile unit may be needed for screening programs and health assessment clinics staffed by community health nurses.

For service areas encompassing great distances, where it is not feasible to have a physician, a satellite center can be developed and staffed by nurse practitioners or physician's assistants who relate to the physicians at the primary care center. The method of service delivery refers to the way in which the services will be provided. During the review of the alternative methods of service delivery it will become apparent that changes in the service package may be necessary. A viable method of service delivery should always utilize resources that already exist in the service area. Through consideration of the scope of services of existing agencies, it will be possible to determine the extent to which there may be duplication or overlap in the provision of health services. It will be beneficial to have the plans reviewed periodically by a program developer or administrator in health services, who may be able to make recommendations based on experiences of other similar communities.

Several alternative plans will no doubt have to be discussed and reviewed, giving consideration to area needs, cost, resources, relationship with other health providers in the area, if any, and possible cooperative arrangements with other area services. A written program plan will serve as a document for discussion, revision, and compromise in the group. The plan then can be made available to the service area to help gain citizen support.

The next procedure in the program planning must give consideration to the development of an organizational structure appropriate to the program chosen, policies and procedures to follow, facilities needed, recruitment of physician and nursing personnel, outside support, approvals, marketing and program variations such as use of satellite clinics.

In the structure for delivery of services there are four general categories or models: (1) community-based, (2) hospital-based, (3) private group, and (4) public agency. This paper is concerned generally with the community-based model where there is formally established through the board a nonprofit community corporation with an ongoing responsibility for the design and delivery of a program of primary care services. The board representing the service area is directly involved in the administration of health care. It participates both directly and indirectly in employing health care personnel, buying equipment and supplies, securing funds, and giving other necessary support on a continuing basis. Of course there are various degrees of cooperative arrangements between the providers of service and a community organization in the development of programs adapted to local conditions.

In the search for rural health manpower it almost becomes imperative that the program be geared to an area-wide health care system. The small towns involved have an opportunity to assist in the search for some members of the health team. They can identify their own nurses, active or retired, technicians, teachers who have health skills, or others who can be trained to perform relatively simple but nonetheless critical services. A nurse with special training or other specifically trained assistants can relieve physicians of many time-consuming professional activities.

In planning a system of comprehensive health care delivery, the greatest investment is made by those who will be served. They will provide the resources—time and money—that make it work; eventually they will become the consumers. Their cultural base is important in determining how human and natural resources are treated. The key focus is on community consciousness.

The operation of the community health care system will be reviewed under the section, Organized Primary Care.

EMERGENCY MEDICAL SERVICES

Special emphasis should be given to emergency care in a rural service area. Emergency health services often are inadequate in rural communities. In addition to farm and home accidents about two thirds of highway fatalities occur in rural areas. One study indicated that people injured in rural counties are almost four times as likely to die of their injuries as those injured in urban counties, despite the occurrence of less severe accidents and more survivable injuries.[2]

There are four basic components to an effective emergency care system:

1. Thorough training for on-the-spot first aid
2. A communications system that provides prompt response to the need
3. Fully equipped emergency vehicles, staffed by trained emergency medical technicians who can provide all necessary life support at the scene and during transportation
4. High-quality emergency care facilities, equipment, and staff

These four basic components should be coordinated with the goal of quality care for emergency victims. Currently an area may fall short of these standards. The reasons may be many: failure in any one of the four basic components, fragmented efforts, lack of coordination, and public or private apathy.

The first step in upgrading an emergency services system is to secure the cooperation as well as the involvement of all appropriate community agencies and health facilities. To improve the area's emergency care system, the board should work toward meeting the criteria developed for designating a rural hospital as an emergency facility:

1. A two-way radio capable of contacting other hospitals and all emergency ambulances, with a trained staff on hand 24 hours a day.
2. A nurse or physician extender who is adequately trained in emergency procedures in the hospital and is available to the emergency room 24 hours a day.
3. Protocols to cover emergency proce-

dures while the physician is en route to the hospital.

4. A physician trained in emergency medicine on call or in the hospital 24 hours a day and available within 15 minutes.
5. Laboratory and X-ray technicians available in the hospital, or on call and accessible within 30 minutes 24 hours a day.
6. Minimum equipment available including examining tables with safety belts, oxygen, suction, resuscitation items, splints, sutures, cardiac emergency equipment, and an incubator.
7. An emergency department committee that is active and meets at least four times a year and has the authority to review operations and make recommendations.
8. Strategically located, distinctive, easy-to-read signs that identify the location of the hospital as well as the emergency center within the hospital.
9. A primary schedule for all of the physicians who will be carrying out basic coverage as well as for backup specialists.
10. A readily available plan in the emergency room, which covers the types of patients to be provided with basic emergency care preceding transfer to the hospital and the necessary procedures and arrangements to be made with ambulance and ambulance personnel as well as with the hospital receiving the patient. Accompanying the patient should be a patient record outlining problems and recommended treatment during the transfer.
11. The patient's record of problems, care, and outcome on file that allows for easy and comprehensive review.[3]

An important resource in emergency medical services is the Department of Health, Education, and Welfare Emergency Medical Services programs. The board should coordinate and explore linkage with and possible support from the department.

ELEMENTS OF A RURAL HEALTH CARE SYSTEM

Since a health care system should attempt to meet the health needs of all people in the area, the essential elements of the system must be coordinated to achieve its goal. A model is an ideal system that can be used to evaluate progress. It must be remembered that no one community or area will have all the elements listed in an ideal system. There are many experimental models for the delivery of rural health services that are being tried in our nation. Following are suggested elements of a rural health care delivery system:

I. Personnel
1. Two or more physicians representing primary physician skills such as family practitioner, internist, or pediatrician
2. Nurse, dentist, and laboratory and X-ray technicians
3. Health aides recruited from local area
4. Nurse practitioners and/or physician's assistants
5. Community health nurse—outreach and follow-up
6. Social worker
7. Administrator and staff
8. Receptionist and other office staff
9. Medical specialties staff—either visiting or by referral

II. Services: one door for all economic levels
1. Preventive, curative, and rehabilitative—medical and dental
2. Social services
3. Mental health services
4. Health and patient education

5. Transportation to and from clinic and to referral source
6. Home health care
7. Outreach case finding
8. Appropriate technology
9. Satellite clinics where needed
10. Administration
11. Mobile unit where needed
12. Evaluation and medical audit
13. Central records, master family records, and established referral and report-back procedures
14. Adequate physical facilities
15. Emergency medical services, well-equipped ambulances with trained crew, and two-way communication between ambulance and hospital, and hospital that meets standards for an emergency facility
16. Provision for primary, secondary, and tertiary care
17. Linkage to other health agencies in area and to medical school where possible

III. Community relationships
1. Community health board representing total area
2. County and state health department
3. Medical and dental societies
4. Community college for training aides
5. Health systems agency
6. Voluntary health agencies
7. Medical and nursing schools for referral and source of students and residents
8. Elementary and secondary schools
9. Cooperative extension service
10. Mental health center
11. Citizen health education service

IV. Funding: Multiple method approach
1. Fee for service
2. Prepaid and/or capitation—health maintenance organization
3. Sliding scale
4. Public funding for nonreimbursible services

ORGANIZED PRIMARY CARE

The establishment of three distinct but complementary levels of health care—primary, secondary, and tertiary—provides the basic potential for the development of a model system in comprehensive health services for the people of a rural service area.

Primary care refers to the routine medical care and services people receive on first contact with the health system for a particular health incident such as prevention, maintenance diagnosis, limited treatment, management of chronic problems, and referral. Primary care represents from 75% to 80% of the care that people need and is usually provided by physicians, nurse practitioners and physician's assistants, and dentists and their staff. These health care professionals should function together as a team. Each member of the health care team should provide that portion of the health care services for which he or she is responsible in a coordinated way.

Secondary care encompasses most medical and surgical diagnosis and therapeutic health services such as diagnostic radiology and laboratory studies, referrals for consultation, general surgery, most medical and pediatric disorders requiring hospitalization, and all but the most unusual obstetric problems. It is desirable that the secondary care site be not more than 60 minutes driving time from the primary care facility.

Tertiary care is provided at major hospital centers for patients requiring diagnostic, therapeutic, or rehabilitative services that transcend the capabilities of the average community hospital. Such care is normally available in large teaching hospitals or university medical centers. Helicopters and other aircraft may be used to link rural areas to tertiary care centers.

Substantial community support is a key factor in the success of a rural primary health care center. Local people with accounting, legal, management, and organizational abilities have proven to be indispensable in the community development of a primary health care system. Health education and preventive services are important elements in primary care. Health education programs should be planned carefully to meet the needs of the people. The programs must be linked to other community resources and included in the financial plan.

Where medical schools are available, linkages may be established for speciality consultation, continuing education opportunities, staff support, and training opportunities for students and residents.

In the operation of the primary health care system, the major components are personnel, financial management, administrative management, patient management, clinical policies and procedures, statistics and information, and quality assurance. Rationally developed policies and procedures should be written for each of these areas.

A staffing pattern indicating the desired number and kind of health professionals should be developed. It is estimated that a physician can effectively manage 1800 to 2000 patients and a nurse practitioner or physician's assistant can increase a physician's productivity by 50% to 75%. To ensure the necessary support, the center will need to provide two to three nursing, clerical, and/or medical-technical personnel per primary care physician.

More and more the business and management side of medical practice requires the employment of an administrator. Such a person would be responsible for management of the center and must be skilled in setting up management systems, as well as in evaluating and adapting them as required. Financial skills are especially important. The adminis-

trator should handle budgeting, accounting, and fund raising; oversee personnel and record keeping; and manage capital improvements and maintenance.

Job descriptions should be formulated for each staff member; the description should include duties, performance requirements, and relationship to other positions. Next an organizational chart should be drawn up. The personnel program also involves the development of a wage and salary schedule. Personnel policies may include a history of the program, recruitment policy, job requirements, salary administration, discipline and rules, and safety procedures. There is also a need to develop performance evaluation and plans for staff meetings.

A smoothly running health care delivery service involves a carefully developed patient management system. Consideration must be given to appointments, reception and registration, information to the patient, encounter form, hours of operation, patient flow, telephone calls, coverage and emergencies, referrals and consultations, patients' rights, and grievances and complaints.

Quality of primary care and continuity of care are two important factors in any provider-patient relationship. Malpractice is another important concern for all health providers. A well-organized health care delivery system and well-trained staff will avoid most of the problems of malpractice.

ACTION THROUGH COMMUNITY ORGANIZATION

An example of a community health care services organization is Southwest Minnesota Health Care Enterprises (SMHCE), a nonprofit, citizen-controlled health system designed to serve 15,000 people in two counties. The towns of Lamberton and Jeffers are a part of this system, which explains why there are two primary care physicians working in this area after so many doctorless years.

In July 1971 several concerned individuals from a six-community, doctorless area in southwestern Minnesota banded together in an effort to recruit physicians. They secured financial support from the Regional Medical Program. The Department of Family Practice and Community Health of the University of Minnesota Medical School did a survey of rural health services and assessment of needs. A U.S. Department of Agriculture official, who was superintendent of the University of Minnesota Southwest Experimental Station in the area, was a key leader in the community organization.

Utilizing the findings of the survey as well as new concepts in group dynamics and medicine, the University medical school designed a health care system for SMHCE. The planners of the health care system realized that long-term survival would require an organization that was actually part of the structure of the communities involved. They knew that regional approaches to health care planning had often failed because they were not successful in providing effective and ongoing participation by the people involved.

Rural Minnesota traditions extend far beyond the routine needs of caring for the ill. Those who have a concern for the health of animals and plants have a much broader outlook on life. The real strength of SMHCE lay in its developing plans for improving the health of all the people.

The health care system used innovative approaches to solve the problems of practicing in a rural area including:

1. Creating an area-wide basis for a health system that would eventually evolve into a health care system serving the multicommunity
2. Utilizing the County Extension Service to involve citizens
3. Securing a financial commitment from the people in the six communities to fund the system until it could be self-supporting
4. Developing the ambulatory concept that uses the hospitals and works closely with physicians already available in the larger region around the six communities
5. Placing the administration of the system in the hands of a board of directors
6. Establishing a long-range school and a community health education program
7. Embodying health care in a system of which the physician is an integral part. (More than shortage of physicians, we have a shortage of rural health care systems.)

Most symbolic of the success of the model is the fact that 22 area towns and townships joined together in March, 1974, to form the Health Services Board of Southwest Minnesota, the first rural joint-powers agreement in the state. Now that they have created a central group representing all of the people in the area, they are able to work together even more effectively in planning a medical delivery system based on their needs as they see them.

UTILIZATION OF SERVICES

The greatest untapped health manpower resource in this country is the individual consumer. Needed is an informed and "activated" citizen who can take his own initiative in personal health—approaching and utilizing the health care system properly for all of the services required in his personal health management program.

An important and promising avenue for encouraging this appropriate, active response is through a broader program of consumer health education. For such a program to succeed it must have an appropriate and high-quality, substantive base. This must be coupled with a pervasive delivery and access system that will ensure widespread involvement as well as methods of effectively dealing with personal motivation.

The greatest potential for improving our

health lies in what we do or fail to do for and to ourselves. The choice is up to us. It can be said that a significant reduction in sedentary living, overnutrition, hypertension, alcoholism, and cigarette smoking would save more lives in the age range of 40 to 64 years than the best current medical practice. It would also add to national productivity by reducing absenteeism and illness.[5] The lower incidence of cancer among Mormons and Seventh-Day Adventists as well as their lower mortality rates are evidence of the preventive effects of healthful life-styles such as abstention from tobacco and alcohol and maintenance of a diet comparable to the degree of their physical activity.[6] In addition, these healthful life-styles are reflected in lower medical care expenditures; for example, total federal and state personal health care expenditures per capita in 1969 in Utah were significantly below what would be expected for a state of its per capita personal income and its welfare load.[6]

Given the present demand for health care, a rural health care system should put forth a major effort directed at consumer health education as well as patient education in the physicians' office and in the hospital. The county and possibly the area Cooperative Extension Service can assist in the health education effort.

People must get involved in their own health promotion and become concerned about the health care delivery problems in their own communities. People have to become interested and confident in solving health problems—those problems that they themselves define.

The principal resource of any area is its people, and the ultimate goal of any program is to raise the level of human well-being. Remedial health services are indispensable to the pursuit of that goal. But in the long run,

self-maintenance of health and prevention of disease are just as necessary.

Education for health then is a fundamental aspect of community health services and is basic to every rural health care system. The objectives of health education are to interest each individual in his own health as well as in the means to improve it, to teach him where health services are available, to motivate him to use these services intelligently, and to teach him what aspects of personal behavior and environment will affect his health. In rural areas particularly, the environmental impact on health is critical and apparent. Community health education can lead to community organization around such problems as adequate sanitation and improved water supplies.

We must recognize that health does not exist in a vacuum. Health is but one aspect of the quality of life which includes all of the socioeconomic, ecological, and educational factors that make for a satisfactory living situation. To improve rural health we must also address the totality of deficiencies in rural living today.

REFERENCES

1. Moe, E. O.: Nature of today's community. In Reinhardt, A. M., and Quinn, M. D., ed.: Current practice in family-centered community nursing, St. Louis, 1977, The C. V. Mosby Co.
2. American Medical Association Council on Rural Health: Emergency medical services: widening the road to access, Rural Health News, January-February 1974.
3. Waller, J. A.: Urban-oriented methods—failure to solve rural emergency care problems, J.A.M.A. **226:** 1441-1446, Dec. 17, 1973.
4. Fuchs, V. R.: Who shall live? New York: 1974, Basic Books.
5. Wynder, E. L.: Nutrition and cancer, Fed. Am. Soc. Experiment. Biol. **35:**1309, 1976.
6. Kristein, M. M., Arnold, C. B., and Wynder, E. L.: Health economics and preventive care, Science **195:** 459-461, February 4, 1977.

10

The nurse and the adolescent in today's changing social structure

Miriam S. Rosenberg

Adolescent health care in the community has been a challenge to all those concerned with the health care of young people. This ·chapter will address itself to the historical development of adolescence in our society and the resulting health needs. Our working definition of health is that of the World Health Organization: "a state of complete physical, mental and social well being and not merely the abscence of disease and infirmity." We accept the premise that in meeting these health needs, the practitioner who has a holistic framework and uses a general systems theory will be more effective in meeting the total needs of the adolescent.[1-3] Some models of adolescent health care that attempt to meet the needs of this age group will be presented. These models recognize that the health system is only one part of a complex, open system that has evolved over a period of time. The community or interacting subsystems are the school, family church, work place, and law enforcement groups. They are continually acting and reacting with one another. The youth in search of self affects all of these groups in society, and they in turn help or hinder the growth of young people.

DEFINITION OF ADOLESCENCE

Webster's definition of adolescence is "a state or process of growing up from childhood to manhood or womanhood; youth or the period of life between puberty and maturity, extending in legal use to the attainment of full legal age, or majority."[4] The term "growing up" must also include a definition that takes into consideration the biological, sociological, and psychological variables.[5]

Biological variables

Biological variables are the anatomical and physiological changes that begin in early adolescence with the onset of secondary sex characteristics. They result from endocrine changes, which in turn are determined by an interplay between heredity and environment. This interplay leads us directly into the wide variability in the physical development of the maturing adolescent. Tanner[6,7] has repeatedly demonstrated this variability in physical maturation in both boys and girls. Such a biological timetable is accelerated in our culture so that pubertal development occurs earlier; that is, there is an earlier and faster maturational process. Another factor that probably affects the rate of maturation is nutritional status; that is, an earlier onset of menstruation is associated with better nutrition. Other findings indicate that there is an association with early menarche and a stout physique, and late menarche with a slim body. Because there is confusion in describing the pubertal stages of adolescence, Tanner's classification system is recommended and accepted (Table 6) as the common guide for determining maturity.

There is a direct correlation between the anatomical-physiological changes and adolescents' sense of self; it is thus helpful to share the observed physical changes with adolescents while taking histories and performing physical examinations. It is reassuring to

Table 6. Tanner pubertal stages

Boys: Genital development

Stage 1: Pre-adolescent: Testes, scrotum and penis are about the same size and proportion as in early childhood.

Stage 2: Scrotum and testes are enlarged. Skin of scrotum reddened and changed in texture. Little or no enlargement of penis is present at this stage.

Stage 3: Penis is slightly enlarged, which occurs at first mainly in length. Testes and scrotum are further enlarged.

Stage 4: Increased size of penis with growth in breadth and development of glans is present. Testes and scrotum larger; scrotal skin darker than in earlier stages.

Stage 5: Genitalia adult in size and shape.

Girls: Breast development

Stage 1: Pre-adolescent: Elevation of papilla only.

Stage 2: Breast bud stage: Elevation of breast and papilla as small mound. Enlargement of areola diameter.

Stage 3: Further enlargement and elevation of breast and areola, with no separation of their contours.

Stage 4: Projection of areola and papilla to form a secondary mound above the level of the breast.

Stage 5: Mature stage: Projection of papilla only, due to recession of the areola to the general contour of the breast.

Both sexes: Pubic hair

Stage 1: Pre-adolescent: The vellus over the pubes is not further developed than that over the abdominal wall: i.e., no pubic hair.

Stage 2: Sparse growth of long, slightly pigmented downy hair, straight or curled, chiefly at the base of the penis or along labia.

Stage 3: Considerably darker, coarser and more curled. The hair spreads sparsely over the junction of the pubes.

Stage 4: Hair now adult in type, but area covered is still considerably smaller than in the adult. No spread to the medial surface of thighs.

Stage 5: Adult in quantity and type with distribution of the horizontal (or classically 'feminine') pattern. Spread to medial surface of thighs but not up linea alba or elsewhere above the base of the inverse triangle.

Stage 6: Spread up linea alba.

Source: Tanner, J. M.: Growth and endocrinology of the adolescent. In Gardner, L. I., ed.: Endocrine and genetic diseases of childhood, Philadelphia, 1969 W. B. Saunders Co.

young people to know how development unfolds in general, the uniqueness of each individual, and the fact that the uniqueness is normal. Their preoccupation with the body, and its development and beautification is related to the feeling that any one who appears different from the group's norm will be rejected or teased. This preoccupation has resulted in adolescents' concern with their weight, their breast or penis size, and their skin condition in relation to their sexuality.

Psychological variables

Stress and conflict are set into motion by the search for identity, as described by Erikson.[8] This sense of self is part of a developmental process of a person that has been going on since birth. The adolescent period in our culture has no rituals that clearly define for young people when they are adults. On the other hand, not all adolescents go through a troubled time; for some, the transition is made easier by their acceptance of family values, which demonstrate stability and consistency. It is curious that very little is studied or written about young people who present no problems. Erikson believes that adolescent problems erupt either when a young person is not able to establish firmly his identity or when he chooses an identity that is deviant from accepted norms. Another significant contribution has been made by Kagan[9] in summarizing the major developmental tasks of adolescence:
1. Resolving uncertainty about sexual adequacy
2. Interpersonal power
3. Autonomy of belief and action
4. Acceptability by peers

From the health care worker's point of view it is important to note that the adolescent who is nonconformist usually will not conform to the standard models of health care. Therefore these youths in the community must be identified and creative, nontra-

ditional modes of health care must be established so that we do not further abandon them (see description of the Door).

The struggle for autonomy and the importance of peers are two factors that have led to the development of peer group health teaching. Peer group leaders have been trained to lead discussion groups on drugs, sexuality, contraceptives, and any other area of identified importance. In one community a cadre of both adults and teenagers were trained in techniques of the group process, as a direct result of an escalating drug problem. These groups of adolescents and adults were established to facilitate communication and understanding between the two. There were coleaders in each group, one adult and one adolescent. The experience was considered positive by the participants, but its impact on the drug problem is indeterminate. The hard-core drug abusers were rarely involved. After a period of time (2 years) interest waned—which is typical for these types of groups—and funding ceased. This type of rap group is useful as it promotes the sharing of feelings among adolescents as well as among adults and adolescents. The capacity of adolescents to profit from this type of rap session is a result of their ability to deal with abstractions, as described by Piaget.[10]

Other factors besides nonconformist behavior can lead to a profound reluctance to use a health setting that adolescents do not trust. These youths, especially the poor ones, have learned to ignore their health needs as professionals define them. This may be due to a low priority given to health care, lack of information related to maintaining health, and/or fear of the unknown. They also may have accepted limited health care as part of life, thus reflecting the attitudes of their parents who do not seek health care because of the low priority they have assigned to it. The health needs of adolescents living in poverty are clearly tied to economic and social conditions such as poor housing, poor schooling, poor sanitation, lack of jobs, and just trying to "get by."[11] One's ability to explore "Who am I?" is looked upon by such youths as a luxury in a society where they must find jobs in order to help themselves and their families survive.

Sociological variables

Sociological variables have contributed to the diversity of the adolescent experience in our society. Changes have been so rapid and constant that the values and norms of the past have not been able to keep pace.[12] During the 1960s the accelerated rate of social change and the complexity of life led to a heightened awareness of the problems young people were facing. According to Kett,[13] "Every generation of intellectuals since 1820 has been convinced that an acceleration of the velocity of social change has disrupted traditional harmony and has had a calamitous effect on youth." Some scholars feel that our perception of youth says more about adults than young people.

Kett[13] describes the historical evolution of adolescence. He points out that in the nineteenth century individuals did not have an adolescence per se, but went directly from childhood to adulthood, from child to worker. This contrasts with the twentieth century where there is a prolonged period of adolescent dependency characterized by extended schooling for a technological society. For those young people who go on to graduate study, economic dependency on family and society is prolonged until their late 20s.

It is clear from the above that the young person of the twentieth century spends much more time at school than his counterpart of the 1800s. Therefore the school setting rather than the work place becomes a major socializing force. His work experience is limited by the paucity of jobs, and the educational program has little relevance to real work. Young people are basically consumers rather than producers. Their social setting, the school, is controlled by adults. These adults are the ones who provide an educational experience intended to give some purpose to the lives of young people. This is particularly true since the increasing collapse of the extended and nuclear family. In other words, the adolescent often does not have the family as a support system in time of need. This places a greater burden on the school and other community agencies to provide the limits and guidance that many adolescents need. Unhappily it is still true that many schools have become wastelands as far as any sort of meaningful education is concerned. Ideally, since the school is the social institution in which our adolescents spend most of their time, it is the natural setting for the provision of health care, utilizing the professional nurse as a provider of primary health care. Primary care in the schools should include the following:

1. Health appraisal
2. Treatment
3. Referral
4. Follow-up
5. Preventive health education[14]

In reality this has rarely been the case; however, there have been some encouraging developments in this direction. These programs will be discussed in the section on models of health care.

MODELS OF ADOLESCENT HEALTH CARE IN THE COMMUNITY

The role of professional nurses in relation to providing adolescent health care in a variety of settings will be presented in this section. I recognize that the general deficiencies of the health care system will also apply to the health care of the adolescent. These deficiencies include fragmented, physician-dominated, illness-oriented, uncoordinated, and inadequately utilized services bound by tradition. The role of professional nurses and their contributions in meeting the needs of the adolescent consumer will be the focus of the models of health care to be presented. The models of health care will include the following:

1. School health programs and the utilization of school nurse practitioners
2. An alternate comprehensive environment that attempts to meet the needs of the inner-city adolescent

3. Comprehensive health care facilities in the community with in-hospital back-up

School health programs

There has been growing concern about the quality and effectiveness of school health throughout the country. Most programs in public schools are fragmented and inadequate. The school nurse spends most of her

Table 7. Leading causes of death as percentages of all deaths, ages 12 to 19: 1973*

Accidents

0%	50%	100%

58.1%

Homicide

0%	50%	100%

7.3%

Malignant neoplasms

0%	50%	100%

7.1%

Suicide

0%	50%	100%

5.4%

Major cardiovascular diseases

0%	50%	100%

3.5%

Congenital anomalies

0%	50%	100%

2.1%

Influenza and pneumonia

0%	50%	100%

2.0%

*Maternal and child health project, MSRI, using data from National Center for Health Statistics. Cited in Millar, H. E. C.: Approaches to adolescent health care in the 1970's, DHEW Publication No. (HSA) 76-5014, Washington, D.C., 1975, U.S. Government Printing Office.

Table 8. Percentage of 12 to 19 year olds using alcohol and tobacco: 1972*

Alcohol

33.4%		
0%	50%	100%

Tobacco

22.8%		
0%	50%	100%

*Maternal and child health project, MSRI, using data from National Center for Health Statistics. Cited in Millar, H. E. C.: Approaches to adolescent health care in the 1970's, DHEW Publication No. (HSA) 76-5014, Washington, D.C., 1975, U.S. Government Printing Office.

Table 9. Percentage of 12 to 17 year olds who have ever used marijuana and other drugs: 1972*

Marijuana

23.6%		
0%	50%	100%

Glue and other inhalants

6.4%		
0%	50%	100%

LSD and other hallucinogens

4.8%		
0%	50%	100%

Cocaine

1.5%		
0%	50%	100%

Heroin

0.6%		
0%	50%	100%

*Maternal and child health project, MSRI, using data from National Center for Health Statistics. Cited in Millar, H. E. C.: Approaches to adolescent health care in the 1970's, DHEW Publication No. (HSA) 76-5014, Washington, D.C., 1975, U.S. Government Printing Office.

time doing clerical work and first aid. Health programs in nonpublic and private schools are either absent or minimal.

The school health program should be primarily preventive in nature. In New York state the school health program has been defined as those coordinated activities delivered by or through the school for school-age children to improve, maintain, and promote health, especially as it relates to learning and social functioning.[15] Ideally this type of program will do the following:

1. Reduce the mortality and morbidity rates for youths attending school (for example, accidents, alcohol, and drug abuse) (see Tables 7 to 9).
2. Improve the health status of youths after they enter school, because the quality of care delivered in well child clinics stops once the child enters school, except for a yearly or biyearly physical.
3. Provide continuity of care by using professional nurses who render primary health care. In recent years school nurse practitioners have assumed this role. To date it is not clear whether they are viewed as professionals or as extensions of physicians.

School nurse practitioners in New York. The School Health Project Bill (s.10060-A/ A.I2869-A) was signed by Governor Carey on May 31, 1978—which is a step in the right direction. It appears, that at the time of this reporting, the State Education Department has limited utilization of this law to approved health demonstration projects; this reflects a lack of understanding of the professionalism of nursing. The passage of the School Health Project Bill was necessary to ensure New York State's eligibility for funds from the Robert Wood Johnson Foundation, which states that there must be a law authorizing a designated state official to negotiate contracts with school districts to provide specific health services. The bill describes nursing services in the following manner:

The health services which may be performed by such registered professional nurses in collaboration with a licensed physician shall include diagnosis of illness and performance of therapeutic and corrective measures, including issuance of prescriptions for drugs, other than controlled substances, and immunization against preventable diseases. Such nurses shall, either before or after licensure, have satisfactorily completed educational preparation for these health services in a nursing program registered by the State Education Department or in a program determined by the department to be equivalent. Nothing in this act shall be deemed to limit the practice of the profession of nursing as registered professional nurse pursuant to Article 139 of the Education Law or to deny any registered professional nurse the right to do any act now authorized by such an article.[16]

It appears that the debate in the New York State Legislature continues in relation to the role of the professional nurse. Despite this, innovative school nurse programs have been established in Harlem and other parts of the country.

School health program in Harlem. With the decentralization of school districts in New York City and greater input from the community, the School Board identified health as an important factor in the children's lives and in 1969, with limited funding, established a health team. Initially it focused on screening for visual and auditory problems with aggressive follow-up to ensure further diagnosis and follow-up. Unskilled community residents were trained and supervised by a public health nurse to perform these screening tests and make follow-up visits. In 1970 funds were terminated and another program, this time in conjunction with the Division of Community and Social Pediatrics of Harlem Hospital, was established. In 1972 a comprehensive health program was established. It serviced two public schools with a staff of two public health nurses and four community health workers. Parents were informed by letter of the program and initial medical histories were obtained; written consent was also requested for all examinations and for taking children to other health facilities as indicated. The program consisted of the following:

1. Vision and hearing screening
2. Height and weight measurements
3. Physical examination
4. Dental screening
5. Laboratory examination
6. Tuberculin skin testing
7. Immunizations
8. Referral and follow-up

Health education was thus extended to the children, their parents, and the teachers.[17]

School nurse practitioners in high school. Another example of professionalism in nursing is demonstrated by the school nurse practitioner program in the San Diego, California, school system. The school district has committed itself to implementing a health maintenance program that provides a physical examination and health conference consisting of the following:

1. Reviewing the history with the student, focuses on helping the student learn about his health needs.
2. Physical examinations are given, along with an explanation of the procedures and an explanation of the findings (including self-breast examination and Pap smears).
3. Laboratory tests include those that are appropriate for this age group, such as tuberculin skin tests; they hope to add cultures for gonorrhea.[18]

Educational program for school nurse practitioners. The University of Colorado Medical Center School Nurse Practitioner Program is geared to the registered nurse.[19] The program consists of 4 months of theory and clinical experience. It is flexible enough, however, so that some nurses can complete the program over two summers. At the end of this advanced educational experience, they are able to do the following:

1. Take health histories from children and or parents

2. Give complete physical assessments including lab tests
3. Administer immunizations
4. Test and evaluate the child's physical, cognitive, social, and emotional development
5. Diagnose and treat children with injuries at school, referring to a physician when necessary
6. Provide health education to groups or individuals—students, teachers, or parents
7. Monitor the school environment for health hazards
8. Provide evaluative and rehabilitative counseling to handicapped children and their families and teachers
9. Work on an interdisciplinary team in the school setting

It is hoped that more baccalaureate nurses will be prepared so that they have primary care and change agent skills, independence, colleagueship, accountability, assertiveness, analytic ability, concern for individuals and their needs, an understanding of normal growth and development as well as deviations from health, and therapeutic management.

Center of alternatives and multiservice center for youth

The Door is a model comprehensive center for inner-city youths from 12 to 21 years of age.[20] It is the result of an identified need in the community and is based on a wholistic approach to adolescents and their needs. The staff recognizes that more is needed than to dispense birth control pills, provide abortion counseling, and treat diseases that are prevalent among all sexually active people. The Door is a place where adolescents can go to get help with immediate problems that may be related to school, legal issues, health questions, and pregnancy or abortion counseling. These services are all free and do not need parental consent.

The health center is one component of the

total center. The comprehensive facilities are housed in a building in Manhattan. Its 55,000 square feet are arranged in units that provide areas for an adolescent-run cafeteria, photography, graphics, sculpting, dance, theater, karate, vocational and educational aid, legal counseling, a health center that has its own laboratory and pharmacy, group discussions, and mental health counseling. The night I visited there, group discussions in relation to vegetarian diets and sex education were going on.

This center evolved from the needs of the inner-city youth—needs not being met by traditional settings. The major emphasis is to establish a sense of trust in the team with whom the young person works. The nurse practitioner is a member of this team and performs within the areas that are the domain of family nurse practitioners, recognizing that expertise in family planning is an essential component.

The Door has been able to provide comprehensive health services in a humane manner because of the dedication and understanding of all the people involved. The major problem is one of funding. As this is being written, funds from the federal government, the state, and/or contributors may be in jeopardy. This type of financial crisis detracts from the energy spent developing programs that will help these alienated youths develop that sense of "Who am I?"

The center and its professionals have demonstrated what can be done; now it is up to the communities to develop and fund similar programs. Legislation and the allocation of money by the federal government indicates that it is committed to supporting the teenage single mother but not programs that allow the adolescent to realize that as an adolescent there are other tasks to be achieved. Too many young people feel that they have no choice in establishing a sense of identity besides having a baby. The staff at the center attempts to help these young people arrive at the realization that there are other alternatives in life than being pregnant or giving up and resorting to drugs and alcohol. This center is a model for those who are interested in meeting the total developmental needs of the adolescent.

Traditional medical center models

There are two outstanding examples of the more traditional medical center models that offer adolescent health care in a more innovative manner. The outreach programs of the Division of Adolescent Medicine in the Department of Pediatrics at Montefiore Hospital [21] in New York City is an illustration of how a traditional medical center delivers health care to the adolescent in the community. Following are some of the ways in which they have reached out to the adolescent:

1. Walk-in ambulatory adolescent clinic in the outpatient department
2. Primary health care in youth detention facilities
3. Establishment of a separate adolescent unit in a federally funded comprehensive health care facility in the community
4. Outreach to schools for health teaching

Whenever possible the young people have a voice in identifying their health needs to the professional staff. This positive consumer input allows adolescents to feel that they are contributing something meaningful. It also allows youths to be exposed to the various careers that are open in the health field.

Another adolescent health care center in New York City is at The Mount Sinai Hospital Medical Center. It has a multidisciplinary approach and has the following goals:

1. Provide a walk-in clinic for youth.
2. Assign each patient a primary physician.

3. Develop an outreach program into the adjacent community.
4. Use an approach that is interdisciplinary and a model of primary care.[22]

These two health services are attempting to do more than meet the health problems of venereal disease and pregnancy. The problem is that to date the Department of Health, Education, and Welfare tends to fund programs that focus on a specific problem to utilize limited funds and manpower. Possibly this is one of the reasons that adolescent health problems are escalating. The question we have to ask ourselves is How much of a commitment do we want to make to preventive health care and education?

Many traditional health care facilities in the inner city recognize that children reared in poverty enter adolescence facing a positive experience with a comprehensive health care facility where their needs have been met with continuity of care by a health team. Preventive health care, health maintenance, and well child management with a focus on prenatal care and the preschool aged child are abandoned once the child enters school. The quality of health care of school aged children cannot be compared to that in the preschool years. Possibly the outreach of these facilities to the schools will serve this population. Some adolescents prefer to be cared for outside their school setting because they are concerned with confidentiality; therefore the adolescent clinics in the community must have hours so that young people can attend after school.

THE FUTURE

With a greater commitment to preventive health care, using the primary care model, it appears that the school is one of the major places to develop adolescent health care programs. The professional nurse will make a significant contribution to emerging models of adolescent health care in a variety of community settings provided that the program meets the following three conditions:

1. There is an awareness of the physical, emotional, social, and economic status as well as the cultural and environmental backgrounds of individuals, families, and communities.
2. The health care system is made accessible to the client.
3. A single provider or team of providers, along with the client, is responsible for the continuing coordination and management of all aspects of the basic health services needed for individual and family care.[24]

REFERENCES

1. von Bertalnfry, L.: General systems theory, Main Curr. Mod. Thought 11:75-83, March 1955.
2. Rogers, M. E.: An introduction to the theoretical basis of nursing, Philadelphia, 1970, F. A. Davis Co.
3. Muhich, D. F., and Johnson, B. S.: Youth and society, Pediatr. Clin. North Am. 20:771-777, November 1973.
4. Webster's new international dictionary, ed. 2, unabridged, Springfield, Mass., 1956, G. & C. Merriam Company.
5. Feinstein, S., Giovanchini, P., and Miller, D., eds.: Adolescent psychiatry, vol. 1, New York, 1971, Basic Books, Inc., Publishers.
6. Tanner, J. M.: Growing up, Sci. Am. 229:34-43, September 1973.
7. Kagan, J., and Coles, R., eds.: Twelve to sixteen: early adolescence. New York, 1972, W. W. Norton & Co., Inc.
8. Erikson, E.: Identity, youth and crisis, New York, 1968, W. W. Norton & Co., Inc.
9. Kagan, J.: A conception of early adolescence, Daedalus 100(4):997-1012, Fall 1971.
10. Beard, R. M.: An outline of Piaget's developmental psychology, New York, 1972, The New American Library, Inc.
11. Fielding, J. E., and Nelson, S. H.: Health care for the economically disadvantaged adolescent, Pediatr. Clin. North Am. 20:975-989, November 1973.
12. Toffler, A.: Future shock, New York, 1970, Random House, Inc.
13. Kett, J. F.: Rites of passage: adolescence in America, 1970 to the present, New York, 1977, Basic Books, Inc., Publishers.

14. New York State Planning Commission: Policy recommendations on school health, unpublished draft, 1977.

15. New York State Nurses Association: report, Official Newsletter, 9:5-6, July-August 1978.

16. Rogers, S. C: Innovative school nursing in Harlem, Am. J. Nurs. **77:**1469-1476, 1977.

17. Blust, L. C.: School nurse practitioner in a high school, Am. J. Nurs. **78:**1532-1533, 1978.

18. Silver, H. K., and Igoe, J. B.: The school nurse practitioner, Am. Educator **2:**31-33, Fall 1978.

19. McGivern, D.: Baccalaureate preparation for the nurse practitioner, Nurs. Outlook **22:**94-97, 1974.

20. Millar, H. E. C.: Approaches to adolescent health care in the 1970's, DHEW publication No. (H.S.A.) 76-5014, Washington, D.C., 1975, U.S. Government Printing Office.

21. Morgenthau, J. E., ed.: Adolescent health care: a multidisciplinary approach, Westport, Conn., 1976, Techomic Publishing Co.

22. Federal Register, vol. 41, No. 16, January 23, 1976.

SUGGESTED READINGS

Moore, T. D., ed.: Adolescent gynecology: report of the 7th Ross Roundtable on critical approaches to common pediatric problems in collaboration with the ambulatory Pediatric Association. Columbus, Ohio, 1977, Ross Laboratories.

Caldwell, L. R.: Use of the social readjustment rating scale combined with the P.O.R. in a college health setting, Nurse Practitioner **3:**24-28, February 1978.

Caplan, G., and Lebovici, S., ed.: Adolescence: psychosocial perspectives, New York, 1969, Basic Books, Inc., Publishers.

Cigarette smoking among teenagers and young women, DHEW publication No. (N.I.H.) 77-1203, Washington, D.C., 1977, U.S. Government Printing Office.

Clasky, K. K., et al.: The school nurse and drug abusers, Nurs. Outlook **18:**27-30, December 1970.

Congressional report urges more money for nutrition education for students school cafeteria workers, Adolescent Med. **9:**3, January 1977.

Hayes, J., and Littlefield, J. H.: Venereal disease knowledge in high school seniors, J. School Health **46:**546-547, November 1976.

Head, F. P., ed.: Adolescent gynecology, Baltimore, 1966, The Williams & Wilkins Co.

Hill, P. M., et al.: Screening for scoliosis in adolescents, Maternal Child Nurs. **2:**156-159, May/June 1977.

Hoffman, A. D., and Pilpel, H. F.: The legal rights of minors, Pediatr. Clin. North Am. **20:**989-1003, November 1973.

Jaffe F., and Dryfus, J.: Fertility control services for adolescents: access and utilization, Fam. Plann. Perspect. **8:**172-179, 1976.

Jekel, J. F.: Primary or secondary prevention of adolescent pregnancies, J. School Health **47:**457-461, October 1977.

Joint Practice: a new dimension in nurse-physician collaboration, Am. J. Nurs. **77:**1466-1468, September 1977.

Jones, A.: Overview of a nursing center for family health services in Freeport, Nurse Practitioner **16:**55-58, April 1968.

Kreutner, A. K., Kessler, J., and Hollingsworth, D. R.: Adolescent obstetrics and gynecology, Chicago, 1978, Year Book Medical Publishers, Inc.

Lopez, R. I.: Adolescent medicine topics, New York, 1976, Spectrum Publications.

Mathis, J. L.: Adolescent sexuality and societal change, Am. J. Psychother. **30:**433-440, July 1976.

McAmarney, E. R., et al.: Development of an adolescent maternity project in Rochester, New York, Public Health Rep. **92:**154-159, March/April 1977.

Mitchell, J. J.: The adolescent predicament, Toronto, 1975, Holt, Rinehart & Winston of Canada, Ltd.

Needle, R. H.: Factors affecting contraceptive practices of high school and college age students, J. School Health **47:**340-345, June 1977.

Normal adolescence: formulated by the Committee on Adolescence, Group for the Advancement of Psychiatry, New York, 1969, Charles Scribner's Sons.

Sheffield, R.: Team health service employs team approach, Hospitals **50:**93-98, December 16, 1976.

Torre, C. T.: Nutritional needs of adolescents, Maternal Child Nurs. **2:**118-127, March/April 1977.

U.S. Department of Health, Education, and Welfare: The association of health attitudes and perceptions of youths 12-17 years of age with those of their parents. DHEW publication No. (H.R.A.) 77-1643, Washington, D.C., 1977, U.S. Government Printing Office.

White, K. M., and Speisman, J. C.: Adolescence, Monterey, Calif., 1977, Brooks/Cole Publishing Co.

Zeltzer, L. K., et al.: The adolescent clinic: a model and profile, Clin. Pediatr. **16:**426-430, May 1977.

11

Medical care for the rape victim

Charlotte R. Platt,† Dorothy J. Hicks, and Denise M. Mori

The understanding that forcible rape is a crime and not an act done for the purpose of sexual gratification is a concept that has come into being only recently. Sexual assault is the result of violence, hostility, and the need for power rather than the need for sexual satisfaction. This new attitude is probably the direct result of the feminist movement, although most people working in the field, both law enforcement and medical personnel, accept it. The task remains to educate the general public.

The Rape Treatment Center at Jackson Memorial Hospital is the outcome of a group of feminists literally marching down the main street of Miami, Florida, in 1971 and demanding that the county establish a center for the treatment of rape victims. The County Commission finally heard them, and in January, 1974, the Rape Treatment Center was opened at Jackson Memorial Hospital. The first patient was seen during the ribbon cutting ceremony.

The need for treatment centers is crucial. It is an accepted fact that the majority of rapes are not reported; most workers estimate that only one in four is reported to the authorities. In 1977, 63,020 forcible rapes were reported to the Federal Bureau of Investigation, an

increase of almost 200% over the number reported in 1960. However, this figure includes only forcible rapes and attempted forcible rapes; it does not include rape homicides and sexual assaults on children. If only one rape in four is reported, it means there were about 252,000 forcible rapes last year in the United States or one rape every 2 minutes. The need is there.

Any program for victims of sexual assault should be comprehensive and include both medical and psychological care not only for the victim but also for any significant others in her sphere. Ideally victims should be separated from the mainstream of an emergency room setting. They are extremely sensitive about having been raped and usually feel guilty that something like that happened to them, because for centuries women have been taught to believe that if they had not been seductive or "available" no one would have raped them. "Good girls" are never sexually assaulted. We know this is not true. All that is necessary for a female to be the victim of a rapist is for her to be in the wrong place at the wrong time. Rapists look for someone who is vulnerable, someone to overpower. Their sole purpose is to humiliate and degrade, not to get sexual satisfaction.

The rape victim needs empathy, not sympathy, from those who come in contact with

---

†Deceased.

135

her. Sympathy can be degrading. No one should judge the actions of the victim before the assault. Medical personnel should accept her history of the attack without question. It is the job of the police if they are involved to decide the accuracy of her story. Actually the details of the crime are not needed by those examining the patient. All that is needed by the medical team is a history of what happened so that they can best treat her medical problems and the psychological trauma that has occurred. Too much detail in the history may jeopardize the case in court because patients are upset at the time of the medical examination and often have their facts wrong.

The patient should be seen and taken care of as soon as possible after her arrival at the treatment center. It is desirable to have a special area and specially trained personnel to care for these victims because they are not "emergencies" in the usual medical or even psychiatric sense, although the way in which they are cared for will influence the degree of their recovery and the speed with which they recover.

Our center is located in a double house trailer adjacent to but not a part of the hospital emergency room. A rape treatment center should have the resources of a general hospital nearby. Patients may be injured and need more than "first-aid." Occasionally the trauma is so severe it is necessary to take them to the operating room immediately.

We use a "floating team" concept to be sure that the personnel are trained and willing to care for rape victims. The team is composed of a gynecologist who has been specially trained to examine these victims and a nurse from the hospital emergency room. The third member of the team is a crisis-trained social worker who works during the day, Monday through Friday, from 10 A.M. to 6:30 P.M. Originally a crisis counselor was a part of the team, but we found that few patients need crisis counseling at the time of the assault. Usually they are very quiet and may even refuse to talk about their experience. Most of the victims are exhausted after the assault and are more receptive to counseling the next day. If the nurse or physician thinks that the patient is sufficiently upset to need immediate psychological counseling, the psychiatrist on call for the emergency room is asked to see the patient. This is a judgment decision of the people who are doing the examination.

The examination should be tailored to the circumstances of the attack. If the patient has been severely beaten, she should be seen in the surgical area of the emergency room, and the necessary trauma procedures should be done before the "rape examination"; indicated X-ray films are taken, lacerations are sutured, and so forth. On several occasions in our center the forensic examination was done in the operating room while the patient was under anesthesia.

The nurse is usually the first person to see the patient. Her role should be a supportive one and, unless it is in the protocol, the nurse should not ask for any details of the attack. Our nurses ask only those questions needed to initiate a chart for the patient. Asking the patient to tell and retell the story of the attack can contribute to further psychological trauma. Even the physician should get the details from the police if they are present and then ask only those questions necessary to fill out the report. If the patient wants to talk about the incident, the nurse should listen and then tell the physician what she has learned about the attack. The physician should not ask the victim for facts already told to someone else. The patient should be spared as much as possible having to repeat her story.

It is important that the patient be given control of her life as soon as possible after the attack; therefore she should be allowed to make the decisions as to the kind of examination and treatment she is to receive. If she does not give the desired responses, the personnel should try to guide her to the appropriate answers, but at no time should she be forced to do anything she does not want to do. Most patients will be very cooperative once they feel secure and realize that the people caring for them understand the traumatic experience they have had and the problems they face.

The nurse should always be present during the examination of the patient and should be supportive and empathetic. In all cases, the physician looks for any external signs of trauma such as bruises and lacerations and documents these carefully both as to size and location. If there has been a struggle and the patient has scratched the attacker, the fingernails should be examined. An orange stick should be used to remove the material from under the nails and the stick, and any material found is placed in a clean paper envelope. If a nail has been broken, the distal portion of the nail should be cut off and placed in another envelope so that the edges can be matched if the broken piece is found. Photographs should be taken if there is visible trauma.

The remainder of the examination is tailored to the areas involved in the attack. Extensive, all-inclusive examination of the victim is not essential in every case, and only those procedures necessary for the case in point should be done.

Venous blood in a red-top tube should be drawn for screening VDRL in almost every case. A pelvic examination is indicated in all cases of rape. The pubic hair should be combed, and both the comb and combings placed in an envelope. A Pederson speculum should be used for the examination whenever possible because these patients are usually tender in the vaginal area. The narrower speculum is more comfortable because only water may be used to lubricate the instrument before it is inserted into the vaginal

canal. Any other form of lubrication such as jelly will interfere with the forensic tests. Cotton swabs should be used to remove material from the distal vaginal wall and from the area of the vaginal vault. Air-dried smears on glass slides are made from these smears. Both the swabs and the smears should be sent to the laboratory. Two milliliters of sterile saline are injected into the vaginal canal and retrieved with a plastic transfer pipette; this fluid is labeled "vaginal aspirate." Next a cotton swab is placed in the endocervical canal, left in place for at least 20 seconds, removed, and used immediately to innoculate a Transgrow agar culture plate, a culture for gonorrhea. A Papanicolaou test should then be done. The culture and Pap test should be done in that order and are the last tests done because they may cause bleeding and the blood will interfere with the forensic tests.

The vaginal aspirate should be examined as soon as possible after the examination is completed. The presence or absence of sperm should be noted as well as whether or not they are motile and their anatomical integrity. Usually sperm are not motile for more than 4 to 6 hours in the vaginal canal because of its acidity, although they may remain active in the cervical mucous for a much longer period of time. If sperm are present it is not necessary to test for acid phosphatase, an enzyme found in high concentration in semen, because sperm are one of the components of semen.

When indicated, cotton applicators moistened with saline are used to retrieve semen from skin surfaces. These areas may be easily identified with the light from a Woods lamp because semen will fluoresce.

If the oral cavity has been invaded (fellatio), it should be examined for the presence of semen and a culture for gonorrhea taken from the pharynx.

If there was rectal intercourse (sodomy), the anal canal can be washed with 2 ml of

FILE COPY

RAPE TREATMENT CENTER

JACKSON MEMORIAL HOSPITAL   UNIVERSITY OF MIAMI SCHOOL OF MEDICINE

ADDRESS_____

PLACE OF EXAM_____TIME_____

PERSONAL HISTORY

PARA __ __ __ __ GR. _____

LMP: DATE_____NORMAL ABNORMAL

LAST COITUS: DATE_____TIME:_____

CONTRACEPTION: YES NO TYPE:_____

DOUCHE BATH DEFECATE VOID SINCE ASSAULT

VENEREAL DISEASE: YES NO TYPE_____RX_____

HEPATITIS: YES NO WHEN_____RX_____

HISTORY OF ASSAULT_____

DATE:_____TIME:_____

LOCATION:_____

NO. OF ASSAILANTS_____RACE: B W L O UNK

ATTACKER: KNOWN_____UNK_____RELATIVE_____

THREATS: YES NO TYPE_____

RESTRAINTS: YES NO TYPE_____

WEAPON: YES NO TYPE_____

	ORAL	ANAL	VAGINAL	DIGITAL	FOR. BODY
TYPE OF SEX:	____	____	____	____	____
PENETRATION:	____	____	____	____	____
EJACULATION:	____	____	____	____	____

COMMENTS:_____

BIRTHDATE_____RACE_____ M S W D SEP

POLICE DEPT._____CASE #_____

OFFICER_____

GENERAL EXAM: (bruises, trauma, lacerations, marks)
NO HISTORY

PELVIC EXAM: (include signs of trauma, bleeding, foreign bodies)

VULVA_____

HYMEN_____

VAGINA_____

CERVIX_____

FUNDUS_____

ADNEXAE_____

RECTAL_____

JMH-02-5862-6
8-1-78

PAGE 1	**SEXUAL BATTERY FORM**

Fig. 8. Sexual battery form.

FILE COPY

RAPE TREATMENT CENTER

MIAMI, FLORIDA

JACKSON MEMORIAL HOSPITAL   UNIVERSITY OF MIAMI SCHOOL OF MEDICINE

PHYSICIAN_____ NURSE _____ COUNSELOR_____

TESTS   **TREATMENT**

GC CULTURE: ORAL ANAL CERVICAL OTHER_____   V.D.-PROPHYLAXIS: YES NO TYPE_____

VDRL: YES NO (5cc venous blood - red top)   PREGNANCY PROPHYLAXIS: YES NO TYPE_____

PAP TEST: YES NO   TETANUS: YES NO OTHER MEDS:_____

EVIDENTIAL SPECIMENS, TESTING AND RECEIPT

RESULTS OF PRELIMINARY TESTS: A.P.: NEGATIVE WEAK MODERATE STRONG

SPERM: NONE 1-5   6-10   10+   MOTILE   NON-MOTILE _____

SPECIMENS OBTAINED:	**GIVEN TO POLICE**	**OTHER TREATMENT**
10 cc VENOUS BLOOD (red top)_____	_____	X-RAY_____
FINGER NAIL SCRAPINGS _____	_____	SURGICAL CONSULT _____
PUBIC HAIR COMBINGS _____	_____	PSYCH. CONSULT_____
VAGINAL { SMEAR_____ SWAB_____	_____ _____	OTHER: (Explain)_____
CERVICAL { SMEAR_____ SWAB_____	_____ _____	_____
VAGINAL ASPIRATE _____	_____	_____
RECTAL { SMEAR_____ SWAB_____	_____ _____	_____
ORAL { SMEAR_____ SWAB_____	_____	_____
SALIVA SPECIMEN _____	_____	GIVEN TO POLICE
CLOTHING (number)_____ { TYPE_____ CONDITION_____		_____
FOREIGN BODIES (number) _____ { TYPE_____ LOCATION_____		_____
OTHER SPECIMENS_____	PHOTOGRAPHS: YES NO TAKEN BY_____	

TOTAL NUMBER SPECIMENS   **TOTAL TO POLICE**

RECEIPT OF EVIDENCE: THE ABOVE EVIDENCE HAS BEEN RECEIVED BY ME ON (DATE) _____ AT

(TIME)_____   (OFFICER'S SIGNATURE)_____

PHYSICIANS SIGNATURE:_____

WITNESS SIGNATURE_____

JMH-02 5662 6
8 1 78

PAGE 2 | **SEXUAL BATTERY FORM**

Fig. 8, cont'd. Sexual battery form.

saline and the fluid can be recovered, or swabs can be inserted to retrieve evidence of semen. A culture for gonorrhea should be done.

If the case is to be prosecuted, venous blood should be drawn and a sample of the patient's saliva should be taken. The saliva sample is easily obtained by having the victim chew a small square of clean cloth or by putting a few drops of saliva on a clean filter paper. This can be tested to see if the victim is a "secretor." Secretor substances are found in about 85% of the population and may be identified in all body fluids if the patient is a secretor; therefore it is important that no one but the patient touch the material used for this test.

Any clothes worn during the attack should be placed in a sack and saved for the police. All specimens collected must be carefully identified and placed in paper sacks. Plastic should not be used because the moisture that collects will result in the overgrowth of bacteria and destroy the evidence.

Everyone involved must initial the specimens so that the "chain of evidence" is kept unbroken. Ideally the evidence is then handed directly to a police officer who signs a receipt for each item.

The treatment offered the patient will vary with the circumstances of the attack. If she has been exposed to venereal disease, prophylactic treatment should be given because only about 50% of these patients will return for follow-up care. Protection against pregnancy should be offered if the patient is not already pregnant and will consent to an abortion if she should conceive in spite of the medication. If there is any question, a pregnancy test should be done before the drug is prescribed. Protection against tetanus should be given if there has been trauma. Medication may be given for symptomatic relief, that is, analgesics and sedatives.

For prophylaxis against venereal disease we use the dosage regimen of the Center for Disease Control in Atlanta:

A. If the patient is not allergic to penicillin:
1. Probenecid, 1 gm orally, plus Aqueous procaine penicillin G, 4.8 million units intramuscularly.
2. If high-concentration penicillin is not available we substitute LA Bicillin, 2.4 million units intramuscularly, plus ampicillin, 3.5 gm by mouth stat.

This will protect against incubating syphilis and will treat gonorrhea.

B. If the patient is allergic to penicillin: Trobicin, 2 gm, intramuscularly.

This will not protect against syphilis but will treat gonorrhea.

Injections are preferred over oral medications for protection against venereal disease because not all patients can be relied on to take the full course of oral medication.

Although the risk of rape-related pregnancy is thought to be about 1%, few patients wish to take that chance. For prevention of pregnancy we offer them the "morning after pill": diethystilbesterol, 25 mg orally twice a day for 5 consecutive days.

This must be started within 72 hours of exposure to be effective. Nausea is often a side effect of DES medication so we offer antiemetics to be taken before this medication. We withhold medication if the patient is adamant in refusing menstrual extraction or abortion should pregnancy occur, because DES will damage a fetus.

The formal counseling session usually occurs after the medical examination, although it may be done before if the patient is very upset. In actuality, however, the counseling begins from the moment the patient is met by a member of the treatment team.

Forcible rape precipitates a personal crisis and all victims will have some degree of psychological trauma; therefore the treatment of the rape victim is not complete without assessment of the psychological state of the victim and the significant others in her sphere.

Oftentimes the most significant trauma suffered by a rape victim is internal and may go completely undetected by those around her. Even some professionals in the psychiatric field are unaware of the unique emotional reaction experienced by victims of sexual assault. It is most important for the victim's emotional recovery that we recognize the psychological aspects of this crisis and help her to resolve it.

What actually happens to a victim of sexual assault? How does she feel during the rape and after? What kinds of issues worry her? Do all women react the same after an experience like this? What can we do to help her deal with it?

The following history was taken from a patient seen at the Rape Treatment Center at Jackson Memorial Hospital. Perhaps through this case as well as the following information, these questions will be answered.

Case history

Kathy S. had worked a hard 8 hours at a local hospital as a nurse. As she unlocked the door to her apartment, all that she was thinking was getting to bed. She washed and undressed as usual and it seemed that as soon as her head hit the pillow she was fast asleep. Suddenly she was awakened by a man's hand over her mouth and a dry, raspy voice telling her not to scream. He told her of a knife and that he would harm her if she did not cooperate. Cooperation meant performing various sexual acts, telling this masked man how much she enjoyed it and how great it was. She did all that she was told to do and in a short time, which seemed like hours, the man left, threatening her not to tell anyone. She lay in her bed, silently wishing she would wake up only to find that this was all a nightmare. However, within seconds, she realized that it was not. Now it was necessary for her to make some decisions. Should she call the police, her family, her boyfriend? . . . Would Jason ever understand? She knew she was really frightened and wished that someone would come and rescue her but there was a slim chance of that. Therefore Kathy decided to call Jason—he would help her.

About 1 hour later, Kathy was brought to the Rape Treatment Center by her boyfriend, Jason. There she was examined and questioned. She tried to remain calm, answering all that was required but each time reliving the experience—each time wondering if this was really happening to her.

For Kathy and many women who have experienced rape, the reality of the event is difficult to accept. Most people live in a protective bubble, denying that they would ever be victims of crime. This is the way that they live in a society laced with the criminally active without being in constant fear. They accept the "It won't happen to me" philosophy that effectively shields them from the "seedy" side of life, and for most it works rather well. However, for those who must face the reality of victimization, this denial no longer works. The rape victim must face that she has been and can again be a victim of a crime, and the fear is overwhelming. It is a fear that is not easily dealt with because it is a fear of the unknown. Like most victims she deals with it by giving messages to those around her that she requires protection and comfort. She must accept her regressive, "Please make me feel safe" behavior as an essential reaction to the event. Once the victim feels safe, then she can contend with other consequential reactions.

Rape victims experience a battery of reactions to the event. How they react is sometimes influenced by their age and their premorbid personality type as well as their external support system. The age of the victim is often critical in determining the postrape reactions. Young children place little significance on the sexual aspects of the event. It has been observed that adolescents seem to be more concerned with sexual issues and peer acceptance. Young adult women who have already established their sexual identity worry more about pregnancy and venereal disease on the medical side and trust and control on the psychological side. Elderly victims appear to dwell on the issues of safety and physical harm.

As has been suggested, the premorbid personality structure also plays a part in determining the postrape reaction. How has the victim handled crises in the past? How does the victim view her self-image? Was she able to develop and maintain relations with others prior to the attack? Does she demonstrate good judgment in making critical decisions? All of these factors influence how the victim reacts to the assault. For example, Dorothy G. had had an almost ideal life. She was properly educated and never worried about daily life problems. She was relatively attractive and reasonably bright. When she was assaulted she had much difficulty dealing with the experience. It became evident that Dorothy never had had an opportunity to question her self-confidence; nor had she ever been exposed to situations that demanded problem-solving capabilities. Her reaction therefore was more acute than were those of people who had handled crises before and had had confidence in their ability to cope with them.

The external support system is also very influential in determining the postrape reaction. A victim who views her peer and family relationships as important places a lot of significance on how these people will judge and support her. If they condemn her for what happened, this may cripple her emotional recovery.

The nucleus of the child victim's response is affected by how those around her view the experience. For the young child the impact of the event itself is usually minimal unless she has experienced severe pain. If the event is handled openly by those around her, a child under the age of 10 will respond with no apparent emotional trauma. In working with the child victim, the parents are the main focus. Often the parents have problems dealing with their own guilt and shame and therefore evade the issue completely. In this instance the child may develop long-range emotional problems. For example:

Case history

Susie, a 4-year-old, was brought to the Rape Treatment Center after having been sexually molested. The parents seemed supportive but were not receptive to counseling. Four months later the parents called the center requesting further treatment for Susie because she was exhibiting some overt sexual behaviors. The child, while at day care, was lifting her skirt asking the boys to touch her genitalia. After a review of the parents' method of dealing with the actual event, it was determined that because of their feelings and since there had been no evident behavioral changes in the child, the parents had decided to never speak of it again. By doing this they had left the child confused as well as curious.

It is critical with a young victim to offer an explanation, to support the child, and not to cast blame. The parents must realize that even a 4-year-old may have found the experience enjoyable and cannot understand why it was so wrong. The parents must explain the significance of the event and how it relates to adult sexual behaviors. They should stress that sex is a healthy expression of love and caring between adults and that the negativeness of this event is due only to the child's age. The parents should try to alleviate blame regardless of how the event occurred. If a child's sexual assault is not handled appropriately, these children as adults may develop such problems as sex-guilt, frigidity, and difficulty developing lasting relationships with men as well as promiscuity.

In working with the adult victim at the Rape Treatment Center, we have found that the responses have often followed the classical postrape syndrome described by Burgess and Holmstrom in their various studies. They have found that the rape victim experiences three stages: the acute stage, the outward adjustment stage, and the integration stage.

As in Kathy's case, the acute phase of

shock, disbelief, and denial is seen in the first days immediately following the assault. The victim has a problem dealing with routine life responsibilities and requires support and empathy from those around her. She feels ashamed, humiliated, and usually guilty about her responsibility in the event. It is very important to help her realize that she is not to blame and that she did nothing wrong.

Once the acute phase has passed, the victim moves into the second phase, which is described as the outward adjustment stage. In this stage the victim is capable of returning to work or school and outwardly appears to be coping with the experience. It is important to know that the victim usually achieves this through suppression of her feelings and that the actual resolution of the assault has not been completed. At the Rape Treatment Center the victims have remained in this stage for months, even years.

Case history

Mrs. K, a well-established business woman, returned to work a week after the assault. She claimed, on initial interview, that she felt fine, complaining only that she was still a little frightened. Also Mrs. K. claimed that her husband was very supportive and perceived no marital problems as a result of this experience. Six months later Mrs. K called the center requesting further counseling. She stated that in the last 2 months she had been experiencing nightmares and headaches. In talking with us about how she handled the period immediately following the assault, Mrs. K. explained that she actively attempted to forget it. She had not discussed such issues as sexual devaluation, shame, or responsibility but rather suppressed her anxiety about these concerns. Her feelings therefore were now being expressed through her dreams. Mrs. K. was now ready to move into the integration period, the third phase, in order to resolve these issues.

The integration period is sometimes precipitated by some event that requires the victim to deal with her feelings, for example, nightmares, irrational fears, or sexual dys-

function. In this stage the victim is usually ready to work on these problems, seeks help with them, and is willing to talk about her experience. Frequently she has gained enough objectivity to express her feelings about the assault without further emotional pain. However, during this stage depression may be evident. It has been observed that the longer the outward adjustment period lasts the more difficult it is to come to a final resolution. At the Rape Treatment Center the victim can deal with her experience through two different treatment modalities; individual counseling as well as group therapy are available.

Regardless of how the victim reacts to being raped, it is evident that she needs the empathetic understanding of all those who care for her professionally as well as within her personal life.

The procedures used in treating victims of rape and sexual assault have improved during the 1970s, and services such as those offered at the Rape Treatment Center may be found in centers in various areas of the United States. In these centers the victim is given a healthy foundation on which to venture forth into society again. However, society passes the final judgment. Most medical and social service personnel have finally accepted as truth the fact that rape is a violent crime and not a sex act; but the mind of the general public still perpetuates the myths about it. Reaching the public is the most difficult task because people are reluctant to acknowledge that the problem exists, let alone try to understand it. Unfortunately rape will never be eliminated; there is no use denying it any longer. We must face it and cope with it, and eventually through the efforts of concerned individuals, the public will be forced to understand it. Health professionals, especially nurses must be aware if we are to accomplish this.

SUGGESTED READINGS

Brownmiller, S.: Against our will: men, women and rape, New York, 1975, Simon & Schuster, Inc.

Burgess, A. W., and Holmstrom, L. L.: Rape: victims of crisis, Bowie, Md., 1974, Robert J. Brady Co.

Federal Bureau of Investigation: Uniform Crime Reports: Crime in the United States, Washington, D.C., 1977, U.S. Government Printing Office.

Halpern, S., Hicks, D. J., and Crenshaw, T.: Rape: helping the victim, Oradell, N. J., 1978, Medical Economics Book Co.

Hicks, D. J.: Rape: sexual assault, Obstet. Gynecol. Annu. 4:447–465, 1978.

Hicks, D. J.: Rape: a crime of violence, Contemp. OB/GYN 11:67-78, 1978.

Hilberman, E.: The rape victim, Washington, D.C., 1976, American Psychiatric Association.

Hirschowitz, R. G.: Crisis theory: a formulation, Psychiatr. Ann. 3:36-47, 1973.

Sutherland, S., and Scherl, D. J.: Patterns of response among victims of rape, Am. J. Orthopsychiatry 40:503-510, 1970.

12

Diagnostic framework for victims of sexual assault

Lora F. Wortman and Anne Curran

Rape, short of murder, is the most extreme violation of the self. It is one of the most dangerous offenses against the person as the potential for death, serious injury or severe psychological damage is present in each assault.[1]

Rape has been the focus of much public attention in the past few years, a fact that can largely be attributed to the work and involvement of the women's movement. The movement brought into focus many astounding facts that delineate rape as the truly heinous crime that it is. Rape is one of the four major crimes in the United States and affects the lives of thousands of women each year.

In 1973 the FBI reported 51,000 founded cases of attempted and forcible rape across the country.[2] The National Opinion Research Center at the University of Chicago found that this crime actually occurs more than three and one-half times the reported rate.[3] Statistics have indicated that from 1967 to 1972 there was an increase of 70% in reported forcible rapes in the United States, and now 43 out of every 100,000 women are subjected to at least one act of forcible rape each year.[4]

The philosophical ideation of the women's movement transcends viewing rape as just a crime and approaches the problem in its most global sense. Brownmiller epitomized this view in her controversial book, *Against Our Will*. She contends that rape is institutionalized in our society as a "constant process of intimidation by which all men keep all women in a state of fear."[5]

The media has capitalized on this issue, subjecting the public to sensational articles, films, and television programs. They typically portray rape as being the ultimate psychological and social devastation for both victim and family. They have exploited such issues as the abusive treatment by the criminal justice system, the insensitive and inhumane treatment of victims by the medical profession, and the belief that rape charges are easy to make but difficult to prove. As a result women have been reluctant to report the crime of rape. After exposure to such negative depictions of rape, many women feel themselves unable to take the risk of losing their families and friends and are most unwilling to risk additional mental anguish resulting from ostracism if they were to identify themselves as victims of rape.

Most people with whom the rape victim comes in contact are unaware of the emotional trauma and unique complications inflicted by such an event. Myths and stereotypes have permeated the issue of rape, and as a result many people have specific preconceived notions concerning how a victim should look, act, and feel. These perjorative attitudes, in conjunction with viewing the rape victim as a political symbol, negate and often neglect the fact that a rape victim is in a state of crisis.

Studies have revealed that many women suffer emotional problems as a result of the assault and the postassault treatment. These problems are often exacerbated by the lack of immediate and effective counseling. For many victims the aftermath of the ordeal becomes more traumatizing than the actual rape itself.[6]

In reaction to this overwhelming social problem, a 1975 federal mandate was issued to all comprehensive community mental health centers stipulating a need to demonstrate involvement in direct or supportive services to victims of rape.[7] Consequently more mental health professionals and paraprofessionals, who are not necessarily specialized or knowledgeable in the treatment of rape victims, are exposed to rape victims in greater numbers.

It is our contention that there is a need for separation of the sociological, political, and mental health aspects of rape. In this article we propose to acquaint health care professionals with the rape trauma. From our study we have identified specific factors found to be necessary for consideration when assessing and treating a victim of rape. A treatment and assessment typology is presented that will promote understanding of the specific needs and problems of rape victims.

RAPE CRISIS SYNDROME

Rape constitutes a crisis in a woman's life. As defined by Caplan, a crisis "is a psychological disequilibrium in a person who confronts a hazardous circumstance that for her or him constitutes an important problem which he or she can for the time being neither escape nor solve with his or her customary problem-solv-

ing resources."[8] In the following study crisis intervention was used as a theoretical base because the basic principles and treatment implications were applicable to victims of sexual assault.[9-11]

Burgess and Holmstrom,[8] Sutherland and Scherl,[3] and Medea and Thompson[12] have conducted studies that described the psychological impact of rape and the emotional needs of the victim. From these works emerged the "rape crisis syndrome." This is defined as the acute and long-term reorganizational process that occurs as a result of a rape.[13] This syndrome is usually a two-phase or three-phase process and closely parallels the stages of a crisis as described in crisis intervention literature. Following is a brief description of the rape crisis syndrome.

Phase one, or the acute stage, occurs immediately following the rape and usually lasts for several days. During this phase the victim's acute reaction may take a variety of forms including shock, dismay, disbelief, or anger. She may appear to be in an agitated, incoherent, volatile state or calm, composed, subdued, or indifferent. This period is also characterized by a great deal of disorganization in thought processes, decision-making abilities, and problem-solving skills. It is during this period that the victim is most amenable to help and intervention is optimal.

Phase two, or the pseudoadjustment phase, is characterized by an outward adjustment. This phase occurs after the immediate anxiety issues have been resolved and the concrete problems, such as the police and hospital, have been appropriately handled. Often in an attempt to gain control over her life and to demonstrate emotional stability, the victim implements psychological defense mechanisms such as denial, suppression, repression, and rationalization. The woman resumes her normal activities and appears to be adjusting to the assault; her interest and motivation in seeking help and talking about the crisis wanes. It is more difficult to engage the victim in treatment during this phase.

Phase three is defined as the period of integration. It is a time when the victim must resolve her feelings about her assailant, her world, and herself. The movement into phase three is often marked by depression and reliving of the rape experience. Phase three may be precipitated by an event related to the incident such as a court appearance, sight of the assailant, or exposure to another threatening incident. The individual is thrown back into a state of crisis and is forced once again to examine her feelings and fears about the original incident. Unfortunately not all rape victims reach this third stage of resolution; some victims remain in stage two because of the impervious defense systems they have developed.

The studies that delineated the rape crisis syndrome were used in designing our Rape Crisis Intervention Program. Rape had been designated as the crisis-precipitating factor in these studies and the emotional needs and reactions of rape victims were identified. These studies provided essential insight into the emotional trauma incurred by victims of rape.

RAPE CRISIS DEMONSTRATION PROJECT

In December, 1975, the Rape Crisis Intervention Program was established in Salt Lake City, Utah, with the following objectives:

1. To develop a 24-hour crisis counseling program for victims of sexual assault
2. To coordinate community institutions, agencies, and other existing resources in a collaborative effort to provide effective intervention
3. To assess the circumstances and patterns of the crime in the Salt Lake County area
4. To describe the demographic characteristics of all rape victims who presented themselves to the emergency rooms of

the two Salt Lake City hospitals participating in the study
5. To determine the emotional and social problems that individuals experience as a result of being raped
6. To evaluate the effectiveness of crisis intervention with victims of sexual assault
7. To utilize research findings and counselor experiences for future policy recommendations in hospitals, police, legislative, and community mental health systems as well as for education, training, and consultation purposes

Protocol for program implementation

A protocol was established to coordinate and integrate the activities of the police department, courts, hospitals, and project staff in cases of rape. The following procedure was implemented:

1. When a rape victim came to one of the two designated hospital emergency rooms, the project counselors were notified immediately via a paging system. We served as the project counselors.
2. A counselor arrived at the hospital within 30 minutes of notification.
3. The counselor acted as liaison between victim and involved systems. They implemented crisis intervention techniques and elicited data for research purposes. A questionnaire schedule was designed to facilitate the recording of data.
4. At the completion of the interview the victim was offered follow-up services, which included assisting victims through the legal proceedings.
5. If victims requested assistance, they were contacted within 24 to 48 hours after the initial interview, and follow-up services were rendered.
6. Follow-up with victims continued until

resolution of the crisis. Counselors referred those victims who required long-term counseling.

Study population

The study population over the 1-year study period consisted of 80 rape victims. They ranged in age from 3 to 83 years. These victims presented themselves to the emergency rooms of the two cooperating hospitals generally within hours after the attack. Of this study population 68% were single, 8% were married, and the remainder were divorced, separated, or widowed; 80% were Caucasian, 11% were Chicano, 8% were American Indian, and 1% were Vietnamese.

Of all the subjects 88% consented to further involvement with the counselors after initial contact; 6% were uncertain at that time, and 6% refused entirely. Of the victims 19% were seen only in the initial contact, although follow-up by telephone was often done. The counselors had between two and six contacts with victims in 44% of all cases; 37% were seen for more than six contacts. The counselors recorded that 81% of the victims were receptive to their intervention on initial contact; 5% were hostile, and 9% were not recorded because the victim was either inebriated or severely emotionally disturbed.

The victims' assailants ranged in age from 14 to 40; 50% were between the ages of 20 and 30, 40% were 30 or over, and the remaining were under 20 years of age. Of the assailants 58% were Caucasian, 15% were Chicano, 8% were black, 1% were American Indian, and for 17% the ethnic identity was unknown.

Research findings

From the research demonstration project we found that (1) the type of rape, (2) the developmental stage of the victim, (3) the victim's social network, and (4) the victim's pre-morbid personality adjustment all had particular relevance in assessment and treatment. These factors were found to determine to a significant extent the emotional style of the individual, the type and degree of involvement of persons significant in their lives, the meaning and importance placed on the rape experience, and the degree of emotional and social imbalance.

The following section includes a descriptive analysis of these four factors. We used the data obtained from this research to support our basic supposition that counselors will intervene more effectively with rape victims if they obtain and utilize information based on the four preceding factors, are knowledgeable concerning the rape crisis syndrome and crisis intervention techniques.

Type of assault. It is essential when analyzing the rape crisis that the type of assault and the specific stresses accompanying it be carefully considered. Burgess and Holmstrom have developed a typology of rape that delineates several categories based on how the assailant gained access to the victim. We have extrapolated from this typology three distinct categories of assault and have applied them to our study and subsequent work: (1) the blitz rape, (2) the confidence rape, and (3) the inability to consent rape.[8] We found that there often existed particular emotional reactions and unique concerns that related directly to the type of assault:

THE BLITZ RAPE. The blitz type of sexual assault occurs randomly, seemingly without reason for the selection of victims. It is a surprise attack with no prior interaction between the assailant and the victim. There appears to be no explanation or understandable provocation for the man's action. In our study 27 of the 80 subjects were victims of blitz rapes. Of these 17 occurred at home. These were generally precipitated by the assailant's breaking into the home or by his hiding on the premises.

The authors found that in 71% of all cases fear was the predominant initial emotional response. What is notable is that this response dissipated after the initial stage of crisis for victims of confidence rapes and inability to consent rapes; this is in contrast to the blitz rape, in which fear permeated all three stages of the rape crisis syndrome. This influenced the behavior of the victim as well as her coping skills. In the blitz rape the major task of the therapeutic intervention was the management of fear and the acceptance of the individual's vulnerability.

Often women who encountered this type of rape experienced a tremendous amount of disruption in their lives. As a consequence of the rape they often secured other living arrangements, changed employment, withdrew from social interaction, or became extremely dependent on others. We believe that such pronounced fear disruption emanated from the following factors:

1. In 88% of the blitz rapes the victim had little identifying information about the assailant. This made apprehension and legal prosecution more difficult. Consequently the rape victim was faced with the knowledge and fear that her assailant was free and could possibly attack again.

2. The randomness and utter senselessness of the attack often propogated a feeling of paranoia. This seemed to be predicated on the victim believing herself vulnerable and fearing that the event could occur again. Victims tended to generalize these fears of senseless acts of violence to other situations.

3. Of the blitz rapes 63% occurred within the victim's home. As a result, many of these victims moved, had someone move in with them, or made security changes in their homes.

4. A weapon was used in 52% of these rapes, which was true for only 20% of the confidence rapes. It is likely that this use of a weapon contributed to the element of fear.

THE CONFIDENCE RAPE. In our study, 42 of the 80 subjects were victims of the confidence rape. According to Burgess and Holmstrom, "the Confidence Rape is an attack in which the assailant obtains sex under false pretenses by using deceit, betrayal and often violence."[8] In the confidence rape there is some degree of trust and relationship established between the victim and assailant prior to the attack. The victim may have sought assistance with her car or hitched a ride, or the assailant himself may have asked to use her telephone. On the other hand, the assailant may be a date, past boyfriend, relative, or close family friend. In all cases the victim, for whatever reasons, trusts the assailant and places herself unknowingly in a vulnerable position.

In the confidence rape, self-blame and guilt were the overriding predominant emotional reactions. Of all rape victims who experienced self-blame 70.4% were victims of the confidence rape. These feelings became the prevalent issue in the counseling process, for they interfered with the individual's ability to adequately and realistically assess the situation.

We believe that these feelings were premolded and supported by a variety of factors. As previously stated, many erroneous myths and misconceptions exist in the area of rape. Attitudes that women ask for or provoke rape and secretly enjoy it are pervasive in our society. Many people assume that, once stimulated, a man is unable to control his sexual urges. Consequently the woman is held responsible for having urged him into such a situation. The study found that women who experienced the confidence rape often accepted the responsibility and blame for the act. This belief may have been reinforced by the fact that in 49% of all the confidence rapes the victim was using alcohol or other drugs.

It is interesting to note that 68% of all confidence rape victims reported that their families would have negative feelings toward them as a result of the rape. Of all victims reporting uncertainty as to how their families would react, 52% were victims of the confidence rape, as opposed to 19% of the victims of the blitz rape. We found that often the major therapeutic task was one of confronting both the victim and her family's irrational beliefs and assumptions concerning the role of responsibility in the rape.

We found that guilt was often used as a defense against the individual's vulnerability. By accepting responsibility the woman could believe that not only did she play an integral part in the experience but that her behavior determined the course of events. Thus she could believe that if she changed her behavior, she would gain control over her life and ensure herself against the recurrence of such an event. By accepting responsibility the victim was able to avoid and deny the acknowledgment that life can be threatening and that she cannot always have control over all threatening external factors.

We found that 68% of all patients referred to long-term counseling were victims of the confidence rape, in contrast to 18% for blitz and 14% for inability to consent. The high percentage of referrals in confidence rapes may reflect the fact that this victim is more vulnerable to challenging her self-worth and self-esteem.

THE INABILITY TO CONSENT RAPE. According to Burgess and Holmstrom, victims of this type of rape in some manner aided or contributed to the sexual activity. The victim's collaboration comes about because of her inability to consent because of her stage of personality or cognitive development.[8] In all cases the assailant assumes a stance of power in his interaction with the victim. Eleven victims out of our total sample population experi-

enced this type of rape. The majority of these victims were children ranging from the ages of 3 to 9 years. The remaining four victims were either mentally retarded or emotionally incompetent. In 82% of these cases the assailant had been known prior to the assault, often being a friend of the family or a relative.

Burgess and Holmstrom have delineated the following three methods by which the assailant gains access to his victims: (1) by pressuring the victim to take material goods, (2) by pressuring the victim to accept human contact, and (3) by pressuring the victim to believe that sex would be appropriate and enjoyable.[8]

Four of the victims in this category were coerced into sexual activity with material goods of money or candy. One collaborated with the assailant because of her own need for human contact and love. Three of the victims were led to believe that sex between themselves and the assailant would be appropriate and pleasurable. The remaining three victims were difficult to categorize because their ability to relay information about the incident was marginal.

There were several factors in these cases that influenced the therapeutic role of the worker. As previously stated, the victims were either children or impaired adults and almost all were totally dependent on the support of their family. The major thrust of intervention was often with the entire family system. The major tasks were to discern the meaning the rape had for the client and to help the family work through the guilt and responsibility they often felt. Parents often became embroiled in their own crisis and believed themselves inadequate. They tended to shift the focus of attention from the victim, often neglecting the victim's needs and concerns. We found it necessary to work with the family, educating them to the needs of the child as well as helping them to deal with the conflicts they were experiencing.

Developmental stage. A developmental theory was employed in this study because it provided a useful conceptual framework whereby behavior could be observed and analyzed. An adequate understanding of this theory provided insight into the individual's motives, abilities, social systems, and defenses.[8] These elements were essential for placing the behavior of a victim into the proper perspective, thus enabling the counselors to assess adequately and intervene appropriately in the crisis.

To a significant degree the developmental stage determined the emotional style of the victim, the degree of involvement of significant others, and the meaning the rape had for the individual. The following is a discussion delineating how the developmental stage influences these three areas (see Table 10 for the developmental stages of the victims in the study).

EMOTIONAL STYLE. As stated previously, there is no one reaction that constitutes a typical response to rape. A wide variety of reactions were exhibited by the study population. Some women were expressive and extremely verbal, exhibiting their anger, fears, and frustrations, while others appeared stoic, controlled, and at times indifferent. Of our sample population 60% exhibited a controlled emotional style, 35% appeared expressive, and the remaining 5% were incapacitated by drugs or alcohol.

The emotional style of the individual was significantly determined by developmental age. Obviously a 4-year-old child exhibits behaviors quite different from those of the adolescent or the young adult. Often people who are initially involved with the rape victim make erroneous assumptions that the behavior exhibited reflects not only her emotional reaction but the extent of the trauma incurred. We found this to be particularly pertinent to both the young child and the adolescent in our study population.

For the child under 6 years the discernible characteristic was a sense of withdrawal and a reticence to speak. Most people coming in contact with these victims were extremely sympathetic and supportive. A difficulty occurred when others assumed that the quick, silent behavior reflected minimal emotional trauma. Often the significant others involved with the victim reinforced this behavior because of their own inability to deal with the situation and their need to minimize the trauma. Consequently the child was often denied the opportunity to express and work through her feelings and fears.

The adolescent faces more judgmental attitudes from her family, the medical staff, and police than any other victim. Her behavior often seems incongruent and inappropriate to the situation. It was not uncommon for an adolescent to giggle or be preoccupied with her appearance. During a pelvic examination one 15-year-old girl vacillated between tears, embarrassment, and concern for her looks, while showing the counselor pictures of her boyfriend and friends. Behavior such as this was often interpreted to indicate either a rape had not occurred or the victim was minimally upset. We found that such behavior reflected the embarrassment and self-consciousness

Table 10. Developmental stages of victims in study

Stage	Age range (years)	Number of victims in study
Infancy or early childhood	0-6	5
Middle childhood	6-12	4
Adolescence	12-18	27
Young adult	18-25	28
Adult	25-40	13
Middle age	40-60	0
Later life	50 and over	3

the adolescent experiences during such a crisis.

THE MEANING. The meaning of the rape experience was different for each of the victims, seeming to depend on the biological age, maturational development, and cognitive level of the victim.

The young child, because of her cognitive and emotional development, placed little sexual significance on the rape experience. The predominent feelings she associates with the event were harm and betrayal, not those of a sexual violation.

The victim in middle childhood was found to be more cognizant of the sexual implications of the rape experience than the child under 6 years. This child felt both fear and hurt along with a sense of sexual violation. She had a strong need for protection and support from her significant others. In addition, there was a need for clarification of the sexual implications for the child to be able to gain cognitive mastery over the situation.

The adolescent, because of the inherent conflicts of that stage, was faced with a multitude of issues, which often complicated the meaning of the rape experience. The meaning was essentially discerned through the interplay of three factors: (1) her newly formed sexual identity, (2) her peer relationships, and (3) her relationship with her parents. In addition, the adolescent, like the younger child, had to work through many fears directly related to the experience.

The discernible meaning for both the young adult and adult centered around the issues of power and control. Most people with whom the victim came in contact made the assumption that the sexual violation was the focal point of the emotional trauma. Contrary to this belief, most of the adults regarded the sexual violation as secondary to the feelings of helplessness and loss of control. These victims often needed to work through the power issue, which often con-

fused those significant others who believed the main issue was sexual.

The women over 60 in many respects viewed the rape as did the young child. The feelings of fear and betrayal appeared to take precedence over the sexual implications.

A woman's prior sexual experience, or lack of experience, was found to be an important factor in analyzing the meaning of the rape for each woman. Women with some prior sexual experience appeared to be better equipped to cope with the sexual implications of the rape, whereas women without any prior sexual experience appeared to have more conflict and experienced more confusion. Of our study population 75% had prior sexual experience; 29% of the victims felt the rape would hinder future relationships with men, and another 26% were uncertain.

THE DEGREE OF INVOLVEMENT WITH SIGNIFICANT OTHERS. The degree of involvement with significant others was primarily dependent on the developmental stage of the victim. The reactions these individuals displayed had a profound effect on either facilitating a resolution or adding to the conflict for the rape victim. It was important for the counselors to ascertain this degree of involvement, for it often determined which individuals other than the client should be included in the treatment process.

For the child and young adolescent living at home, intervention was focused on the entire family system. In many instances, the adolescent was found to have already existing conflicts with her parents. The rape experience often exacerbated these conflicts and frequently the crisis shifted to become a family crisis. The counselor's role became that of mediator, clarifying the needs and issues of both victim and family.

The young adult and adult were faced with the decision of whether or not to involve family members. Unlike the younger client, these individuals were able to receive medical and legal services without parental permission; consequently the family was minimally involved. Often the significant others included in the treatment process was the significant man in the client's life, either husband or boyfriend. Conflicts often evolved between the victim and significant man from the different meanings, values, and judgments the two people had about the experience.

For all three of our subjects over 60, the degree of involvement of significant others, primarily their grown children, was particularly significant. All of these victims were widowed and living independently at the time of the assault. The families, in reaction to the crisis, attempted to force the victims into nursing homes or into the family dwelling. Like the families of the young children, these significant others tended to negate or neglect the victim's needs by attempting to overprotect her.

Social network. Each individual victim needed to deal with a multitude of systems, the more significant ones being the family and the medical, law enforcement, and legal systems. Because of the victim's emotional state she was found to be highly susceptible and vulnerable to the impact of these systems. This impact was often dependent on the values, beliefs, and behavior exhibited by the personnel contacted within these systems. Consequently each played a distinct and vital role in the victim's experience.

FAMILY AND SIGNIFICANT OTHERS. As stated previously, the reactions of the significant others had a tremendous impact on the victim. We previously examined the degree of involvement of significant others within the context of the developmental framework. In addition, we found three types of relationships that existed between family and victim that influenced the victim's ability to resolve the crisis. These relationships often determined the type of intervention implemented.

The victim whose family responded negatively to the rape was faced with additional conflicts. Such reactions often influenced the victim's view of herself as well as of the rape. Her belief that she was either responsible for or guilty of precipitating the assault was often supported by such reactions. At other times a victim's defensive response to negative reactions cut her off from the protection and support she needed from her family. In this instance the counselor's role became one of facilitating communication between the victim and the family members. The needs and concerns of both victim and family were clarified in an attempt to make each more sensitive and supportive of the other.

The family that offered the victim positive support increased her chances for a positive, healthy resolution of the crisis. The worker's role with this family often became one of mobilizing the family members and helping them direct their support and concern in a constructive manner. Though the family's involvement and participation was encouraged, members were cautioned against overprotecting and fostering unnecessary dependencies in the victims.

The victim with little support and few significant others posed a very different problem for counselors. Such a victim had to face the crisis and trauma alone. She did not have the opportunity to rely on the support and love of others. In these cases the counselors often found themselves compensating for this lack of support. There was a tendency to become more involved with these clients, contacting them more frequently. Unlike the other victims, for whom the counselor's role was one of minimizing the conflict within the support systems, the role here was one of facilitating relationship skills for the purpose of helping the individual establish relationships.

LAW ENFORCEMENT, MEDICAL, AND LEGAL AGENCIES. The recent wide-spread publicity on rape has enumerated many instances in which the medical, legal, and law enforcement agencies handled the victim inadequately. Such publicity has suggested that these systems place the victim through unnecessary humiliation and mental anguish. Of the victims participating in our study 74% reported that they felt the police were understanding and sensitive to their situation, and 91% related that the police were helpful and supportive in their intervention, and 83% expressed the belief that the hospital staff was understanding and helpful. These statistics directly contradict the belief that the majority of rape victims are maltreated by the police and hospital staff. It is difficult to discern whether these positive attitudes reflect the impact of the liaison work of the program, are just unique to Salt Lake City law enforcement and medical authorities, or are a combination of both.

In the community of Salt Lake City we found that the medical, legal, and law enforcement agencies involved with rape victims were exceptionally willing to improve their services and were extremely receptive to our input and intervention. It was necessary for the counselors to work closely with these systems, developing a collaborative arrangement, because 64% of our subjects had definite questions concerning the police and legal procedures surrounding their rape experience; 50% asked for direct help and support in dealing with these systems, and 32% expressed uncertainty about their need for assistance at the time of the initial contact with counselors.

The victims in our project were educated by counselors about the judicial process not only for their own emotional well-being but also for the purpose of improving the legal status of the case. It was found that when the victim was sufficiently educated about these systems, and when the systems were educated to the needs and reactions of the individual, both were better able to carry out their prescribed functions more efficiently and humanely.

Premorbid personality adjustment. Premorbid personality adjustment relates to the level of functioning an individual had prior to the sexual assault. According to Rapaport, "Some appraisal of basic personality structure and identification of basic defenses as well as habitual adaptive patterns is relevant and important in crisis intervention in order to be able to designate more sharply both appropriate goals and techniques for intervention."[16] Crisis intervention, because of the crucial factors of time and the need for immediate intervention, does not lend itself to exhaustive systematic psychosocial appraisals. The workers needed to be aware of and able to evaluate the marginal clues communicated either subtly or overtly by the victim. This enabled the counselors to ascertain not only the unique significance the rape experience has for the individual but also her general adaptive capacities.

When assessing an individual's premorbid level of adjustment, we looked at the following constellation of factors, which was derived from direct observation and reports from both client and significant others:

1. Was the victim comfortable and satisfied with herself prior to the attack? What was her degree of self-worth, self-esteem, and self-confidence?

2. What was the victim's ability to relate to others prior to the attack? Was she able to establish and maintain satisfying relationships with peers, family, employment, and so forth? Did she have a reasonable amount of trust in herself as well as in others?

3. Was the woman able to meet the daily demands of life prior to the attack? Did she master the tasks of previous and present developmental stages? Is her behavior governed by impulse or is she able to delay gratification? Is she able to

adapt to societal demands or is she unrealistic in her expectations? Does the woman demonstrate good judgment? Does she weigh the consequences of her behavior? Does she have adequate coping skills?

In our study 43% of the women reported that prior to the attack they were experiencing some type of emotional conflict; 35% were referred for long-term counseling. These referrals were made when counselors ascertained that prior problems were precluding resolution of the crisis.

We found that 14 of our 80 victims had previously been sexually assaulted. This was found to have a great affect on the victim's ability to resolve the crisis. The past sexual assault often became intertwined with the present crisis. The counselor's role thus was one of separating the two incidents, thus allowing the victim an opportunity to realistically resolve both.

SUMMARY

We believe that a clear conceptualized framework is necessary when working with a victim of rape. We have suggested that this framework needs to be comprised of an adequate understanding of (1) crisis intervention and treatment techniques, (2) the rape crisis syndrome, and (3) the four factors delineated, namely, the type of rape, the developmental stage of the victim, the victim's social network, and her premorbid personality adjustment.

We wish to stress that, although there exists a specific constellation of factors that influence the rape crisis, rape is a unique experience for each individual woman. The only absolute in working with a victim of rape is that the sexual assault was the precipitating event.

REFERENCES

1. International Association of Chiefs of Police Investigations: Training information pack, Gaithersberg, Md., International Association of Chiefs of Police, Inc., undated.
2. Burgess, A. W., and Homstrom, L. L.: The rape victim in the emergency ward, Am. J. Nurs. **73**:1741, October 1973.
3. Sutherland, S., and Scherl, D.: Patterns of response among victims of rapes, Am. J. Orthopsychiatry **40**:503-511, 1970.
4. Federal Bureau of Investigation: 1972 Uniform Crime Report, Washington, D.C., 1973, U.S. Government Printing Office.
5. Brownmiller, S.: Against our will: men, women and rape, New York, 1975, Simon & Schuster, Inc.
6. Rowan, C. T., and Mazie, D. M.: The terrible trauma of rape, Reader's Digest **104**:198, March 1974.
7. Federal Mental Health Center Act of 1975, Public Law 94-63.
8. Burgess, A. W., and Holmstrom, L. L.: Rape: victims of crisis, Bowie, Md., 1974, Robert J. Brady Co.
9. Parad, H. J.: Crisis intervention: encyclopedia of social work, ed. 16, New York, 1971, National Association of Social Work.
10. Rapoport, L.: The crisis state: some theoretical considerations, Soc. Serv. Rev. **36**:214-217, 1962.
11. Smith, L. L.: Crisis intervention theory and practice: a source book, Millburn, N.J., 1975, F. R. Publishing Inc.
12. Medea, A., and Thompson, K.: Against rape, New York, 1974, Farrar, Straus & Geroux, Inc.
13. Burgess, A. W., and Holmstrom, L. L.: Rape trauma syndrome, Am. J. Psychiatry **131**:981-986, September 1974.
14. Coleman, J. C.: Abnormal psychology and modern life, Glenview, Ill., 1964, Scott, Foresman & Co.
15. Rapoport, L.: Personality development, Glenview, Ill., 1972, Scott, Foresman & Co.
16. Rapoport, L.: Crisis intervention as a mode of treatment. In Roberts, R. W., and Nee, R. eds., Theories of social casework, Chicago, 1970, The University of Chicago Press.

13

Home health care services for the family with an elderly parent

Ellen M. Scheel

Home health care services for the family with an elderly parent poses several questions at the very onset: (1) What does the parent plan for himself/herself? (2) Is the parent ill? (3) Is the illness acute, chronic, debilitating, or terminal? (4) What are the rehabilitation potentials? (5) Will the parent remain in his/her own home or be moved into the family home? (6) What community resources are available to help make this decision and to help in carrying out the plan? (7) What will the cost be and how will it be financed? As Colt et al. remind us,

Many elderly persons who are not acutely ill but have chronic conditions or disabilities and limited normal function in activities of daily living can remain at home with supportive home health care services.[1]

Community services available to families vary from one community to another but could well include home nursing services, which also provide home health aides and homemakers, physical therapists, occupational therapists, and speech therapists. If an agency is too small to have these services within its boundaries, contracts with these specialists for part-time assistance can usually be obtained. Hospitals are most helpful when

they share their specialized personnel, thus increasing the number of services available to the family and parent. The family physician and pastor are also vital members of the care plan team.

The home health care agency should be available on a 24-hour basis. This does not mean the service is continuous for 24 hours: the availability of the intermittent care covers the panic situations that may arise in a terminal condition or a sudden change in a chronic condition. Home health aides or homemakers may be put into the homes on a continuous basis for 4 to 8 hours when the situation is not of a serious medical nature. A home health care nurse should remain with the dying patient if death is imminent and the family so wishes; a special kind of nursing care and support is needed at this point.

Through the Commission on Aging, services for the family and parent includes visitor services, telephone reassurance to the home-bound, escort services, marketing services, and mobile meals. Sitter services are available through the employment of senior citizens who wish to work for short periods or take part-time jobs.[2,3]

Equipment for home care is available through the Jaycett's Loan Closets, drug stores, hospitals, and small equipment loan outlets. The kinds of equipment available to home care are wheelchairs, hospital beds, bedside tables, stands, commodes, Hoyer lifts for the car and home, bed rails, trapezes, oxygen, IPPB machines, and suction machines.

In special cases the kidney dialysis machines are used in home settings. These are not rented but are purchased by the family or presented to the family from a community charity source. Smaller items for home care may be purchased or improvised from existing articles found in the home—a valuable source of surprise helps.

FEASIBILITY OF HOME CARE

Home care is effective in the convalescence and rehabilitation of the elderly parent if the home is physically adaptable and the family is willing to accept the challenge of the care. The following quote from the General Accounting Office report includes the time given by friends and relatives and should be read with this in mind to clarify the meaning: "We do not believe that a decision to institutionalize an individual who wants to remain at home should be based on cost comparisons alone."[4]

For a family that brings a parent into their home there is an element of "prestige" that is soon worn thin by the problems that can occur, such as lack of privacy due to crowded conditions. Friends and relatives who were enthusiastic about offering help in the beginning of care gradually withdraw for personal reasons or because of their own family commitments. Therefore it is necessary to make long-term plans for the parent and the family with existing agencies that will carry the parent through the entire time that care is needed.

If the parent needs to be placed in the family's home for a short period, temporary arrangements can be made in the home without much trauma to all concerned, because the physical facilities usually are adequate for a short period. However, long-term plans must be given special consideration not only for the parent but also for the entire family, especially if there are young children in the home.

The relationship of the elderly parent to the family is a determining factor in long-term compatibility. Is the parent the husband's close relative or the wife's? What might be contrary to most thinking, parents of the husband are welcomed into the home for a longer period. This may be due to the wife's desire not only to help the parent but also to extend her love for her husband to the elderly parent.

Today more homes are being built with separate bath and bedroom combinations. Such a separate unit is ideal for the elderly parent. Homes that are too small may have adequate land on which a mobile unit can be placed. This close proximity enhances privacy for both the family and the parent, but allows the proper attention to be given to the needs of the parent; for example, nutrition is an important factor in total health care, and meals from the family unit can be brought to the parent.

If a child is asked to give up his room for the elderly parent, the arrangement should be temporary, and the child should be given this information along with the assurance that in fact it is a temporary situation.

Some homes do not have bedrooms or bathrooms on the first floor for the elderly parent's area. A less frequently used room or den may become a temporary elderly parent's quarters. If the home arrangement is to be disrupted by furniture moving, the complete cooperation of the husband and wife is essential for the best acceptance of the circumstances. Help from an experienced home health care agency nurse lessens the tension of this transition for the homemaker and her family.

In some instances the families are proud to have equipment such as a hospital bed in their home. Some families think it represents caring to those who come to visit. However, a twin bed works out fine. The amount of bedside care that needs to be given by the family and others may dictate the kind of bed best for the situation. A twin bed keeps the homelike atmosphere and tends to lessen the obvious problem the family must deal with.

If a home is small and the patient's hospital bed is located in the center of activity, the physical arrangement of equipment and furniture is vital to the aesthetic atmosphere of the home and its normalcy of daily living.

The following example is an extremely negative one—a condition that occurred before the home health care agency was called in to help:

Case history

A couple in their 30s had one child whom they loved so much that the child's bedridden condition made the mother want to keep the child's bed in the dining room, the very center of activity. The love factor lost its reasonableness when the meals served in the dining room became so unpalatable to the husband that he removed himself from the home. He sought help from his physician and pastor who called in the home health care service to change the arrangement and to give supportive care to the mother, helping her to accept the change without too much feeling of child rejection. In a few months the father returned to the home and a semblance of normalcy resumed.[5]

There are conditions that apply in evaluating a home for feasibility of home care when, for example, a wheelchair becomes a permanent part of the elderly parent's life:
1. Type of dwelling:
   a. Apartment
   b. Private home
   c. Housing project
2. Entrance to dwelling:
   a. Number of steps
   b. Handrail
   c. Width of doorways

   d. Elevator
3. Living quarters:
   a. Width of doorways
   b. Size of bedroom to manipulate wheelchair
   c. Height of bed
4. Bathroom
   a. Space adequate to transfer from chair to toilet
   b. Height of toilet
   c. Height of tub
   d. Type of tub rim
   e. Space to maneuver a Hoyer lift
5. Kitchen
   a. Room to get wheelchair in the room and maneuver it inside
   b. Sink, stove, and refrigerator accessible to a patient in a wheelchair
   c. Height of cabinets accessible with wheelchair
   d. Sink height
   e. Electric outlets[6]

This kind of information can become as sophisticated or as simple as is needed for appropriate planning.

CARE PLANS

Plans for home care are more complex than in an institutional setting where the environment does not need to be planned. Home care is done in a private, uncontrolled environment not meant for continuous health care needs.

The plans must include, in addition to medical and rehabilitative needs, housekeeping, nutrition, and sociological and recreational opportunities. Each of the above items must be considered in light of the ethnic and religious beliefs of the family in the particular home. Amount and duration of privacy required by both the family and the parent should be well understood prior to bringing a parent into the family home.

Privacy is every person's right. The following example focuses on such a need:

Case history

An elderly couple living alone in their own home wanted to stay in this comfortable environment. The elderly mother had bilateral upper mid-thigh leg amputations. Rehabilitative efforts had failed for crutch walking and prosthesis. The condition had existed a number of years before the home health care agency became involved. The wife spent most of her time sitting in a comfortable chair near a sunny window. She began to prefer to stay in the chair night and day. She could experience some privacy at night when her husband slept in the bedroom. The concerned husband spent all his waking hours attending to her needs. If he had to leave the home to shop or to run other errands, he prevailed on a neighbor to be in attendance during his absence.

The home health care agency had assigned a home health aid homemaker to the family to assist in personal care and nutritional planning. The home health care nurse made supervisory visits at regular intervals. On one of these visits, the wife begged the nurse to get the husband to leave her alone when he had to be away. A conference with the husband resulted in granting the wife's wish with the stipulation that the phone be easily accessible to her from her chair.[5]

The plan worked so well the husband found occasional enjoyment eating his noon meal with other senior citizens at the Commission on Aging center in his community, thus giving his wife more time for privacy so that she might visit with her friends by phone during her "husband-free" hours. At the

---

CARE PLAN FOR HOME HEALTH AIDE/HOMEMAKER*

This form becomes a part of the patient's record and a copy is given to the family for clarification of the duties expected.

Name of patient _____

Blood pressure _____ Temp _____ Pulse _____ Respirations _____

Details: Bath _____ Skin care _____ Nails _____ Hair _____

Treatments: Range of motion _____

　　　　　　　Enema _____ Other _____

Toileting: Bed pan _____ Commode _____ Toilet _____

Oral hygiene _____

Moving: In bed _____ Walk with crutches _____

　　　　　Bed to chair _____ Walker _____

　　　　　Walk with canes _____ Wheelchair _____

Feeding _____

Meal planning _____ Food preparation _____

Specially prescribed diet _____

Housekeeping: Make beds _____ Dust and vacuum _____

　　　　　　　Wash and dry dishes _____ Defrost refrigerator _____

　　　　　　　Keep bathroom and kitchen clean _____

　　　　　　　Check laundry to send out _____

　　　　　　　　　　　Signed by: Nurse _____

　　　　　　　　　　　　　　Family member _____

*From Wausau Visiting Nurse Association: Problem-oriented medical records. Wausau, Wis.

same time the husband found the care of his wife less confining, all of which made the entire situation more tolerable for both persons.

In the case of a chronically ill or terminally ill parent the social life of a family should be kept as nearly normal as possible. If the husband in the family has a regular working schedule, if the wife belongs to a church circle or if she has a certain day for shopping, this private time should be changed as little as possible.

The purpose of a phone at the bedside of the parent is similar to that of the hospital call bell. Relatives can print their phone number in large digits next to the phone, along with those of the home health care agency, and the fire and police departments.

If the parent is apt to panic he should be instructed to just dial the telephone operator who will do the rest. Alerting the telephone operator of this condition gives both the parent and family member a more secure feeling. Fire departments in some areas ask that a symbol (which they provide) be placed on the outside of the bedroom window frame so that in the case of fire they can find the invalid immediately.

Too often a family feels bound to "wait on" the elderly parent; many times the parent wants to wait on the family members as much as his disability will allow. The family often becomes more concerned when there are other sons and daughters; there may be criticism from those not involved in the direct care. The other sons and daughters should be included in the plans before the care at home is begun. Critical siblings should be invited to take over the care if this element is present.

TRANSFER OF HOSPITALIZED PARENT TO FAMILY HOME

The home health care agency should be alerted as early in the hospitalization as possible when the parent will need extensive care.

Assessment of the home facilities can be made prior to the teaching process and preparations made for the patient and his family during the hospital stay. Ideally the referral from the hospital is most complete with medical directives and any necessary information. Information concerning the condition leading to the hospitalization, progress made in the hospital, and progress expectations makes for continuity of care with the best results.

Keeping problem-oriented medical records, if used by both hospital and home health care agency, results in less time-consuming communication at the point of referral. At present most referrals are accomplished by a form developed through cooperation of the hospital and agency (p. 161).

An evaluation visit to the family home includes inventorying what equipment may already be in the home and making arrangements for securing additional equipment that may be needed. It is important that everything be in readiness on the patient's arrival to ensure a smooth transition from hospital to home. The degree of preparation can mean the acceptance or nonacceptance of the situation by the family; the hour of the day that the parent is brought into the home can be another factor leading to greater acceptance.

It is recommended that the nurse be in the home at arrival time of the parent if the care needs complex equipment that must be set up properly and put into use, for example, oxygen equipment. The proficiency of the professional nurse is very visible at this point.

An example of the referral information given the agency is shown on the next page.

All equipment used in the home should be kept aesthetically pleasing and kept hygienically clean. The home health care nurse teaches the family member who has become her "helper" how easily cleanliness can be achieved. Family members often are afraid to

REFERRAL INFORMATION*

Name of patient _____ Discharged from _____

Address _____ Address _____

City _____ City _____

Age _____ Birth date _____ Sex _____ Marital status _____

Telephone _____ Dr. in charge _____

Medicare no. and letter   Plan   Social Security Number

_____   _____ _____

Other insurance   Responsible relative/guardian

_____   _____

_____   Address and phone _____

Primary diagnosis _____

Secondary diagnosis _____

Prognosis _____

Physician's order and instructions _____

Was diagnosis told patient? _____ Family _____

Date _____ Physicians' signature _____

Self-care status: Areas where help is needed _____

Independent in what activities? _____

Date of last enema _____ Incontinence _____

Bowel and bladder program _____

Catheter _____ Type _____

*From Wausau Visiting Nurse Association procedure manual. Wausau, Wis., 1978.

touch some of the equipment and need supportive teaching to eliminate this fear.

All medications for specific use by the elderly parent should be kept in one place—on a tray in the patient's room or in a dresser drawer if small children are not around. Preferably medications in any home should be kept in a locked cupboard. The bathroom medicine chest is a poor place not only because of the easy accessibility of the drugs to all family members but also because the heat and moisture will impair the effectiveness of the drugs.

The drug list of the elderly parent should be reviewed by the home health care nurse on each of her visits. There are times when neighbors, friends, and others feel that they must assist by advising the parent to try a drug they use with "good results." The family members should be alerted to this possibility and be taught to give only prescribed medications.

The home health care nurse must be alert to prescriptions from former doctors—prescriptions that may be 10 or 12 years old. New precautions are now being taken by limiting the number of times a prescription can be refilled but the problem is not as yet completely controlled. There is also the possibility that an old prescription is the same as the new, with the result that double doses are liable to be taken by the parent.

Information concerning the patient's medications given to a responsible family member must include the importance of spacing the doses as well as adverse reactions to watch for; this includes the restriction against alcohol while taking drugs. Early indications of adverse reactions reported to the home health care nurse will be checked with the family physician for changes in dosage or discontinuance of medication.

The kidney dialysis equipment and supplies present a greater problem than most health situations for they take much more space. It may be necessary to assign an entire room as a treatment and storage area. This room need not be formidable. Quite the contrary, a homey treatment room lends itself to card playing and entertaining friends during the treatment, such diversions are important because of the long, regular, and frequent periods that must be spent in treatment. The family member who takes on this care needs much supportive help from the doctor, nurse, pastor, and counselor. Nutrition plays an important role for the dialyzing parent, and food creatively prepared can be served during the card playing period with friends.*

NUTRITION

Better nutrition is a continuing goal not only for the parent but also for the entire family. The home health aide homemaker

---

*Ann Campbell, Instructor of Community Health Education, and James Campbell, doctoral student, University of Missouri, St. Louis, speaking in Wausau, October 1977. (James now has a kidney transplant after 5 years on the machine in his own home.)

teaches good nutrition through menu planning, marketing for appropriate foods, and learning the "tricks" in making food most palatable for each specific family. It has long been established that the ethnic and cultural foods of one family cannot be forced on another. The health care nurse realizes this in her care plans for each family, as illustrated by the following example.

Case history

An elderly Polish couple was experiencing malnutrition and dehydration. They would not enter a nursing home. Hospitalization was not the answer, for they refused to eat the hospital meals. When they had been taken to the hospital intravenous feedings were administered. Hospital food was completely rejected. A care plan was begun in the hospital with the social worker and the health care nurse included. The home health care agency had a Polish home health aide/homemaker on staff, who could speak and understand the language. She was placed in this home for 4 hours a day. (This service was purchased through the Department of Social Services for far less than the cost of nursing home care.) After listening to the couple's wishes, she asked for family recipes and purchased the necessary groceries. Grocery shopping once a week was sufficient to make one big meal a day with prepared items for the other meals. On occasion the homemaker was able to surprise the family with tasty recipes from her own Polish pantry.

This couple to date has been maintained in their own home for more than 2 years. Medical attention has been needed on only one occasion during an episode of the flu.[5]

SCHEDULING OF VISITS

The knowledge of the daily schedule of family members plays an important part in planning the schedule for the elderly parent. The following excerpt is one example of this type of planning:

If the parent needs to give herself colostomy care which is best done in the bathroom—and should be done as near to the same hour daily—the plan should be to use the facilities after working members of the family are finished with the bathroom. This includes the children's preparation for school.

After the parent becomes accustomed to giving self-care he/she may want to get this chore completed in the very early morning hours before the family activities begin. Elderly persons may have the pattern of very early rising and find this hour to be the best. However when the nurse is teaching the procedure a later visit time must be planned for. This is also true if there is need for a family member to be taught the procedure.[5]

The spacing of home visits is arranged according to the needs of the parent and the family. The visits may be as frequent as three times a day to twice a month, and visits of the nurse and other personnel should be alternated in order to utilize the time well and give supportive care with more continuity.

Some insurance contracts specify the total number of visits per diagnosis with uneventful convalescence that the policy will pay for, with an allowance for more visits if documented complications arise. There is an indication that the number of visits will be limited in future national health care plans. The good judgment of the home health care nurse can be brought into play at this point.

In the case of chronic illness the weekly visit may increase to daily visits until the crisis is over. After the crisis a new plan should be studied and put into practice.

Visits may be entirely discontinued temporarily, but the family should be made aware that the home health care nurse can be reached whenever the need should recur. For insurance reasons, a completed dismissal must be recorded when visits are discontinued; however, admission to service may recur immediately at any time there is need.

The care plan schedule is developed to include primary care nursing but does not include the physician's home visit. If a doctor is making a home visit, the nurse should be in attendance in most cases. Good communication between the doctor and the nurse results in better management of medical directives

and care plan, thus making the home visit more satisfying for all concerned.

If the doctor's visit includes such things as the debridement of a wound by cautery or a surgical procedure, the nurse can be of assistance. The procedure may need sterile equipment and dressings, which the nurse can prepare in advance.

PRIMARY NURSING CARE

Primary nursing care should be adequate and appropriate to avoid "self-care" from becoming no care at all. A dedicated home care nurse must believe in bedside care. The trend to earlier hospital dismissals of patients demands more and better nursing in the home. Nursing in its fullest meaning is needed to raise the quality of care for the patient above its present profile: the typical statement, "Anyone can do home care!"

Primary nursing care includes the therapeutic bathing of a patient who is seriously ill and bedridden. This is most true in the care of a dying person suffering from a terminal illness such as cancer.

In a recent newspaper article the "news" was that a small group of nurses and doctors were teaching nurses the therapeutic value of "laying on of hands." The article claimed that 3000 nurses have taken this course. A primary care nurse has learned this valuable tool through her own growth in her professional work. Where did this part of nursing get lost?

The article goes on to say there is a magnetic or electrical field area between the hands of a caring nurse and the patient. This is not "news": any nurse who has held the hand of a dying patient has felt the strength drawn from her own hands.

Patients are often sent to their homes to die. A dignified death is the right of every person. To die in familiar surroundings and within the family circle is a calming experience; it does not need to be a traumatic climax to any person's life.

Death is a part of life's total process, and preparation of the family and patient for death is a part of the responsibility of a primary care nurse. In a prepared situation death can be a beautiful and rewarding experience. This is not to say there will not be sadness and grieving; intelligent acceptance is the key.

A home health care nurse with public health education and real commitment to patient care has an unbeatable combination for judging what is the best for the patient and his family. The full use of this knowledge leaves no doubt as to what nursing is—complete care plus appropriate teaching. Teaching families and their infirmed member is an excellent goal and should be a continuing effort, but the situation must be carefully analyzed in each situation according to the degree to which the family members can use what they are taught. This is not a simple process; nor is it a static one. The approach to teaching may need to be changed from day to day, from visit to visit; some days there may be a regression, which needs more reinforcement than other days. Home care nursing differs from hospital nursing where responsibilities are shared by many; in a home situation one or two may carry the entire load.

Community service personnel entering the family home should be identifiable by a well-groomed appearance in the uniform of the agency. A "uniform bag" of the agency, containing all equipment needed for the nurses work, will add to the family's acceptance of help.

QUALITY ASSURANCE

Accreditation and certification are tools to evaluate the quality of care. Certification for Medicare and Medicaid eligibility is done on a state level. Accreditation, a more sophisticated evaluation, is done jointly through the National League for Nursing and the American Public Health Association.

Accreditation is an on-going surveillance of the total home care agency in four areas: (1) organization and administration, (2) program, (3) staff, and (4) future plans.

There is some duplication in the certification requirements and efforts are being made through the federal government, the National League for Nursing, The American Public Health Association, and other interested organizations to make the accreditation the accepted requirement for all home care agencies. Accreditation is a voluntary commitment as of this writing.

FINANCES

Who pays for all of this home care?

Insurance companies have always had a concerned interest in home health care—in the actual nursing care and the preventive health teaching given by a prepared home care nurse. From 1909 to 1953 the Metropolitan Life Insurance Company provided home nursing in areas throughout the United States and Canada. Statistics gathered from this care proved that home care was a deterring factor to multiple hospitalizations and untimely deaths. After 1953 this visiting nurse service continued under local sponsorship in the communities that had learned the value of such service.

Other sources of finances are the United Way, or Community Chest funds; Medicare; Medicaid; private insurance; Veterans Administration; other health organizations such as the Wisconsin Lung Association; and private foundations. In addition, the private family may be a source of payment for service received.

In 1965 the federal government enacted the Medicare program for payments to all health care providers. Home care was a minor part of the expense experienced by the government due in great measure to the paucity of home care agencies. Records show that only about 1% of the total national health care money was spent on home care. This picture is changing as new agencies are developing and their use is proving effective.

Persons eligible for Medicaid funds tap this source usually only after Medicare payments are used up. Medicare and Medicaid payments are often made through the same insurance company in a given state and the policy is to use Medicare funding first.

As home care programs have become more available, private insurances are developing an interest in controlled, quality home care. Accredited home care agencies have caught the attention of concerned insurance companies. Insurance companies involved in Workman's Compensation programs used qualified home care agencies even before Medicare came on the scene.

In the case of medically indigent families free care is given or an appropriate sliding fee schedule is used. One agency reports that Medicare pays 53.6% of their receipts; Medicaid, 10.8%; United Way, 19%; and private sources, 12.4%. The agency reporting these figures has other programs such as maternity classes and visits, which are separate from the home care nursing program per se.[7]

In this cold, electronic, and mechanical world, the home health care agency remains the nucleus for tomorrow's knowledgeable, compassionate care for the family and the elderly parent.

REFERENCES

1. Colt, A. M., et al.: Home health care is good economics, Nurs. Outlook **25**(10): 632-636. October 1977.
2. North Central Community Action, Inc.: Community resources, Wausau, Wisc., 1976, North Central Community Action, Inc.
3. Marathon County Commission on Aging: Annual report, Marathon County, Wis., January 1978, The Commission.
4. General Accounting Office: Home Health Line, II, Issue 12, Washington, D.C., December 1977, U.S. Government Printing Office.
5. Wausau Visiting Nurse Association: Problem-oriented medical records, Wausau, Wis., 1976, The Association.
6. Wausau Visiting Nurse Association: Procedure manual, Wausau, Wis., 1976, The Association.
7. Wausau Visiting Nurse Association: Annual report, Wausau, Wis., November 1977, The Association.

14

Occupational health nursing

Margaret L. Hornyack

The employed adult is one of the primary supportive structures of the family and of the community. Professional nursing assists in maintaining that supportive structure by promoting health, preventing disease, and determining and implementing nursing measures in the cure and rehabilitation of ill persons. Community health nursing and occupational health nursing attempt to accomplish the same objective but from different perspectives. Where community health nursing focuses on the individual in his family and community, occupational health nursing focuses on him in his working environment.

The earliest provision of occupational health nursing service in the United States was made by the Vermont Marble Company in 1895, which employed Ada Mayo Stewart, R.N., to provide care for its employees. One facet of that care required visiting employees in their homes. During these visits she was able to assess the family unit and/or significant others as a part of the plan for providing total health care for the employee. Thus a link to community health nursing was established.

This link has become more viable and vital as the general public, special interest groups, environmentalists, businesses, and communities that have experienced unique problems have become aware of the effects of working conditions on the health of the person, the family, and the community. As a result the employed adult is more frequently being included in health care now that emphasis is being placed on health conservation and promotion. An ever-increasing number of health professionals as well as community health nurses are changing commitments from the "treat and patch" approach to preventing disease and injury. The combined efforts of these groups and occupational health nursing can now develop into more meaningful, comprehensive health care for the employed worker.

Keeping the employed adult on the job as a healthy, productive member of the work force is the primary purpose for any occupational health nursing service. This purpose accomplishes the goal of the employer who wants a work force that can produce for the company without the excessive costs of injury and illness, increased absenteeism and diminished production. The occupational health nurse realizes the satisfaction of achieving that goal and the goal of contributing to the quality of life for the employees entrusted to her care.

Nursing services for the worker are most appropriately delivered at the place of employment but health services for employed adults are now being offered more frequently in physicians' offices, clinics, hospitals, universities, and union facilities. Occupational health services directed by physicians at these alternate locations may range from diagnostic studies to specific treatment of trauma or disease to total preventive health programs in relation to the work environment.

While the occupational health nurse applies all of the basic nursing principles, there are unique blocks of knowledge and functions applicable only to the practice of occupational health nursing. Basic nursing principles and procedures are used in routine activities such as preemployment, preplacement, periodic and special physical examinations, acute illness and injury care, management of chronic disease conditions, health education, mental health counseling, community resource referral, and rehabilitation.

Preemployment physical examinations determine the general health status of an applicant according to criteria established by the employer, determining whether or not the job can be performed without causing harm to the worker or others, and recording baseline data. Preplacement examinations ensure that the employee is not placed in a position that would jeopardize his or her health and safety because of preexisting conditions or hypersusceptibility. For example, a person susceptible to cold would not be placed in a position that requires working in a frozen food locker in a food processing plant but would be assigned to another job where such a hazard does not exist.

Periodic physical examinations are performed on a scheduled basis for health maintenance. Special examinations are done because of particular exposures that require health monitoring. Biannual physical examinations for executives are an example of the first type; examining for lead poisoning is an example of the second.

Acute care encompasses not only injuries

or illnesses that are job related but also those occurring off the job—those that can be remedied to enable the employee to continue working, and those that require immediate emergency first aid and referral for further medical care.

The management of chronic disease conditions permits the employee to remain on the job under prescribed orders of a physician and within the parameters of company policy. An example of such management is blood pressure monitoring of a hypertensive employee.

Health education activities may be conducted individually or on a group basis. These activities might include instructing workers on wearing ear defenders to protect against hearing loss, providing information packets, or conducting classes on obesity, diabetes, cancer, cardiovascular disease and so forth.

Mental health counseling is an important aspect of providing preventive health care. The complexity of living in an urban industrialized society, in many cases without benefit of support from family and close friends, creates feelings of isolation and helplessness when problems of everyday living begin to accumulate and are not resolved. These are the stresses an employee may bring to the job. These stresses, compounded by a highly competitive or demanding position, coupled with prolonged periods of overtime required to complete a scheduled project, can result in an overload on the central nervous system. When usual problem-solving techniques do not work, the employee may appear at the health service unit exhibiting such physical symptoms as headaches, gastrointestinal disturbances, "flu" symptoms, or other vague complaints. Assessment and intervention by the nurse assist the employee in finding solutions to his problem prior to the crisis stage— actions that prevent further complications and subsequent faltering job performance.

During periods of high stress in the work place, whether it permeates the entire location or is confined to one department, the number of employee visits to the health service unit will increase. Accident rates usually go up, morale and productivity decrease, absenteeism increases, the use of alcohol and drugs increases, and disturbances in interpersonal relations result. All of this information should be documented in the daily report. On analysis, as in an epidemiological study, a pattern may begin to emerge; the nurse presents the pattern to management. Informing management of the developing problem and recommending methods to reduce the stress and eliminate the symptoms are another responsibility of the nursing service.

Community resource referrals are vitally important in assisting the employee to enter the medical care system at the most beneficial point. This eliminates or reduces loss of time from work while seeking assistance, facilitates the solving of the problem by the employee, and reduces the cost and ineffectiveness of redundant or inappropriate care. Referring an employee to a pain clinic when traditional care has not diminished symptoms would be an example; referring an employee suspected of alcoholism or drug abuse would be another example.

The above has served to outline those activities that occupational health nursing has in common with general nursing; as has been mentioned, there are challenges that are specific to occupational health nursing. An extremely important starting point in occupational health nursing is obtaining a thorough knowledge of the work place. This includes the physical layout—a schematic drawing of every floor and/or department as well as adjacent structures—the equipment and processes used in producing the product, including all materials; the operations' schedule for each department, especially if there is shift work; and a demographic profile on all employees such as number of men and women, ethnicity, ratio of salaried to hourly workers, type of union if present, and the information communication network.

This type of information is essential when planning an occupational health program. In emergency situations, for example, time cannot be lost in consulting maps or drawings. When preparing a health education program, levels of education and cultural values must be considered. The range of salaries influence plans for developing a referral system and planning further care; for example, an employee earning $4 per hour and needing mental health services would not be referred to a psychiatrist who charges $75 an hour when a psychologist charging $15 an hour would be adequate or when other appropriate services can be arranged. Nursing care plans may be influenced by salary classifications also; for instance, a salaried employee whose pay will continue when advised to stay home from work may accept that recommendation, thus facilitating his recuperation. For an hourly worker who does not have this benefit, recommending time away from work will increase his stress and lengthen the period of convalescence; it may even contribute to the further deterioration of his health.

Since an occupational health nurse is frequently the only health care professional at a place of employment, she will have multiple roles to perform, including that of an industrial hygienist, health services administrator, safety professional, toxicologist, and health physicist. At times these activities will blend into one another, and yet each professional activity retains its own identity.

All of the above roles, including that of the medical professional are an essential part of an occupational health and safety program; consequently a reasonable understanding of the principles and practices in each of these areas must be obtained. A point of clarification is that while one may function in any of these roles many nurses do not, and they recognize their own limitations in skill and knowledge. However, the key to discharging the responsibilities concerned with occupational health, especially if one works alone, is to recognize when the services of other professionals are needed and to arrange for obtaining their expertise. Preparing the worker to perform his job in a healthful manner is the single most important aspect in preventing occupational disease.

As mentioned before, special knowledge in addition to nursing is required of the nurse practicing occupational health; for example, a knowledge of toxicology is essential. Paracelsus, the "Father of Toxicology" (1493-1541), stated: "All substances are poisons; there is none which is not a poison. The right dose differentiates a poison and a remedy." Industrial toxicology involves the study of the toxicity of materials and chemicals and the mechanisms by which they produce their effects, so that their hazard and impact on the worker can be predicted. Within this area of study is a branch called behavioral toxicology, which deals with toxic effects on the nervous system and their behavioral manifestations that interfere with the productive functioning of the employee. The nurse must be able to recognize the signs and symptoms of a toxic episode, and, just as important, she must relay educational material and information concerning the potential hazards of the toxic substance to the worker during preplacement physicals or other periods of care or contact.

Occupational health physicians are board certified or have been thoroughly trained in the concepts and practice of occupational medicine. They, too, are becoming more and more dedicated to preventing disease and injury, and are devoting time and effort to epidemiological studies and preventive medicine programs, which include evaluating life-

styles that are detrimental or beneficial to the health status of the worker. Many physicians practicing in the community do not fully understand occupational medicine but serve employed patients; frequently they overlook conditions or diseases related to the work place. Unless these physicians are extremely astute or have opportunities to learn about occupational diseases, they treat many patients for signs and symptoms associated with common chronic diseases. Consequently quantities of data that would be useful in developing profiles on groups of workers are lost. This may be one explanation for the delay in recognizing the cases of glioblastoma associated with work exposure in a single industry in Texas City, Texas, reported in 1979.[1]

Rapport must be developed by the plant nurse with physicians in the community so that data regarding the worker can be relayed to foster continuity of care, to educate the physician regarding the work processes that affect the worker and may influence treatment plans, and to facilitate communication when the physician needs to converse with the employer or the nursing service.

Another important field is industrial hygiene—the science of recognizing, evaluating, and controlling environmental factors or stresses that may cause sickness, inefficiency, or impaired performance of the worker. The occupational health nurse should be able to recognize potential hazards, but evaluation and control are more appropriately discharged by a professional industrial hygienist. This knowledge, which leads to recognition of the problem, permits the nurse to alert and advise management of areas that may cause serious illnesses or accidents and to recommend the services of a practicing industrial hygienist where needed.

The safety professional is another prominent member of the occupational health team. This discipline employs the principles of accident prevention and occupational health hazard control, utilizing engineering, education, and enforcement techniques. Job performance, machine and product safety, and compliance with safety rules, regulations, and laws form the basis of this specialty. Ergonomics—the study of the relationship between man and machine—is sometimes included in this profession also.

It is evident that all of these disciplines, including occupational medicine, interact and blend at times, yet still retain their individuality. Nevertheless, the team members have a common goal: protecting the worker while facilitating the accomplishment of the employer's goals.

The occupational health nurse, the occupational physician, the industrial hygienist, the safety professional, and the toxicologist are all part of the in-plant health team. Yet there are other professionals outside of the plant who exert great influence on the health of the worker. These are comprised of members of the judicial system—attorneys, legislators, lobbyists, and special interest groups. They have a great impact on society since it is they who draft and pass laws and regulations and adjudicate claims.

In addition, insurance companies, both Worker's Compensation and private health policy companies, influence significantly the injured employee. One influence, although seldom considered, is the insurer's philosophy concerning the interpretation of the laws and regulations pertaining to the processing of claims. Their philosophy may range from providing whatever is required to return the claimant to optimum health following an incident to providing the minimum benefits under the law. Since many workers are unaware of their rights and may not understand the complexities of the law, they may not receive all of the benefits to which they are entitled.

Other difficulties are that not all states require Worker's Compensation of employers; nor are adequate benefits provided through existing programs. Companies that sell Worker's Compensation insurance policies usually demand a certain level of health and safety practices to promote a good working environment. They also attempt to control the number and cost of claims. This is advantageous for all concerned, since the severity and the cost of accidents are reflected in the premiums paid by the employer. If these are kept to a minimum the company pays less in premiums, the insurance company continues to realize a profit, and the worker remains gainfully employed, uninjured, and healthy.

Private health insurance companies usually exert their influence through the medical treatment and billing processes. Occasionally there are disputes over coverage, which may delay or interrupt plans for treatment and rehabilitation of the injured worker and quite frequently leave the injured employee without a source of income for living expenses and medical care costs until such time that decisions are made. As a result of the traditional method of completing and filing insurance claims to facilitate payment for medical care, the injured worker and the treating physician will ignore the correlation between the illness and the work place, sometimes through ignorance, sometimes through fear of the loss of a job, and sometimes to circumvent the additional paperwork and reporting procedure that is required for work-related incidents.

Traditionally labor (the worker) has been rather subdued in voicing its concerns about the healthfulness of the work place. Recently, through a movement gaining in popularity and visibility, the unions have been teaching and encouraging members to take responsibility for their own health. The Oil, Chemical and Atomic Workers Union, for instance, has a very active health and safety unit. They employ industrial hygienists, health educators, and others to accomplish the goal of educating workers. Activities such as educational programs regarding the hazards associated with the chemicals with which they work, personal protective equipment, personal hygiene, and rights and responsibilities under the Occupational Safety and Health Act (OSHA) are conducted at the local level. Work places are monitored, and health and safety clauses are included in negotiations and contracts; toxicological studies, physical examination programs, and epidemiological studies are also supported. Liaisons with universities, organizations such as the American Cancer Society and the March of Dimes, and professional associations such as the Society for Occupational and Environmental Health have been formed to facilitate these endeavors.

Administrative skills are of primary importance in a health service program. The ability to communicate authoritatively with management, which usually identifies productivity, not health care, as the ultimate objective of the business, is of vital importance. Skill in planning the health program must clearly convince management and other departments that the health program's budget, policies, authority, and functions are an essential part of the productive business organization.

The budgeting process is critical in occupational health as there are no third-party payers into the system, and the health program and the funds allotted toward its operation are parts of the master plan for the entire organization. The budget cannot be extravagant; yet it must be sufficient to cover all eventualities of 12 calendar months. The budget exemplifies that the nurse must be knowledgeable about the fundamentals of business operations, including being able to speak and understand the language of industrial relations, personnel, production depart-

ments, procurement department, and so forth. It is essential that she know the fiscal as well as the operational aspects of the place of employment in as much detail as possible.

The requirements for record keeping and its uses are numerous; this includes medical records of all employees and the records and reports mandated by legislation, such as the OSHA records and reports and Workers' Compensation. In addition there are monthly and annual records required by management. These serve as both internal and external information sources and may be used for managerial information as well as for therapeutic communication. The administrative reports supply information to management; such information identifies the operation of the unit and provides data that encourage their support and enable them to recognize the value of the program. The reports are also used for planning additional services or evaluating the effectiveness of the activities presently being conducted within the unit. Employee records facilitate all aspects of care provided to each individual and at times are essential in gaining the cooperation in the departments when extenuating circumstances occur, for example, when assisting a recovering alcoholic.

A written company policy is necessary for the health service to function properly. Daily operations must be planned, and arrangements must be made for physical maintenance, staff relief, and coordination as well as for ordering supplies and equipment and maintaining inventories. Moreover, communication, interactions, and collaborative functions must be developed and implemented with the various departments of the organization. The nurse working alone will carry out all of the activities; however, in a multiple-nurse unit the duties and responsibilities will usually be distributed among several colleagues.

Medical directives as well as standing

orders signed by a physician under contract to the company are needed for medicolegal purposes. A nurse usually is covered for malpractice under the employer's general liability insurance policy. However, it is highly recommended that a professional nurse carry private malpractice insurance also. This insurance is available through the American Association of Occupational Health Nurses as well as through private insurance agencies.

The traditional activities of an occupational health service have not been described specifically, since more detailed information is available through other sources. A comprehensive list of references concerning occupational health is available in a recent publication entitled *The New Nurse in Industry*.[2]

The following discussion proposes present and future impacts on occupational health that are or are becoming important.

The passage of the Occupational Safety and Health Act of 1970, (Public Law 91-596) has resulted in a resurgence of respect, recognition, and acceptance of occupational health nursing. This legislation has mandated safe and healthful working conditions for all men and women. To comply with this law many places of employment and public health departments have implemented or expanded existing occupational health services. Schools of nursing and schools of public health have recently initiated graduate programs in occupational health nursing through funds appropriated by Congress and administered by the National Institutes of Occupational Safety and Health (NIOSH). In some schools of nursing, new course offerings in occupational health nursing as well as continuing education programs are being provided. Thus the number of professional nurses in the field is increasing, as is the introduction of knowledge into other fields of nursing regarding the complexities of the industrial setting and the stresses of the working population.

There exist several definitions of occupational health nursing. The American Association of Occupational Health Nurses, Inc., and the American Nurses Association as well as governmental agencies and collegial professional organizations all have different versions, yet it would not be unusual to have each occupational health nurse define the practice of nursing according to her own experiences. The value and effectiveness of the health service have also been evaluated according to the perceptions of these various organizations. That is not to say that management or immediate supervisors have not exerted considerable control over policies; however, the actual nursing components are usually not evaluated by an objective, knowledgeable person. This is especially true for the one-nurse unit. Because of the diversity of work places and processes in the United States, these personal experiences still influence the present practice of occupational health nursing. It is only recently, as mentioned before, that the specialty is beginning to be taught in structured programs within the university again. The two earlier graduate-level programs in existence—one established in 1950; the other, in 1959—were both phased out by 1964.[3]

Consequently there are many nurses who are practicing on the basis of their early training in hospital settings; that is, they are concentrating on illness and disease, not on the promotion of health. The theories of epidemiology were not taught; nor were evaluation or recognition—the cornerstones of effective occupational health programs. These cornerstones laid the foundation for the future emphasis on occupational health, looking at groups rather than individuals and promoting the health of workers in their environment.

This concept must be accepted and incorporated into existing programs. The cost of occupational illnesses, diseases, and injuries in terms of human suffering; the potential for damage to future generations; the diminished standard of living; and the escalating financial drain on employers and employees demand new directions for occupational health programs.

Nurses provide a major portion of occupational health care. The employers must make provision to use these concepts of epidemiology, industrial hygiene, and health promotion; and the nurses must see that they have the skills to implement these ideas. To accomplish this a few problems that need to be solved are identified:

1. Insufficient numbers of qualified nurses are available to relieve or temporarily replace permanently employed nurses for educational endeavors.

2. Economic factors and job security must be considered prior to the nurses' beginning an education process.

3. Age, remaining work years, and other responsibilities and motivation may be deterrents for embarking on an educational venture.

4. Nurses who have been out of an educational institution for a period of time must be willing to reevaluate their ideas; they should be aware that technology and basic knowledge and educational theories have changed, and considerable effort will be required to accomplish an educational goal.

5. The management of corporations, governmental agencies, and other places of employment must be educated to accept the new and modern concepts of occupational health; they must be convinced that these concepts will be beneficial when integrated into an existing program, especially if a nurse returns to her position on completion of the educational process.

6. Legislation and enforcement of the regulations by the OSHA will have to include all places of employment. At the time of this writing, employers with 10 or fewer employees were exempt from the provision of the OSHA. Innovative methods of providing nursing services to these small employers must be devised.

With the rapid technological changes that have occurred in the field of occupational health, as well as the social, economic, and environmental changes that have had a significant impact on the specialty, it is a challenging, exciting time for anyone interested in the health of the worker. Health care specialists anticipate that much more emphasis on the development of more definitive and specific preventive measures in occupational health will occur. Environmentalists, concerned health care financial analysts, members of communities involved in occupational health problems, and large segments of the population are demanding these measures because they believe that "health is a right." The recent passage of legislation also has involved the government substantially in regulating occupational health. Most influential, however, has been the awareness of the occupational health care specialists. Dissatisfied with the state of the art, they are looking for new and better ways of preventing chronic disability from long-known diseases that are still occurring and from diseases that are just being identified because of the advances of technology.

More emphasis will be placed on the role of nutrition in health within our working population. Questions and hypotheses are being formed to consider the relationship of nutrition to occupational disease. The question has been raised as to whether or not diet and/or food additives act as a catalyst, which, in conjunction with some occupational exposures, might generate conditions that enhance inherent carcinogenicity of chemical and physical agents. Since the most susceptible segment of the working population is pregnant women, more research must be done on the effects of these entities on the fetus. The steady increase of women who are taking jobs, who are entering the heavy industry, and who are working in the chemical industry with its suspected mutagens, presents unusual and under-investigated areas for study. These areas include the effects on unborn children, reproductive capabilities, musculoskeletal systems, and mental health aspects as well as the societal implications for working women.

Modern methods of measuring stress are developing rapidly in relation to people in the work place. The proliferation of studies is increasing the concern for certain groups of workers. Researchers in this field are directing more of their attention to the problems of occupational stress, thus increasing information that reveals both the advantageous and the deleterious effects on human health. These studies contribute to the realization that the working population is an integral part of the overall ecosystem.

Particular attention will be focused on the effects of chemical exposures on both men and women in relation to reproduction and sexuality. Examples include permanent sterility in males in the manufacture and application of the pesticide 1,2 dibromochloropropane (DBCP),[4] gynecomastia in men associated with the manufacture of hormonal products,[5] the effects of irradiation of ova, which are never replaced but present at birth,[6] and the increased fetal wastage associated with workers exposed to vinyl chloride.[7]

Occupational health specialists must be concerned with the developing and resurgent alternatives to traditional health care. What are the implications of holistic health care, acupuncture, auriculotherapy, rolphing, group therapy, and religion-based treatments on the present-day provision for health care under existing legislation? What do these mean for the existing nursing services within

the plant? How will the nurses counsel, interpret, or refer employees who seek these modalities?

Nurses in industry should pay particular attention to employees' descriptions of their signs and symptoms. Some of the old-time descriptions of work-related conditions— "grinder's rot," "phossy jaw," "painter's colic," "chromic itch," "miner's phthisis,"— were indicative of occupational diseases. Recognition of early symptoms of exposure could prevent serious and permanent disability. Alice Hamilton, the first recognized occupational health physician in America, in her writings mentioned workmen's descriptions of their current exposures at work, and many of these descriptions are still applicable to modern day work exposures.

National health issues are an important concern for occupational health nursing. The catastrophic diseases and their cost to family members have profound effects on the working man or woman. Many times this causes functional impairment leading to severe accidents, debilitating reactions, absence from work, and emotional crises. These situations require counseling on the job within the health service. The assistance offered by the nurse also influences the subsequent receptivity for and implementation of health education efforts in other health matters such as diabetes and hypertension. Questions brought to the nurse concerning referrals for abortions, family planning, drug abuse, and alcoholism must be considered and answered objectively.

Incorporating the concept of health maintenance organizations into existing health care plans and assisting employees to use them effectively is an emerging duty. Current knowledge in all these matters is a professional responsibility.

Accountability, a relatively new word to the health field, is especially applicable to occupational health nursing. The demand is coming from management, the employees, physicians, employees' families, union representatives, insurance representatives, lawyers, nursing associations, and peer groups. The expectation that nurses are responsible for their own actions includes the quality of care that is expected of them. Quality care incorporates the most current knowledge and methods in the practice of nursing. When a nurse is the only health care member in a place of employment, she accepts an enormous responsibility and must be prepared to be accountable for the care delivered.

In the specialty of occupational health, the care encompasses an understanding of all of the factors related to the work place that impinge on the health of the worker, for example, the toxic effects of chemicals and the signs and symptoms of acute and chronic exposure to chemicals, and the recommended treatment. Most important though, the nurse must effectively teach employees to participate actively in protecting their health. This instruction should begin on the first day of work and should continue on a consistent basis throughout the worker's career.

The proliferation of information regarding occupational health has propelled the nurse into the spotlight. Where she once was a kind, gentle, "good old soul," she now must not only be kind and gentle but also a progressive, competent professional, possessing the latest knowledge and skills of a nurse prepared for this expanded role and all that this implies. The need for more occupational health nurses increases daily because the majority of present occupational health nurses are near retirement age. The university-trained adult nurse practitioner will find that occupational health nursing provides an atmosphere where advanced skills are utilized to their maximum.

New methods must be designed and integrated into preventive occupational health care. One of these is the developing field of cytogenetics, a method of examining chromosomes to determine the presence of chromosomal breakage or consequent abnormalities that would preclude any employee's working in a position that would or could be detrimental to his health.

Cytogenetic testing is used to detect environmental situations that can affect the human genetic material and to identify those individuals who are hypersensitive to particular materials. This method of identifying actual or potential hazards and their effects on man is extremely valuable because in many situations data from laboratory and animal studies must be applied to man, a difficult and at times questionable task. Studies incorporating cytogenetic monitoring can be expected both to verify existing standards and to provide reliable information about changing toxicological safety data.

Many geneticists propose that man's genes are his most precious heritage, to be protected against erosion within each generation so that the quality of life will not be diminished in the present or subsequent generations.[9] Researchers believe that 25% of our health burden is of genetic origin. Thus the study of genetics and the use of cytogenetic testing in industry would seem to be of particular significance to occupational health. But demonstrating the precise cause of chromosomal damage is difficult because of the great variety and environmental ubiquity of agents known or suspected to cause chromosomal breakage or consequent abnormalities. Drugs, chemicals, viruses, and physical agents such as radiation are some of these agents.[10]

Carcinogenesis in man may involve the interaction of genetic and environmental forces and mutations, whether germinal or somatic, seem to be involved in the origin of many, perhaps all cancers.[11] There is a positive correlation between malformed offspring mediated by mutated germ cells on the one hand and malignancy as a consequence of somatic mutations on the other hand.[12]

The three most frequently encountered chromosomal mutants in man, which are readily visible under an ordinary light microscope by cytogenetic testing, are Down's syndrome (mongolism), Klinefelter's syndrome, and Turner's syndrome.[13] One out of 17 persons with Down's syndrome will develop leukemia. With the present equal employment opportunity regulations and the encouragement to hire the handicapped, employers may well interview applicants who have Down's syndrome or other conditions associated with chromosomal anomalies. These applicants must never be placed in positions where they will be exposed to radiation or other substances known or suspected of causing chromosomal abnormalities.

It has been documented that dose-related exposures, increased cancer incidence, and increased in vivo chromosomal aberration are all correlated in workers employed as radium dial painters,[14] uranium miners,[15] and in plutonium production,[16] as well as those exposed to benzene,[17] vinyl chloride,[7] and epichlorohydrin.[18]

Neoplasms such as acute and chronic myelocytic leukemias, chronic lymphatic leukemia, meningioma, and others are also associated with chromosomal anomalies.[19]

The research conducted on the atomic bomb survivors of Hiroshima documented radiation dose and resultant chromosomal aberrations.[20] A recent study reported by Najarian and Colter in 1978 revealed that a review of the death certificates from 1959 to 1977 of workers exposed to radiation at the Portsmouth Naval Shipyard revealed an excessive proportion of leukemia and cancer mortality.[21] Evans et al. studied nuclear dock workers in the United Kingdom and concluded that workers exposed to ionizing radiation below the acceptable maximum permissible levels of 5 rems per year demonstrated a bio-

logical effect at the chromosomal level.[22] Brandom et al. at the University of Denver found abnormal chromosomes in plutonium workers at Rocky Flats.[16] Although the consequences of the effects of low-level radiation on chromosome abnormalities are unclear, the linking of cancer and chromosomes aberrations is exerting influence to consider reexamining the standards for radiation exposure.[23]

Throughout this discussion the point seems clear that cytogenetic testing should be a part of every physical examination but most certainly it should be done in preplacement examinations where known exposures to chromosome damaging chemicals are possible.

Cytogenetic monitoring using an epidemiological approach can be readily accomplished within occupational health programs because there is a sizable population, the work force is relatively stable and healthy, and there is known exposure to diverse chemicals. Cytogenetic monitoring will ensure that appropriate protective measures will be taken on early identification of genetic risk and before overt damage has occurred. Perfecting this system of screening to a practical monitoring method is an ongoing effort in several laboratories and universities between nurses, physicians, epidemiologists, geneticists, technicians, and employees—another example of a team approach to solving the problems of occupational health.

An occupational health program can be as miniscule or as encompassing as the knowledge, capabilities, and dedication of the nurse and commitment of management.

We cannot expect to solve tomorrow's problems with yesterday's knowledge and today's methods, but progress will continue by building on the experience of yesterday, the knowledge of today, and the imagination, ingenuity, and foresight of tomorrow. Protecting, preserving, and promoting the health of employed adults—the basic support structure of the family and community—is the commitment of the exciting, challenging specialty of occupational health nursing.

REFERENCES

1. OSHA, NIOSH, Industry investigating high rate of brain cancer in Texas plant, Occupational Safety and Health Reporter, Bureau of National Affairs 8:1519, March 1979.
2. Lee, J. A.: The new nurse in industry, DHEW (NIOSH), Publication No. 78-143, Washington, D.C., 1978, U.S. Government Printing Office.
3. Brown, M. L.: Nursing in occupational health, Public Health Rep. 79:967-972, 1964.
4. 1,2 Dibromochloropropane (DBCP), Occupational safety and health reporter, Bureau of National Affairs 8:337, August 1977.
5. Gambini, G., Farina, G., and Arbosti, G.: Gynecomastis, Clinical Lav. L. Devoto (Univ. of Milano, Med. Milano) 67:152-157, 1976.
6. Balinsky, B. I.: An introduction to embryology, Philadelphia, 1970, W. B. Saunders Co.
7. Picciano, D. J., et al.: Vinyl chloride cytogenetics, J. Occ. Med. 19:527-530, August 1977.
8. Hamilton, A.: Exploring the dangerous trades, Boston, 1943, Little, Brown & Co.
9. Committee 17: Environmental mutagenic hazards, Science 187:503-514, 1975.
10. Kilian, D. J., Picciano, D. J., and Jacobson, C. B.: Industrial monitoring: a cytogenic approach, Ann. N.Y. Acad. Sci. 269:4-11, 1975.
11. Knudson, Jr., A. G.: Environmental carcinogenesis and genetic variability in man, Human genetics: Proceedings of the 5th International Congress of Human Genetics, Mexico City, 10-15 October 1976, pp. 404-408.
12. Schmid, S.: Mutagen/carcinogen-induced chromosome damage in human and mammalian cells in vivo and in vitro, Human genetics: Proceedings of the 5th International Congress of Human Genetics, Mexico City, 10-15 October 1976, p. 53.
13. Department of Health, Education, and Welfare, Subcommittee on Environmental Mutagenesis.: Approaches to determining mutagenic properties of chemicals: risk to future generations, Washington, D.C., April 1977, DHEW Committee to Coordinate Toxicology and Related Programs.
14. Polednak, A. P., Stehney, A. F., and Rowland, R. E.: Mortality among women first employed before 1930 in the U.S. radium dial painting industry, Am. J. Epidemiol. 107:179-192, March 1978.
15. Langhma, W. H.: Biological implications of the transuranium elements for man, Health Physics 22:943-952, 1972.
16. Brandon, W., et al.: Chronic irradiation effects in blood lymphocyte chromosomes of plutonium workers. Paper presented at the Second International Congress on Environmental Mutagens, Scotland, July 11-15, 1977.
17. Tough, I. M., et al.: Chromosome studies on workers exposed to atmospheric benzene: the possible influence of age, Eur. J. Cancer, 6:49-55, 1970.
18. Kucerova, M., et al.: Mutagenic effect of epichlorohydrin. Part 2: Analysis of chromosomal aberrations in lymphocytes of persons occupationally exposed to epichlorohydrin, Mut. Research 48:355-360, 1977.
19. Mulvihill, J. J.: Congenital and genetic diseases. In Fraumini, J., Jr., ed.: Persons at high risk of cancer, New York, Academic Press, Inc. pp. 3-37, 1975.
20. Awa, A. A.: Cytogenetic and oncogenic effects of the ionizing radiations of the atomic bombs. In German, J., ed.: Chromosomes and cancer, New York, 1974, John Wiley & Sons, Inc.
21. Najarian, T., and Colton, T.: Mortality from leukemia and cancer in shipyard nuclear workers, Lancet 1:1018-1020, May 1978.
22. Evans, H. J., et al.: Radiation-induced chromosome aberrations in nuclear-dockyard workers, Nature 277:531-533, February 1979.
23. Holden, C.: Low level radiation: a high-level concern, Science 204:155-158, April 1979.

SUGGESTED READINGS

Brown, M. L., and Meigs, J. W.: Occupational health nursing, New York, 1956, Springer Publishing Co., Inc.

Kilian, D. J., and Picciano, D.: Cytogenic surveillance of industrial populations, Chemical Mutagens 4:321-339, 1976.

Reinhardt, A. M., and Quinn, M. D.: Family-centered community health nursing, St. Louis, 1973, The C. V. Mosby Co.

Rogers, Martha E.: Reveille in nursing, Philadelphia, 1964, F. A. Davis Co.

15

School nursing
problems and prospects

Susan J. Wold

One of today's least understood and appreciated community nursing roles is that of the school nurse. Although the school nurse's role originated as a public health nursing specialty of unquestioned value, Hawkins[1] has concluded that withdrawing nurses from school systems "would entail no immediate apparent loss for either themselves or the schools." The present status of school nursing tends to support Hawkins' conclusion. Over the past 50 years the role of the school nurse has diminished in scope and value. It has emphasized episodic care and record keeping at the expense of preventive care, health education, and community involvement. Consequently today's school nurse faces an uncertain future. School nursing services have been severely curtailed by some school districts and completely eliminated by others. The questions to be answered now are, How did the problems confronting the school nurse develop? What are the problems facing today's school nurse? What are the prospects for the future? To answer these questions, the remainder of this chapter will do the following:

1. Trace the historical development of the school nurse role in this country

2. Elaborate on those problems that continue to plague the school nurse today
3. Discuss the future needs and prospects for the survival and expansion of the school nurse role

HISTORICAL DEVELOPMENT OF THE SCHOOL NURSE ROLE

The problems facing today's school nurse can be fully understood only by examining their "roots" and historical evolution. Therefore the remainder of this section will highlight the development of the school nurse role and the problems that evolved with it.

The first school health services in the United States began in Boston in 1894. These early school health services consisted of medical inspections for the purpose of identifying and excluding from school those children with serious communicable diseases such as scarlet fever, diphtheria, whooping cough, chickenpox, and mumps. These inspections were later broadened to include screening for parasitic diseases such as scabies, impetigo, and ringworm.[2] However, since no follow-up was done, many of the children who had been excluded never returned to school.

Frustrated by the increasing numbers of

truant children, Lillian Wald, founder of the Henry Street Settlement in New York City, persuaded city officials to allow her to place a public health nurse in selected schools on an experimental basis. This first school nurse was Lina Rogers Struthers, who began working in the schools in November, 1902. Her health education efforts and follow-up of individual cases resulted in dramatic reductions in the length and number of exclusions. Shortly thereafter 25 more nurses were hired by the Board of Education. Statistical comparison of the number of students excluded for communicable disease in the New York City schools before and after the hiring of school nurses reveals a startling difference: in September of 1902, 10,567 students were sent home, whereas in September of 1903, only 1101 students were excluded.[3] Thus the impact of school nursing was clearly demonstrated.

As illustrated in Table 11, the role of the school nurse evolved through three phases during the 1920s and 1930s. In phase I the thrust of the school health program was *medical inspection*, the goal of which was to prevent the spread of communicable diseases through periodic inspection of children in their classrooms and home visits for follow-up of known cases.

Later, *medical inspection*, which was defined as "the search for communicable disease" was replaced by *medical examination* (phase II), which included "the search for physical defects."[2] This focus on medical examination grew out of the realization that medical inspection as a means of protecting healthy children from those who had commu-

Table 11. Developing role of school nurse in 1920s and 1930s*

Phase	School health program activity	Goal	School nurse's role
I	Medical inspection	Control of contagion	1. Assist school physician with inspection *or* 2. Independently inspect children in the classroom 3. Visit homes for follow-up
II	Medical examination	1. Identification of physical defects 2. Disability limitation through correction of defects	1. Assist school physician with examination 2. Visit homes for follow-up
III	Medical inspection Medical examination	Same as II	Same as II
	Health education	1. Student attainment of responsible health behavior 2. Student and parental attainment of responsible health behavior	Stage 1. Develop and implement own health education program Stage 2. Incorporate health education program into teacher's program Stage 3. Mutual planning of health education program by teacher and nurse

*From Wold, S. J., and Dagg, N. V.: School nursing: a passing experiment? In Wold, S. J.: School nursing: a framework for practice, St. Louis, 1980, The C. V. Mosby Co.

nicable diseases was inadequate because it overlooked the total health of the child. During this phase the role of the nurse was similar to that in phase I: she assisted the physician with the examination and conducted home visits for follow-up of defects.

Recognizing that medical inspections and examinations offered little long-range prevention, in phase III school health workers began a three-stage process or incorporating *health education* into the school curriculum (as shown in Table 11). Their goal was to stimulate students in learning and practicing responsible health behavior. Although the nurse's involvement in health education during stages 1 and 2 (Table 11) was independently planned and executed without input from or collaboration with teachers, the role of the nurse in stage 3 was expanded to include implementation of an integrated health education program.

The role and services of the school nurse continued to expand during the 1930s. However, in their efforts to meet the total needs of school children, school nurses were so overextended they became ineffective. Educators and nurses were shocked when the 1934 survey of public health nursing conducted by the National Organization for Public Health Nursing (NOPHN) showed that the poorest quality public health nursing was that being done in the schools.[2,4] Troop[5] suggested that the poor quality of school nursing stemmed from inadequate hospital-based education.

The need for specialized postgraduate preparation for the practice of public health nursing was recognized as early as 1923, following publication by the Committee for the Study of Nursing Education of *Nursing and Nursing Education in the United States*.[6] This report recommended that nurses working full time in the school setting should strengthen their public health background. However, many school nurses felt more closely allied with educators than with nurses and did not even consider themselves public health nurses. Thus in the 1920s this role confusion resulted in the use of such labels as "school nurse teacher" and "teacher-nurse."[5] Following publication of the 1923 nursing education survey results, state boards of education set up certification requirements for nurses, which helped to improve the quality of school nursing. However, certification requirements were, and unfortunately often still are, unrelated to the education and practice of school nursing.

With the advent of World War II, school health and school nursing services faced reevaluation and possible curtailment. The war required that citizens forego fulfillment of many of their personal needs and wants and focus instead on safeguarding the national interest through diversion of persons and goods to the war effort. Although many domestic services were cut back, the health of school children paradoxically received increased emphasis during this time from both educators and civilians. Palmer[7] cites two reasons for this: (1) because this was a mechanized war, large numbers of healthy young men were needed for the draft; and (2) Selective Service data regarding prospective draftees revealed that approximately one fourth of the registrants were rejected because of physical defects. Thus the discovery that a large number of supposedly healthy young males had physical defects became a potential threat to national security and resulted in a renewed interest in the preventive aspects of school health. Therefore the following services were identified[8] as essential to wartime school nursing:

1. Advisory service to school administrators regarding the school health program and the expanded use of community resources to supplement it.
2. Guidance and inservice for teachers regarding health services they were now expected to perform.

3. Interpretation of student health examination data to parents, teachers, and children with referral to community resources for needed follow-up.
4. Home visiting to interpret children's health needs to their parents, to discover the family's health needs for interpretation to other school personnel, and to assist the family and school to meet these needs.

To enable the nurse to carry out these essential services, those tasks that were frequently carried out by the nurse but that did not actually require nursing skills were delegated to others, including volunteers, aides, and teachers.[7] Dilworth[9] acknowledged the merits of such delegation and urged that this be seriously considered not only as an emergency wartime measure but also as a long-range approach to the improvement of school nursing services. She recommended that older students and interested teachers be recruited as volunteers to whom such tasks as vision and hearing screening, periodic weighing and measuring of children, and daily health inspections could be delegated. This, then, was the origin of the school health aide concept, which some authors[10] in later years have viewed as a threat to the school nurse. It is also interesting to note that during the war years, perhaps as a result of this need to delegate some of the school nurse's functions, involvement of the classroom teacher in the health service aspects of the school health program increased. Not only was the teacher valued for her day-to-day observations concerning changes in students' appearances, behavior, and health,[11] but she was also viewed as the logical person to assume responsibility for emergency care of students. Thus the role of the school nurse in first aid and emergency care became one of inservice educator for the teacher concerning first aid techniques, necessary emergency equipment, and appropriate community resources for emergency medical care.[12]

The trend toward delegation of health service tasks to the teacher freed the school nurse to redirect her time and energies toward other priorities. As a result, during the 1940s school nursing became increasingly identified as a kind of public health nursing; in fact at least half of the available public health nurses, according to a survey by the NOPHN, were practicing in the school. This increased public health focus was reflected in the nurse's renewed concern with family-centered care; thus home visits made on behalf of schoolchildren also focused on other family members including infants and preschoolers.[4]

Communicable disease control and periodic medical examinations continued to be part of the school health program in the 1940s. However, the purpose of medical examinations was gradually modified from emphasis on defect and disease detection and numbers of students examined and referred for follow-up to emphasis on the school medical examination as an educational experience focusing on "health counseling or guidance" for which the *outcome* of referrals and follow-up was most important.[11] The goal of health counseling was now seen as helping students to solve their own health problems and to assume responsibility for protecting, maintaining, or improving their health.

Freeman[13] identified four additional changes in emphasis in the school health program during the 1940s that affected the role of the school nurse:

1. Increased emphasis on the importance of the classroom teacher's involvement in health teaching
2. Increased attention to health as a school subject area
3. Increased acceptance of the need to correlate health instruction and health practice and school and home behavior

4. Increased participation and collaboration by students, teachers, parents, administrators, special health personnel, and community representatives in planning and implementing health programs

Thus during this era responsibility for the school health program was no longer delegated solely to the school nurse and school physician; rather the emphasis was on the sharing of responsibility by teachers, students, and health personnel, and a coordinated and integrated health education curriculum was proposed.[9]

Freeman[13] believed that these developments would free the nurse to take on an expanded role in guidance and consultation but would at the same time add some new responsibilities. For the nurse to help the teacher integrate health content into the curriculum, she would need some understanding of classroom teaching and would need to be familiar with the subject matter included in "health." The school nurse would therefore need some additional educational preparation, including:

1. Increased technical expertise based on accurate and current scientific data
2. Better preparation for leadership, including courses on research methods, decision making, and methods of influencing the behavior of others
3. Expanded background in educational methods and family health guidance
4. Interdisciplinary course work with other school personnel such as teachers, physicians, and administrators to accustom these professionals to group or team problem solving methods on the school

In fact, by the late 1940s efforts were being made to upgrade school nursing by specifying the preparation needed for nurses wishing to practice in the school setting. By 1949, 16 state departments of education required certification of the nurse for work in the school, and 4 other states required a certificate for the nurse if she taught any classes.[14]

The 1950s witnessed expansion and development of the programs and priorities established during the 1940s, with overall emphasis on stabilization of the positive changes that had occurred during the previous decade. Many school nurses were still kept busy with such tasks as exclusion and readmission of sick children because school administrators, wishing to be relieved entirely of that responsibility, emphasized this as the paramount function of the nurse.[15]

By the 1950s, it was generally accepted that "health is the first objective of education" and that the goal of the school health program should be to develop "optimum health" for every school child. Optimum health was now recognized to be more than physical fitness and absence of defects; health included mental, spiritual, and emotional elements as well.[16]

Although the school nurse during the 1950s was still expected to prepare children for the school physician's examinations and to assist with the procedure itself, the physical examination as a learning experience continued to be emphasized. Because school health personnel had finally realized that defect detection was unimportant unless the child could be motivated to correct his problems, they emphasized the child's response to the examination and what he learned from the experience. Thus the belief prevailed that the quality of a school health program was more appropriately evaluated on the basis of changed behavior than on mere changes in statistics.[15]

A related and significant change that occurred during this period was the shift toward completion of students' periodic medical examinations by private physicians instead of by physicians provided by the school. This increased the responsibility placed on students and their parents and created a coordination problem between the school and the family physician. To obtain needed information from the private physician following examination of the child, the school had to develop some kind of reporting form to be filled out by the physician and returned to the school. This in turn raised some ethical questions regarding the appropriateness of sharing information. The complexities of following up known health problems resulted in the adoption of a cumulative health record form for each child in the school. However, this too had its drawbacks; the question that was now raised was Who should keep the records, make them out, and file them?[17] The issue of record keeping continues to be a problem in school nursing today.

The emphasis, then, for the 1950s' school nurse was on health education, which was seen as the most important role for the nurse.[16,18] The school nurse fulfilled her health education role through formal and informal teaching—both one to one and in groups—of students, parents, and classroom teachers. The school nurse was often looked to for leadership in the development of the family life education program, an emphasis that was just beginning to take hold in the school.[15] In addition, the school health program was expanded to include a focus on adequate nutrition and the promotion of positive mental health for school children, which provided further health education opportunities for the school nurse.[19]

During the 1950s the "teamwork" philosophy of the school health program was expanded. Collaboration between teacher and nurse in planning and implementing routine screening procedures was emphasized. This increased interest in teamwork led to the development of the "school health council" concept, which was based on the new philosophy of school health as a responsibility shared by teacher, administrator, and nurse.[16] The purpose of the council was to provide a means for coordinating services of community agencies serving school populations, to formulate policies, to develop programs and services for school-age children in the community, and to participate in the evaluation of the effectiveness of the school health program. Accordingly Wallace[19] recommended that the council include representation from involved community agencies and from the lay consumer group.

The 1960s became an era of rapid and often precipitous social change, characterized by the proliferation of health and welfare programs, many of which were poorly planned and short lived. This growing concern for the health and welfare of American citizens carried over into the school health program. There were now two primary thrusts to the school health program: (1) maintenance of optimal health by the school child so that he might benefit maximally from his educational opportunities, and (2) development of positive health attitudes and practices for the child to ensure a "lifetime of healthful productivity."[10] Within these goals, and in keeping with the national interest in social programs, the school health program, like the educational system as a whole, found itself addressing the issues of "equality of educational opportunity" and special needs of the "culturally deprived" child.[20] Because he was perceived as both culturally and educationally deprived, the handicapped child was the focus of special attention within the school health program. This emphasis on the needs of the handicapped child within the regular school program was continued and further expanded in the 1970s and had a definite impact on the role of the school nurse.

The school nurse faced increasing problems in defining her role and position within the school health program during this era. The nurse's problems in role definition resulted partly from her inability to clarify and communicate her proper role. McAleer[21] suggested that this was due in part to the traditional stereotypic view of the nurse as "a person who took orders but was not supposed to think, question or make any suggestions or decisions." The need for the school nurse to educate her co-workers in the school about her role and to exercise greater leadership in carrying out her responsibilities was emphasized.

Because of her inability to define her role, the school nurse often found herself performing highly inappropriate functions, such as arranging school bus schedules and delivering faculty paychecks.[21] Although the school nurse's lack of assertiveness in role definition resulted in conflicting expectations, research studies during this decade revealed that a significant number of school nurses held less than ideal beliefs about goals and roles for school nursing. In a survey of 614 Illinois school nurses, Fricke[22] and other school nursing proponents were understandably disappointed to learn that school nurses themselves attached more importance to such activities as record keeping and first aid than to activities within the realm of guidance, counseling, advising, and consulting. Fricke's finding that first aid was deemed a relatively important function of the school nurse was supported by Forbes'[23] study in which teachers' perceptions of the nurse's role strengthened the emphasis on first aid activities. Thus though the literature emphasized prevention activities[10] and the importance of the relationships among the nurse, child, family, school health team, curriculum, and community,[24] school nursing became increasingly occupied with more visible functions such as record keeping and first aid.

The discovery that school nurses were engaging in activities that were considered nonessential—such as record keeping, first aid, and attendance monitoring—renewed interest in auxiliary personnel in the school health program, a concept widely proposed during World War II. In addition, the concept of the school health team was being broadened to include other disciplines such as psychologists, counselors, health teachers, and social workers; the school health team was now becoming known as "pupil personnel services."[20,25] Perhaps because of the nurse's limited role perception, the addition of new professionals to the school staff threatened the school nurse's position within the school. The problem of duplicated and overlapping functions surfaced, especially between the nurse and the social worker. Since the school nurse's duties were focused on first aid and record keeping, she had less time available for follow-up activities and made fewer home visits. Thus when the social worker joined the school health team, she assumed responsibility for home visiting, an area that had traditionally belonged to the public health–oriented school nurse. Although the trend toward utilization of nonprofessional assistants to relieve the nurse of nonessential tasks was touted as a cost-effective means to free the nurse for more important activities, Tipple[10] found that such "auxiliary personnel" were serving not as assistants but in lieu of the professional nurse.

Solving the problems that now confronted and even haunted school nurses was recognized as a complex challenge. Educational preparation of the school nurse received closer scrutiny, and there were renewed efforts to encourage the school nurse to obtain at least a baccalaureate degree, preferably including public health nursing, so that her credentials would more closely approximate those of her fellow faculty members. It was also hoped that upgrading her preparation would redirect the nurse to an emphasis on preventive aspects of school health. Some authorities[24,26] advocated further preparation at the graduate level, including maternal and child health nursing, mental health nursing, public health nursing, administration and supervision, and interdisciplinary courses to be taken with the other disciplines that are part of pupil personnel services.

By the late 1960s school districts across the country were facing fiscal problems and sought ways to trim the school budget. Since the benefits of the school health program were generally long-range and less obvious and tangible than outcomes, of other school programs such as athletics, many districts began to regard the school health program as a luxury.[24] This resulted in the reduction, sometimes the elimination, of services that had once been highly valued and indispensable features of the school's program.

The position of the school nurse in the 1970s became more uncertain. Although there was talk about expanding roles, improved educational preparation and increased community health involvement for the school nurse, the budgetary cutbacks that had begun to challenge the nurse's once secure position in the school were increasing, and the school nurse found herself facing role confusion, role reduction, and loss of job security.

At the same time, changes in the health needs and concerns of the school-age child required the nurse to reorder some of her priorities. The school nurse of necessity focused some of her efforts toward problems related to chemical abuse, delinquency, venereal disease, and school-age pregnancy. Too, the national emphasis on equal opportunity for all, which grew out of the civil rights legislation of the 1960s, worked to the advantage of handicapped children. Since it was no longer acceptable to provide "separate but equal" education for them, handicapped children were now "mainstreamed" into regular classes with nonimpaired children. The school nurse became an advocate for these children, working to facilitate their adaptation within the school. The literature continued to emphasize the importance of family-centered care and the role of the nurse in promoting positive mental health through emotional support, crisis intervention, and counseling.[27-29]

During the early 1970s another educational and practice-related trend developed in school nursing: evolution of the school nurse practitioner (SNP) role. Developed in Denver in 1970,[30] the SNP concept required a minimum 4-month postbaccalaureate training program to expand the nurse's skills in such areas as history taking, physical appraisal, and developmental assessment. It was hoped that these expanded skills, coupled with the support of school administrators, would enable the school nurse to participate more effectively and responsibly within the school health program. The SNP could also be expected to have a clear definition of her role, which should help improve her relationship with other members of the pupil personnel services team.

Despite attempts to clarify and expand the school nurse's role during the 1970s, the national trend toward cutbacks in school health and elimination of school nursing positions continued. Among the reasons proposed to account for this were the following:

1. Escalation of educational costs, resulting in close scrutiny and possible elimination of all personnel and services "not directly and demonstratively beneficial to the learner";[31] the intangible and long-range outcomes of school nursing services resulted in school nurses being among the first personnel to be cut.

2. Increased employment of health clerks and school health aides who, as Tipple[10] had predicted, began to replace the nurse, resulting in fragmentation of school health services.

However, perhaps the most honest, accurate explanation for the continued reduction in the number of school nursing positions in school districts around the country was that offered by Ford[32]; her frank opinion was that nursing had failed to demonstrate to the public that its services were *worth* the cost. School nurses had not taken the initiative to "sell" the merits of their services to school boards, administrators, or even consumers. By the time the need to do so was recognized, it was virtually too late: the reductions were well underway.

PROBLEMS CONFRONTING TODAY'S SCHOOL NURSE

Today's school health programs and school nurses have reached a turning point. As noted previously, many of the problems facing school health have evolved gradually and insidiously during the past 70 years. Fiscal problems and budgetary cutbacks in recent years have been jeopardizing the continued existence of school health as a concept and a value. School health faces some weighty problems—problems that may have no obvious or widely accepted solutions. However, there are some solutions for many of these problems, and the prospects for the future of school health and school nursing are not totally bleak. In support of that last statement, this section will identify current problems confronting the school health program and the school nurse in particular, and the following section will present some recommendations for future action.

In their study of health office visits in the Galveston Independent School District, McKevitt et al.[33] noted that there had been at least 60,000 clinic visits within 1 school year. As they point out in the discussion of their study, the school health program must be considered significant by the sheer number of contacts occurring between school health personnel and school children. Indeed if these contacts with school health staff are the primary access to health care for many school children, as they likely are, then the potential impact of the school health personnel and program on these children is staggering. The opportunities for preventive and restorative health education are no doubt enhanced in the "teachable moment" in which the child refers himself to the health office with a specific (or sometimes nonspecific) health concern or problem. But despite this apparent impact of the school health program, for reasons previously cited (primarily financial), the school health program is now considered a luxury. In addition, the health services provided by the school are frequently not integrated into the overall community health plan; the result is fragmented and episodic health care for children.[34] Lack of a community-wide integrated health program can also result in duplication of services and increased costs to the consumer. A frequent example of this is the vision screening routinely done in many schools at periodic intervals. If screening efforts are not planned jointly with the health agencies and professionals to whom students may be referred, the possibility exists of disagreement regarding the criteria used for referral; the result may be inadequate follow-up of some students and an effort by community agencies to discredit the screening program. In this situation unnecessary territorial battles may begin while the needs of the school-age population are not met.

The recent cutbacks in school health generally have affected the school nurse directly. With the decrease in numbers of school nurses, the pupil-nurse ratio has increased; now there are fewer nurses to serve the school-age population. Increased demands on her time resulting from this increased pupil-nurse ratio have made it difficult for the school nurse to build and maintain effective working relationships within the school.

Instead of being assigned full time to one school, today's school nurse typically serves a number of schools on a part-time basis.

The impact of the nurse in the school health program is further lessened by the fact that school nurses have varied preparations for their role; some are graduates of diploma programs that are hospital-based and focused on episodic and acute care, while others have associate, baccalaureate, or master's degrees.[29,35] This diversity of preparation levels and experiences among school nurses increases the role confusion and dissension among nurses themselves as well as between the nurses and other school health team members. In addition, because many nurses do not have at least a baccalaureate degree, their educational preparation is not comparable to that of the teachers, administrators, and pupil personnel services staff with whom they must work. This no doubt diminishes the nurses' status and credibility. And, as discussed in the previous section of this chapter, school nurses need a broad preparation including content from both nursing and education in order to function effectively within the school setting. Nurses with less than a baccalaureate degree do not have that background. Some authorities[24,36,37] believe that preparation beyond the baccalaureate degree is important.

The problems of diverse educational backgrounds for school nurses are compounded by the fact that there are no mandated standards of practice for school nursing. The American School Health Association's *Guidelines for the School Nurse in the School Health Program*[38] have only recently been developed and are not widely known or applied. Indeed, with the variety of nursing and other professional organizations that have vested interests in children, public health, school health, education, and nursing, simply deciding who has the authority to develop

and enforce the standards may well be a sticky problem.

Another problem affecting the quality of school nursing is the wide disparity among states concerning the need for school nurse certification and the criteria to be used. As noted previously, certification became an important concern in the late 1940s. By 1976, 23 of the 50 states had mandatory school nursing certification requirements, 10 states had permissive requirements, and 4 states were in the planning process for certification of nurses.[39] More important than mere numbers of states having certification requirements, however, are the criteria on which certification is based. According to *School Health in America*,[39] a survey of state school health programs conducted by the American School Health Association, the criteria range from those that are relevant and exhaustive to those that are meaningless. An example of the latter is the state that has only two requirements for certification of its school nurses: an RN license and proof (by college transcript or test score) of knowledge of the state and federal constitutions!

Another major problem confronting today's school nurse is role confusion. In his controversial and thought provoking article "Is There A School Nurse Role?" Hawkins[1] explains the problem:

In summary, school nurses perform tasks outside the context of healer and patient, with no clear professional guidelines, under nonmedical norms, and with goals and means for achieving them largely divorced from the basic model of nursing.

He goes on to say that the school nurse is

. . . expected to provide guidance in poorly defined areas, to coordinate activities of which she is only vaguely a part, and to cooperate in health education on terms dictated largely by others.

The nurse's inability to define her role has resulted in difficulties for her within the pupil personnel services team. Thomas'[40] study of the school nurse as a member of the school health team revealed that teamwork was a major problem area for the nurse. The specific teamwork problems that Thomas identified included relationship problems between the nurse and teachers, counselors, school administrators, and parents; breakdown of staff-team communication; and lack of acceptance of the nurse by the school staff. In addition, as previously discussed, these teamwork problems have led to "turf-building," duplication of services, and overlapping of functions within the pupil personnel services team. As a result of these diverse perceptions of the school nurse role, Oda[41] believes that school nurses experience what she calls "interactive role stress."

For a variety of reasons, including lack of leadership skill and assertiveness, school nurses have been underutilized. Because of their limited, often stereotypic, perception of the roles of nurses in general, and school nurses in particular, some administrators have rigidly insisted that the school nurse remain in the school building throughout the school day "just in case" an emergency occurs. Administrators who are concerned about the liability of the school in case of accidental injury are most likely to see this as an appropriate and justifiable expectation. Unfortunately this prevents the nurse from maintaining and broadening her community relationships and thus reduces her effectiveness. For those nurses who obtained additional preparation as school nurse practitioners, restrictive role perceptions and stereotypes held by administrators can make it difficult or impossible to use these expanded skills.

Because of the confusion concerning the role of the school nurse, the nurse all too often focuses on visible functions as opposed to less tangible prevention activities. Thus first aid and emergency care, transpor-

tation of sick children, and record keeping occupy much of the nurse's time and energies. Since these functions can indeed be carried out by a trained, nonprofessional assistant or technician, it is no wonder that administrators and school boards are questioning the cost-effectiveness of school nursing services.

With the role of the nurse limited to these visible yet simple tasks, many school districts, as Tipple[10] had predicted, have begun to replace their nursing staff with school health aides or nonprofessional assistants. Indeed, if first aid and record keeping are the only health services valued within the school, this is an appropriate change to make. It is expensive to employ a qualified nurse whose salary is on the same scale as those of other faculty members if her primary function is to apply Band-aids and transcribe health records, and a school administrator would be unable to justify that kind of wasteful expenditure of the taxpayers' money. However, in districts where the school health program is well developed and where the nurse is utilized appropriately, replacement of the nurse by an aide, while it will decrease the financial outlay for the health program, will also diminish the scope and outcome of the school health program.

Perhaps the greatest problem confronting today's school nurse is the lack of research documenting the *outcomes* of her services. It is no longer adequate or prudent for the school nurse to state her belief that school nursing services "obviously" make a difference in the child's ability to learn effectively. If the nurse is to remain a viable part of the school program, she must be accountable and must be able to present *data* documenting her effectiveness.[42] To accomplish this the school nurse will in many cases need additional education in the form of continuing education or graduate work in the area of nursing research methods.

FUTURE NEEDS AND PROSPECTS FOR THE SCHOOL NURSE

Amid weighty problems such as those presented in the preceding section, it is gratifying to note that school health is about to receive long overdue assistance and support from the federal government.[43] In 1977 the Secretary of Health, Education, and Welfare stated that the government will explore the possibilities for "using schools to provide a full range of services to children and families, including health and social services as well as education." Although the specific actions to be taken remain to be seen, this commitment represents the strongest federal support for school health in recent years.

The idea of using the schools to provide a "full range of services" is consistent with the perceptions and beliefs of some prominent authors.[42,44,45] In their study of community perceptions of health problems, Newman and Mayshark[44] found that community members frequently perceive the school as "a social agency well-equipped to help communities solve many of their pressing health problems." They concluded that schools should place more emphasis on accepting this responsibility to be "community change agents." Chinn[42] believes that the school may in the future become "a practical necessity in health care delivery." Jacobsen and Siegel[45] go on to point out that for the school health program to survive and thrive it must be integrated with the *community* health program. In other words, school health program planning must be part of comprehensive community health planning. This will require close working relationships between school health personnel and community health planners and agencies. Such coordination of efforts will reduce fragmentation of care, prevent duplication of services, promote understanding among health disciplines, and result in continuous, comprehensive, and effective health care for the school population.

To combat the problem of inadequate educational preparation for school nursing and the lack of enforceable standards of practice, the American School Health Association[38] has gone on record as favoring completion of a baccalaureate degree program in nursing with concentration in ambulatory health care and community health nursing as the first step in school nurse preparation. They also recommend that the baccalaureate nurse acquire supervised field experience before beginning employment as a school nurse. Stobo[26] and Tipple[36] agree that preparation beyond the baccalaureate degree is needed. Because the goal of baccalaureate education in nursing is to prepare a basic general practitioner, acquisition of the skills necessary for the practice of a specialty such as school nursing requires graduate preparation. This poses still another challenge for the school nurse. Since there is a dearth of graduate programs in school nursing, concerned school nurses will need to make nursing educators aware of this gap. To further upgrade the quality and accountability of school nursing, the American School Health Association[38] also supports development of school nurse certification requirements at the state level, with input from all groups who will be affected by their implementation, such as nurses, educators, community health personnel, and consumers of school health services.

Obviously improvement of the nurse's educational preparation alone will not necessarily result in high-quality school nursing practice. Since the school nurse does not work in isolation, it is vital that her role be based on effective collaborative relationships. As noted earlier, the school nurse has had problems with teamwork, often finding herself at the bottom of the decision-making pyramid. Hill[34] reiterates the importance of interdisciplinary teamwork in providing comprehensive care to school-age children, and supports the movement away from the pyramid structure in team relationships toward the "pie" concept. Fricke[29] urges the school nurse to take advantage of all opportunities for team participation. She believes that the nurse should be free to align herself not only with pupil personnel services team members but also with other teams in the school and community; this broad base of involvement provides "a larger range of opportunity for meeting the child health needs and promoting positive mental health."

Igoe[46] and Ford[32] emphasize the importance of communication and relationships in improving the effectiveness of the school nurse role. Igoe[46] believes that the misperceptions of the school nurse's role may be due partially to differences in communication styles of school nurses and other health professionals as compared with those of educators. She notes that educators generally learn to communicate in a style that allows them to maintain classroom control and order. Nurses generally learn communication skills designed to elicit the perceptions of the client, which involves more "give and take." These differences in style thus may result in teachers labelling school nurses as "too easy" on students, while nurses may view teachers as authoritarian or "too strict." Whatever the differences in communication styles may be, according to Ford,[32] the improved effectiveness of the school nurse role will depend on the *relationships* she establishes and maintains. The nurse must examine her role in terms of the relationships she needs, not in terms of tasks and functions if further territorial battles are to be averted.[32]

Among the roles that the school nurse is expected to fill is that of manager of health care.[38,47] This role as manager, in which the goal is to participate in planning, implementation, and evaluation of the school health program, provides the starting point for development of all other roles and goals.[47] If she expects to be a vital and viable part of the school health program in the future, the school nurse must begin using management concepts and skills such as planning, prioritizing, organizing, directing and heading (leading), decision making, and controlling (evaluating). Development of strong leadership skills may well hold the key for the nurse's role as manager. The school nurse must become assertive in her communication style and must exert leadership in the community. This includes maintaining good public relations via the press, radio and television, and speaking and writing.[29] If needed health facilities or services are lacking, the school nurse must exercise leadership in promoting their development. Ford[32] envisions the development of school nurse leaders she calls "statesmen" "whose stature and skill in public policy arenas guide and influence the direction of the field and who speak eloquently for the nursing of children in school settings."

Within her role as manager the school nurse needs to plan her time carefully so that she can accomplish those goals that are of highest priority. As noted earlier, the purpose of employing nonprofessional assistants in the school—a concept introduced during World War II—was to relieve the nurse of tasks not requiring her skills and judgment. With the current financial crises facing many school districts and the resultant increase in the pupil-nurse ratio, employment of nonprofessional assistants or school health aides seems like an effective way to "extend" the nurse and free her time for the tasks requiring professional skill and judgment. However, when Randall, Cauffman, and Shultz[48] studied how employment of health office clerks affected the amount of time spent by school nurses following up children with health defects, they found that use of clerical nonnurse personnel did not seem to make a significant difference in the numbers of children receiving follow-up care. In other words, more helpers do not necessarily accomplish more work. The researchers speculated that school nurses may not know how to use clerical and other nonprofessional help effectively, and they may need some additional supervisory skills to improve their utilization of assistants. In contrast, Bryan and Cook[49] found in their study that when relieved of tasks not requiring her skills by employment of a nonnurse assistant, the school nurse will indeed use that released time for activities requiring her expertise; however, the extent to which she will use this release time will vary from nurse to nurse. And, as they note, the willingness of the school nurse to give up "familiar" activities that could easily be done by an assistant is a factor affecting the nurse's ability to redirect her time and energies to more important tasks.

Despite the debate about their impact and the fears that they will "take over" the school nurse's position within the school, nonprofessional assistants are necessary for and an important means of improving the effectiveness of the school nurse. To utilize such assistants effectively the school nurse must be willing to delegate all tasks that do not require her knowledge, skill, and judgment,[29] and she must be willing to provide direct and continuing supervision for the aide.[38] Delegation and supervision are critically important managerial skills that the school nurse must develop and use if she is to utilize her increasingly limited time more productively. Delegation of such activities as first aid and routine transcribing of health records can free the nurse for activities that are more satisfying as well.

Job security and satisfaction for the school nurse also require that she increase her accountability. Dickinson[50] advises the school nurse and other threatened professionals in the school to demonstrate their accountability and their contributions to the school's educational program through the use of behavioral objectives that describe how the student is changed as an outcome of nursing intervention. By writing and evaluating objectives in terms of changed consumer (student) behaviors rather than in terms of the process and intervention used by the nurse, the outcomes of school nursing services can be more readily evaluated. This would enable the nurse to "sell" herself as an indispensable part of the school health program.

Another vitally important means for improving the school nurse's accountability and documenting her effectiveness is nursing research. Chinn[42] decries the lack of substantive research justifying a specific model for school health or school nursing services. She goes on to warn that:

Unless it can be demonstrated that application of nursing skills in the educational setting enhances or promotes learning in the educational process, justification for retaining the traditional school nurse is certainly questionable.

While it is clearly the responsibility of the school nurse, as it is with all other professional nurses, to carry out research, the variation in school nurse preparation levels undoubtedly means that some (perhaps many) school nurses will need additional education in research methods before they can design and implement meaningful studies. This is an area that merits closer attention from nursing schools. Research is needed in virtually all aspects of school nursing practice. Ford[32] stresses the need for epidemiological and demographic studies to identify and prioritize the health needs of target populations within the school and community, from which strengths can be identified and delivery of health services can be planned. Chinn[42] identifies a need for research documenting the appropriateness of the teacher as a "detector and referral agent for health problems," the relationship between health problems and school performance, and the role of the school nurse as it influences educational goals. Igoe[46] emphasizes the need for research to demonstrate the importance of health maintenance, preventive health care, and education to an increasingly skeptical American public.

The SNP role is an innovation that holds a great deal of promise for the future of school nursing. With intensive preparation in such areas as growth and development, physical assessment, family dynamics, health maintenance and education, and community resources,[51] the SNP will bring a broader knowledge base to the school health program. With proper administrative support including availability of nonnurse assistants for completion of functions requiring less skill, the SNP can enhance the effectiveness and efficiency of school nursing services. Qualified school nurses should seek this additional preparation, which may require petitioning schools of nursing and public health to develop an SNP program.

Ultimately the viability of the school nurse will depend on her ability and willingness to expand her educational base, clarify and interpret her role, establish and maintain effective team relationships, delegate "familiar" yet nonessential tasks, and improve her accountability through nursing research and the use of behavioral objectives. She will need to understand and employ planned change strategies as a systematic process for upgrading her preparation and practice. Most important, despite doubts that others might have concerning her competencies and contributions, the school nurse must continually "sell" herself and her service to survive this fiscal era in which health is not necessarily viewed as an essential component of education.

REFERENCES

1. Hawkins, N. G.: Is there a school nurse role? Am. J. Nurs. **71**:744-751, 1971.
2. Gardner, M. S.: Public health nursing, ed. 3, New York, 1936, The Macmillan Co.
3. Gardner, M. S.: Public health nursing, ed. 2, New York, 1926, The Macmillan Co.
4. Wales, M.: The public health nurse in action, New York, 1941, The Macmillan Co.
5. Troop, E. H.: Sixty years of school nurse preparation, Nurs. Outlook **11**:364-366, 1963.
6. Committee for the Study of Nursing Education: Nursing and nursing education in the United States, New York, 1923, The Macmillan Co.
7. Palmer, M. F.: Essentials of school nursing, Public Health Nursing **36**(5):221-222, 1944.
8. Randle, B. B.: Wartime essentials in school nursing, Pub. Health Nurs. **35**:482-483, 1943.
9. Dilworth, L. P.: Essential school nursing in wartime, Pub. Health Nurs. **36**:443-447, 1944.
10. Tipple, D. C.: Misuse of assistants in school health, Am. J. Nurs. **64**:99-101, 1964.
11. Wilson, C. W.: Health counseling in schools, Pub. Health Nurs. **37**:436-438, 1945.
12. Grant, A. H.: Nursing: a community health service, Philadelphia, 1942, W. B. Saunders Co.
13. Freeman, R.: Developments in education of public health nurses for school health work, Pub. Health Nurs. **37**:454-455, 1945.
14. Dilworth, L. P.: The nurse in the school health program, Pub. Health Nurs. **41**:438-441, 1949.
15. Sellery, C. M.: Where are we going in school health education? J. School Health **20**:151-159, 1950.
16. Brown, E. S.: The role of the nurse in the school health program, J. School Health **22**:219-224, 1952.
17. Cromwell, G. E.: Teammates: teachers and school nurses, J. School Health **22**:165-171, 1952.
18. Dierkes, K.: The nurse in a generalized program, J. School Health **21**:131-135, 1951.
19. Wallace, H. M.: School health services, J. School Health **29**:283-295, 1959.
20. Cromwell, G. E.: The future of school nursing, J. School Health **34**:43-46, 1964.
21. McAleer, H. S.: What's new in school nursing, J. School Health **35**:49-52, 1965.
22. Fricke, I. B.: The Illinois study of school nursing practice, J. School Health, **37**:24-28, 1967.
23. Forbes, O.: The role and functions of the school nurse as perceived by 115 public school teachers from three selected counties, J. School Health **37**:101-106, 1967.
24. Fredlund, D. J.: The route to effective school nursing, Nurs. Outlook **15**:24-48, 1967.
25. Dukelow, D. A.: 1960 White House conference recommendations on school health, J. School Health **30**:334-341, 1960.

26. Stobo, E. C.: Trends in the preparation and qualifications of the school nurse, Am. J. Pub. Health **59**:669-672, 1969.

27. Crosby, M. H., and Connolly, M. G.: The study of mental health and the school nurse, J. School Health **40**:373-377, 1970.

28. Brand, M. L.: The potential of school nursing in the '70s. In ANA clinical sessions, Detroit, 1972, American Nurses' Association.

29. Fricke, I. B.: School nursing for the '70s, J. School Health **42**:203-206, 1972.

30. Igoe, J. B.: The school nurse practitioner, Nurs. Outlook **23**:381-384, 1975.

31. Coleman, J., and Hawkins, W.: The changing role of the nurse: an alternative to elimination, J. School Health **40**:121-122, 1970.

32. Ford, L. C.: The school nurse role: a changing concept in preparation and practice, J. School Health **40**:21-23, 1970.

33. McKevitt, R. K., Nader, P. R., Williamson, M. C., and Berrey, R.: Reasons for health office visits in an urban school district, J. School Health **47**:275-279, 1977.

34. Hill, A. E.: Educational preparation for school nursing, J. School Health **41**:354-360, 1971.

35. Marriner, A.: Opinions of school nurses about the preparation and practice of school nurses, J. School Health **41**:417-420, 1971.

36. Tipple, D. C.: Academic preparation of school nurses: implications for the school nurse practitioner, J. School Health **32**:311-315, 1962.

37. Coakley, J. M., and Parker, J. M.: Education of nurses for school nursing, Am. J. Nurs. **65**(11):84-87, 1965.

38. American School Health Association: Guidelines for the school nurse in the school health program, Kent, Ohio, 1974, The Association.

39. Castile, A. S., and Jerrick, S. J.: School health in America, Kent, Ohio, 1976, American School Health Association.

40. Thomas, B.: The school nurse as a member of the school health team: fact or fiction? J. School Health **46**:466-470, 1976.

41. Oda, D. S.: Increasing role effectiveness of school nurses, Am. J. Pub. Health **64**(6):591-595, 1974.

42. Chinn, P.: A relationship between health and school problems: a nursing assessment, J. School Health **43**:85-92, 1973.

43. Califano, J. A.: School health message, J. School Health **47**:334-335, 1977.

44. Newman, I. M., and Mayshark, C.: Community health problems and the school's unrecognized mandate, J. School Health **43**:562-565, 1973.

45. Jacobsen, R. F., and Siegel, E.: Comprehensive health planning in the space age: the role of the school health program, J. School Health **41**:156-160, 1971.

46. Igoe, J. B.: Bridging the communication gap between the health professionals and educators, J. School Health **47**:405-409, 1977.

47. Wold, S. J., and Dagg, N. V.: Philosophy, roles, and goals of school nursing. In Wold, S. J.: School nursing: a framework for practice, St. Louis, 1980, The C. V. Mosby Co.

48. Randall, H. B., Cauffman, J. G., and Shultz, C. S.: Effectiveness of health office clerks in facilitating health care for elementary school children, Am. J. Pub. Health **58**:897-906, 1968.

49. Bryan, S. S., and Cook, T. S.: Redirection of school nursing services in culturally deprived neighborhoods, Am. J. Pub. Health **57**:1164-1176, 1967.

50. Dickinson, D. J.: School nursing becomes accountable in education through behavioral objectives, J. School Health **41**:533-537, 1971.

51. Joint Statement of the ANA, DSN/NEA, and ASHA: Guidelines on educational preparation and competencies of the school nurse practitioner, J. School Health **48**:265-268, 1978.

SUGGESTED READING

American School Health Association, Subcommittee on Educational Preparation for School Nurses of the Committee on School Nursing: Position paper: philosophy and goals for school nurse educational preparation, J. School Health **45**:409, 1975.

16

The dying patient

Joy K. Ufema

EDITOR'S NOTE: The chapter following is unique in style and content. We feel that any attempt to make it conform with the other chapters would dilute the power of its message and detract from its highly personal directness. Ufema speaks with the courage and wisdom born of daily encounters with death as a fact of life. Share in the humanity and humaneness of her words.

No one can teach you anything; however, you can learn from someone. By developing an open attitude toward growing from all experiences and by acknowledging value through interaction with other humans, you can learn lessons that will benefit you professionally and in your development as a sensitive, caring person.

This chapter is my sharing with each of you what I have learned from my experiences with terminally ill patients.

It will be helpful first to explore why we do not like death. One obvious reason is the suffering that we associate with dying. I think we in nursing have a twofold dislike of death: one, we have been taught to be stoic, never to divulge a diagnosis to a patient, never to let him know that we know, either with our words or our emotions—as though we are fearful of losing our professionalism; two, the patient's dying reminds us of our own mortality. For example, you go into a 20-year-old leukemia patient's room and plunk down his

tray and whisk yourself right back out with a sigh of relief that you did not divulge to him any news about his condition, either with your words or your expressions. Unfortunately you did divulge it by your behavior; nurses give cues to the dying. You gave that patient a message that you were uncomfortable in his presence and did not wish to remain in the room. You were fearful that he might grab you by the hand and ask, "I'm dying, aren't I?"

The reminder of our own mortality makes us give a second cue to the patient: "If you know you're dying, I want you to act like you don't, so that I will be more comfortable." This is a difficult thing to ask of the dying because they are at their peak of vulnerability. But we put a second burden on them: "Don't make me uncomfortable. I didn't want to be assigned to you three days in a row; it's not my fault I'm here. I really don't want to be here. Oh, I'll give you a good bath, administer treatments, and rinse your sore mouth, but please, please, protect me from this. I'm not ready; I don't want to think about it, let alone talk about it. I'm only 20 years old; I'm not interested in dying or in any of the pain it takes to die." Our discomfort is not the patient's problem, but ours—and it is a problem we must deal with: 20-year-olds do die; and so do 10-year-olds and so do 2-year-olds.

When I go to see a patient I have these feelings, too. They signal mortality—the thought that I am not going to get out of this world alive. Some days this is very frightening to me. I think it is good for us to start being honest and open about our feelings about death. Sometimes when I go to see a patient I do not know what to say, and I think it is all right to be that totally honest with him, too. It is not unusual for me to visit a person—perhaps one close to my age—an astute, intelligent individual who definitely knows the score and who intimidates me a little. Is he going to judge me on my interviewing skills? Gradually I am learning to be more comfortable with this person. If I do not know what to say, I simply tell him this, and assure him that I care enough to stay. I just do not know if I have the right words at this time—and so I ask him simply if he wishes to share what it is like being seriously ill. If he chooses not to share, I support that right. We forget that this person has never died before. He has no experience on which to draw. Therefore any way he chooses deserves my support. I do not believe in setting criteria for someone else's life, much less his death.

Just because this person happens to be a patient in your hospital and you happen to be assigned to him that day, please do not set criteria for him just to make you comfortable. It is his turn now, and eventually it will be your turn. What I have found successful for me is to find out from every *patient*, not his mate, not his doctor, and not his chaplain, but from the person himself, what it is that he

wants, from whom he wants it, and when. In a sense I am loading him with the correct ammunition. The following two examples are true. The patients were very beautiful people whom I loved, with whom I became emotionally involved, and with whom I cried.

Joan was a 42-year-old with carcinoma of the trachea. She had been in the hospital about 3 weeks, and her condition was rapidly deteriorating. Her husband, perhaps preoccupied by his wife's serious illness, had a minor automobile accident one Saturday. I was called out of my garden by someone at the hospital to say that Joan was hysterical. She did not believe the nurses who told her that Harold was perfectly all right, that he was just shaken up, but not seriously injured. This antagonized her breathing. She kept gasping for breath and got herself in a real frenzy. In my Mickey Mouse tee shirt and wranglers, I ran into the hospital, grabbed an oxygen tank, attached Joan's leader to it, and took her upstairs to see her husband. He was all right—bruised a little, uncomfortable, but not seriously injured. Joan felt much better. I took her back to her room and got her settled in for the night. We thought that Harold would be in the hospital for about 72 hours for observation. Unfortunately, he had a few other minor upsets, so he remained institutionalized for 4 or 5 days. During that interim Joan's roommate was discharged. Because of a shortage of beds, Joan and her roommate were on a gynecologic unit. I suddenly had the idea that perhaps Joan would like her husband as her roommate.

I asked her, "Would you like that?"

Gasping, she looked up, "Yes, could you do that please?"

"Of course," I said.

I went upstairs to see her husband, told him that Joan would like to have him in her room, and asked him how he felt about it.

"Oh, I'd like that. That would be just fine."

He was excited about it, too. However, the supervisor of the gynecologic unit, when asked, said, "Absolutely not."

It seems to me we reach a point in life when no one has the right to make a decision for another person. This is what I felt the supervisor was doing; and she thought she had the right to do it because she was "the supervisor." I discussed the problem with the head nurse and told her that Joan and Harold both wanted this arrangement. The head nurse felt that it would be very bad for both patients: Joan might die in Harold's presence—a possibility that had not occurred to me. I ran back upstairs and asked Harold how it would be for him perhaps to awake and find Joan dead. I was totally honest with him, told him this was a possibility; Joan was critically ill and could die very shortly. What did he want? He said that it would not be pleasant for him, but that he had planned to take Joanie home anyway. He said, "Oh hell, Joy, let's do it."

Waiting for no one else's permission, I scrubbed Harold's bed, transferred him to the seventh floor, and got Harold and Joan settled together in their own room—both of them beaming. Tempers flared throughout the nurses' station, and I probably was not my usual ethical self. I lashed back at all of the nurses, reminding them that Harold was not really a great imposition for them; could they not do something for the patient who was dying? Could they not make it easier for her "turn"? I checked on Joan and Harold the following morning. Joan had gone to sleep that evening at 7:30 and had slept until 7:30 the next morning, with no analgesic or hypnotic. She and Harold had shared breakfast that morning, and she had retained it for the first time in 3 weeks.

This is when you know that you are doing it right. You simply ask the patient what he wants. In doing this, however, you must have the courage of your convictions to follow through in helping the person get what he wants. If you do not care enough, if you ask it flippantly and are not willing to follow through all the way, regardless of the outcome, do not bother asking. I cared enough about Joan to risk my job, to risk everything to do what she needed at this time. It is not necessarily the responsibility of the nurse to the patient—it is a responsibility from one human being to another. We do not always have our white dresses on, we are not always "the nurse," but we are always the human being.

Rose also was 42; she was dying of ovarian carcinoma. I entered the room and found a 60-pound, cachectic, yet still beautiful, school teacher. She and Jack had been married for years and had had no children of their own. On the wall were many little cards made by her third graders with crayons or a little charcoal—get well wishes. How ironic; she would never get well. Rose and I talked for quite a while, and finally the question came up, "What do you want now?"

She said, "Joy, I've got to get home. I've got to get home."

Rose was having projectile vomiting and very bad diarrhea every time something entered her mouth. She was on morphine every 2 hours.

"Rosie, if you go home now you'll probably die sooner than if you stayed here in the hospital. How do you feel about that?"

"I know, Joy, but I've just got to get home."

She had discussed this briefly with her husband, so it was no surprise to Jack when I called him and related her words. He said he was interested in caring for her, although it would be a difficult task.

"Oh gee, Joy," he said, "You know I can't cook, and Rose is having that awful vomiting; I don't know if I can do this."

I helped Jack get nursing care for Rose in his home, and he quit work. One Saturday afternoon, after teaching Jack how to give morphine injections, I got Rose all set in the ambulance; I gave her a big hug and kiss goodbye, along with a bouquet of daffodils stolen from the nurses residence. I called a week later and asked Jack how Rose was.

He said, "She's doing pretty good. I made some homemade vegetable soup and she kept that down."

"I'm pleased, Jack. I called to tell you I have another prescription for the morphine. We were giving it to Rose frequently in the hospital, so I'm sure you're about out of it."

He asked, "you mean that shot medicine in the brown bottle?"

"Yes, Jack, I'm sure it's about empty, so I have another prescription."

"But I haven't used any of it."

I became very anxious that in our haste to get Rose home I hadn't taught Jack well enough. She definitely needed this pain medication. I was afraid that the poor lady was lying there in dreadful abdominal pain and Jack was not astute enough to know that she needed the medication; yet it was right there. He interrupted my thoughts.

"Joy, you know the hospital bed you got us?"

"Yes."

"Well, I don't have Rose in it."

"Where do you have her, Jack"

"Well, she's sleeping in . . . in our bed."

"Where are you sleeping, Jack?"

"I'm sleeping in our bed, too."

I asked, "Are you hugging that girl?"

He answered, "Yes."

This was why Rose had needed no morphine: her hugs were her injections. I was to go up the river to see the family the following Monday. Sunday morning, about 10 o'clock, Jack called and told me that

Rose had just died in their bed. He was there with her, holding her hand.

He thanked me for helping them to be together and he said, "You know, Joy, that was really hard to do—hard to watch her waste away like that. But I want to thank you for helping me. I found out what she wanted and I did it for my Rosie, didn't I?"

"Yes, you did, Jack."

Jack also had the courage, because he had some friends like the visiting nurse and myself who cared to help him help his Rosie, the way his Rosie had wanted it.

I called about a month later to check on him. He was packing to go out West to do some hunting and fishing with his brother-in-law. Jack was all right. He missed Rose; sometimes he still cried about her. But he felt it was okay for him to spend the summer hunting and fishing. He was not being a recluse with the drapes drawn, holding old photographs of Rose. He was not up at the cemetery hovering over her tombstone, guilty about her having had to die in a nursing home. He was okay. This dying was difficult, but I think we as human beings can help each other to do this. It is a simple idea—just ask the patient what he wants, from whom he wants it, and when.

How did I become a death and dying specialist? I was working as a graduate nurse at Harrisburg Hospital 1 year after graduation and, like most recent graduates, was full of idealism. I was working on a urology floor, the 3 to 11 PM shift, and many of my patients were terminally ill. I was very busy doing preops and postops and irrigating TUR setups, giving hypnotics and charting—the whole procedural routine—always promising the dying person that I would return to be with him in a moment. Moments would turn into hours. Four or five times throughout the year I returned to the patient to find him dead. Obviously the patient had died alone.

I decided that since our society has not changed the rules of dying, and we still put dying patients in institutions, I would go to my director of nurses and ask her to change this within our system. I told her I felt that care of our dying patients was abysmal, that we cared only for the living and were interested only in those patients we could save. I asked her to make me responsible for the care of all the dying patients in Harrisburg Hospital. I asked her to free me from my duties as a staff nurse so that I might choose my case load and choose with whom I would spend the time I felt appropriate. To my surprise, she said yes—probably because of an experience she had as a student years before in Philadelphia. There patients were placed in large wards, and when an individual was close to death, the staff would be pressured by the other patients: "Please get him out of here. I'm trying to get better from my operation and I'm not interested in watching this gentleman die in front of my eyes. It's not very conducive to healing." And so she understood what I was talking about, and she agreed to my proposal. I simply changed jobs, though maintaining my usual salary as a staff nurse for the hospital.

I do not know where I learned it, but I cared only for the dying. Obviously I am a product of the same society of people who are uncomfortable with the dying, but I have an affinity for them. I much prefer sitting, holding their hand, talking with them, and wiping away their tears to being an emergency room nurse doing cardioversions and ordering all sorts of machinery and medications.

I think it is an important thing in your career—to study who you are and whether you are the kind of nurse you want to be and then perhaps to seek areas that are most satisfying to you. Somewhere along the line I developed the skill of being a good listener; this comes through genuine caring. It is not that I have to interview a patient and write a verbatim report; it is that I genuinely care that she's 28 years old with a 2-year-old child and that she's dying of breast cancer. My interest is sincere; therefore I think I listen well. Perhaps listening is not the art we think it is. I think it is something that develops in us when we start feeling good about getting involved emotionally with another human being. For years nurses have been taught to stay away from involvement. However, I have been emotionally involved with many of my patients and it has not inhibited my care; perhaps it has heightened it by making me more perceptive. Knowing all of these little things about the patient, I really care; perhaps some patients I have loved. This means that when it is 4:30 in the afternoon and I am supposedly off duty, caring does not stop. This does not mean that I am at the hospital 24 hours a day or on call all that time, constantly with the dying. I need my rest and relaxation and have no qualms about taking it. What it means is that I learn to know my patients. They are other human beings who are touching my life at this time, who come in and out of my life, and I am interested in learning from each and every one of them.

Maybe it is my philosophy of life, that each of us, no matter who, has something to give to the other. Too often we associate that giving with materialism or intellectualism. I have learned a lot from farmers and seamstresses and mothers. I have learned well because I wanted to learn. I have learned to listen well because I want to listen. Caring is very risky: it is painful to be emotionally involved with a patient and then to watch that patient die. It is risky and painful to realize that the patient associates you with death and now that she is moving from the area, she cannot and will not come to say the last good-bye because she needs so much to pretend she is not going to die and every time she sees you it is a reminder of death. But I would not have given up the emotional feelings I had about her or my involvement with her, even knowing that in the near future she would hurt me. Death is like life, with no guarantees of beauty, no guarantees of laughter and of sailing through.

My words in this chapter are not meant to be guidelines for you; they are simply to show you how to do it. If my way is effective for you, very good. I cannot teach you how, but I think you can learn—an important difference. The learning can come by my example. I cannot give you sentences and words that are appropriate in every instance; it never works that way. If I can help you become a little more comfortable with death, especially with your feelings about your own death, then you suddenly will become more comfortable with the death of others—which in turn will make you a little more comfortable with your own; it is a beautiful circle. After reading this, you probably will not always have the dynamic interviews that are found in Kubler-Ross' books. I certainly do not. They are rare. You will not interview dying persons like Dr. Ross does or like Larry LaShan does, or I do. What I am hoping to accomplish is to help you to be as comfortable as possible with death; then your discussions with your patients will simply flow; they will become natural. You do not have to be a psychiatric clinician or a chaplain or a supervisor. All you have to be is a caring human being. And you have the extra advantage of nursing skills; so you can give a luxurious bath, soaking hands and feet in the basin; and you can give a comforting back rub, and stroke the patient's hair, and give soothing mouth care to the dying instead of giving them percodan. It works; I know from experience. My philosophy is not to treat pain but rather to prevent it.

Again, I work by taking cues from the patient himself. Who better knows what he needs than the person who is dying? I usually discount other people's messages because they are often incorrect. They are simply projections and interpretations of what others believe is best for this person, without their having taken the time to ask him.

When I receive a referral—from a physician, nurse, pastor, or stomal therapist, whomever—I enter the patient's room and always sit on his bed. I do this because our discussions often elicit tears, and tears mean "I need you to hold me." I cannot hug the patient; nor can I even touch him if I am sitting in a chair beside the bed; I have noticed that patients tend to move over on their bed to allow room for me to sit down. I think we all need to be touched. However, if the patient gives off cues such as pulling his hand away from mine or turning his back to me, I definitely understand that this means he is uncomfortable with my demonstrativeness. I am very sensitive to his discomfort and share with him how his behavior makes me feel. This gives him an opening cue to say how my behavior makes him feel. I respect him as a human being and respect his right to do this his own way. I accept him where he is. Again, no one has the right to change someone's style of living, let alone the way he dies. So we sit and talk. I ask each patient, each day if he feels like sharing today. Would he like to talk about it? Most patients say yes, and their feelings pour forth—sometimes feelings that they could not share with their wife or their children because they sensed in these people a difficulty in handling the dying situation.

I have noticed how beautiful dying persons are, and I hope I can be as kind and sensitive to others as they are. I have never seen anyone who is dying use another person. I have never seen a dying patient deliberately make another person uncomfortable. I think that when we are dying we put out antennae to pick up cues as to whether someone is uncomfortable with us and whether they are sincere enough to listen. When dying persons get cues that others are not willing to listen, I think they take it easy and carry most of the burden inside. They thus maintain a facade that other people ask them to maintain.

We do not maintain the facade in so many words; rather we do it by plunking the tray down and running out of the room, or we do it by visiting Uncle Frank and telling him he looks wonderful when he knows in his heart he can no longer even hold a water glass by himself. Uncle Frank picks up the cue, and thinks, "You just wouldn't be comfortable if I told you how terrible this is, how sad it is that I can't make my hands work for me anymore."

Many of these patients, I find, are in depression. And perhaps rightfully so. When we have a problem and it stays inside, it doesn't get any better but tends instead to fester and emerge in different ways, in many disguises.

Perhaps the patient gets angry and says, "This food is lousy."

Now we who belong to the "family of the hospital" get defensive: "Well, this is the best we can make around here. This isn't the Hilton, you know."

This is an unkind retort. Many times we do not say it but we communicate it. By having lunch with many of the patients, I act as part-time dietician. I know the food is really lousy—things like very dry pork chops to patients who are receiving 5-FU. These patients have severe stomatitis, but no one thinks about that. So I go out to the kitchen and make a nice warm bowl of cream of wheat and serve this to the patient, and then help him to eat it slowly and gently. This helps his depression for the moment because what it says is, "I can't control your dying. I can't stop that and neither can you. But I can with your help control how you live—because you're not dead yet. So what do you want?"

We talk and I find out that the patient's wife knows the condition, the patient knows his condition, but neither of them wishes to share it with the other. They want to play this game of protection. Usually the motive is kindness, but it is a difficult game for both.

My job is to encourage families to be honest and open with each other, to discuss this final trauma that has affected them all, and to remind the others in the family that once death closes in on them they are never quite the same. I think we all realize that at one point in our life we are going to die. We delude ourselves into thinking that it will not be until we are 98 years old, and it will be with a myocardial infarction, that leaves us dead on the bathroom floor in seconds. It seems that this would be a delightful way to go, but we might miss the loving that can be brought out through the dying process. And I have seen that kind of love, which perhaps was not there before. I have seen patients literally use this final experience to grow by, to become closer. I think that this is a beautiful death. This is when I really feel like I am learning from the patient and perhaps he is setting an example. But again, it means listening to him and then helping him help himself.

I think we probably die fairly consistently with how we have lived. Perhaps we cope with the stress of death the way we have coped with stress throughout our lives. The gentleman who usually drinks, gets "stoned" after he has trouble at work and loses his job, or when he is about to lose his wife and family probably, when he is told that he has a serious illness and that the prognosis is poor, will go out and get drunk. The gentleman who consistently has worked at the steel mill and saved a little money for the kids' college education now discovers he has leukemia. He probably would not snitch the $5,000 savings account and run off to the Bahamas, but would be consistent and cope as he has done through all his life, struggling along day by day—a little chemotherapy here, a little radiotherapy there, clinging tenaciously to life at all costs. This might be helpful, although it is difficult because until we finally get to the dying person, we know very little about him and oftentimes have too little time to find out.

Please remember that the hospitalized patient is a very different animal from what he was before he was admitted. He has brought with him a lot of problems. These problems are grossly complicated by his having to wear Johnny gowns instead of a Mickey Mouse tee shirt. He has to eat meals when and how you say he must; he is not used to doing this. He does not want his shower at 8 o'clock in the morning. These are added stresses for the dying person. We demand much of him, particularly compliance. The fellow who in the past consistently has gone along with what the whole group wanted copes with this and adjusts rather well to institutionalization.

I am sure that you are all familiar with the executive who has the myocardial infarction. We catch him sneaking to the bathroom. We forget what he is saying and what he is doing. Instead we become judgmental; we accuse him of not caring about his own health and its possible outcome regarding his family. What we are really doing is making a judgment about him, and it is very unfair. All he is doing is trying to gain control. Once he becomes a patient in the hospital he has already lost a great deal of control. He can no longer shower when he wants to or eat meals when he wants to. He can no longer decide things for his own life. He has a team of physicians, interns, residents, and nurses—all of whom feel that they know what is best for him. Medically they do.

It is such a fine line in medicine, dealing with ethical and medical decisions. I find that in death and dying we get deeply involved in ethics—perhaps most often when the patient wants to go home, specifically to die. In order to find out what the patient wants, we need to ask him. In asking, we need also to clear the air by giving him some of the facts about his diagnosis as well as some of the facts about his prognosis. I believe that every person has the right to know these facts, so that then they alone can make the best decision for themselves. I can perhaps anticipate some of the questions that come up after one of these discussions, one of which is "What do I do about physicians who do not want their patients to know their diagnosis?"

For the most part I have found these patients to be men with rather domineering wives. The decisions of the physician not to divulge this information to the husband most often comes from his wife. It is she who is having difficulty coping with this serious illness—the idea that her husband is not going to be alive for very long, and her dilemma about how she is going to handle this. I sometimes get angry with physicians for allowing someone else to take control and make decisions for their patient. Sometimes I think physicians too feel uncomfortable about this, and it becomes a good escape hatch for them. They do not know it, but it is the more difficult game to play. Many times I hear reasons such as "Well, I don't think he can take it," or "I'll wait till it gets really bad and then I'll tell him."

Helen was a lovely patient who had carcinoma of the pancreas. I saw her several days before Christmas. I told her who I was—a special nurse dealing mostly with patients who have cancer, and trying to help them and their families deal with this new difficulty in their lives. She thanked me for coming but said that she really did not need me, that the physician had removed the entire pancreas and so got the tumor. I knew this to be an untruth or partial truth but remembered that patients many times hear only what they want to hear or only what they can hear at that time. I decided to clarify the whole thing by speaking with her surgeon who was sitting at the nurses' station writing her discharge. I told him exactly what Helen said and asked him if this was indeed what he had told her.

"Oh, yes," he said. "You know I can't take the whole pancreas out, but I don't want to ram this down her throat."

"But she's packing to go home right now believing that everything is all right."

"Yeah, well she'll be back. You know, this is real bad. She'll be back and I'll tell her then."

So unbeknownst to all of us until Helen did come back 3 weeks later, she went home to elderly parents living in a farmhouse where there was no inside toilet or furnace. Helen was extremely weak, and so were her aged parents—too weak in fact to even open several cans of soup for their meals. Christmas came and went and so did the New Year. And the following week Helen came back to the hospital, quite jaundiced and preterminal. I saw her and we talked a little.

She said, "I had a very bad fever when I was at home, and I think it settled in my bones, don't you, Joy?"

"No, Helen, I don't think that's what it is"; I suspected bone metastasis.

We talked a bit more, and she said, "You know when I had that high fever I took a lot of medicine and that medicine has settled in my bones. That's why I'm having a lot of bone pain and can't walk. Isn't that what you think, Joy?"

"No, Helen, I don't think it's the medicine either." I did not give her information she did not ask for. I simply answered her questions truthfully. If she had said, "He didn't get it all did he, Joy? It's spread to the bones hasn't it?" I would have answered "Yes."

Several days later it was Helen who said, "I can't walk anymore. I think he lied to me."

No one went into Helen's room and told her she had a terrible malignancy with gross metastasis. No one told her she was dying. It was not "necessary"; and it was cruel. In fact, it served no purpose, except possibly for the nurse who sometimes came out of the room feeling rather haughty that it was not she who was dying at that time. Now that you have read these words, do not, I repeat, do not, go bursting into a patient's room anxious for an interview and blurt out things he does not ask for.

Helen became very angry with her physician. He had not lied to her, he just had not told her the whole truth. And so it was her last Christmas—and not a very pleasant one. She had a sister in Philadelphia whom she did not get to see again.

I stayed with Helen late Friday. I realized that she was dying, and wondered if perhaps her parents might like to see her for the last time. I went to the desk to make the phone call. Who was sitting there but her surgeon, who had not visited her for the entire time of her second admission. He kept sending in the resident, and he would write appropriate notes.

I said to him, "Helen's very close to death. I'm going to call her parents."

He answered, "Oh, I don't think you should do that at all. They're elderly and they could have a heart attack up there in that farmhouse all alone."

"Well, I guess that's their decision to make isn't it?"

I called. Helen's mother cried when I told her how serious things were. I asked if she wanted to see her daughter alive, one more time.

She said, "Of course."

They had a neighbor who could drive both of them to the hospital; I promised to stay until they got there late that night.

I left a note with the nurses that they were to call me before Helen died. Saturday morning about 5 o'clock I got a call. She was having Cheyne-Stokes respirations and was very close to death. I hurried to the hospital, stayed with her, and held her hand. Her pulse was 168. Helen died. She never got the chance to say or do the things she had wanted to do. And that, fellow nurses, is an injustice. This is what I want you to fight for.

Fight, not as nurses, not as chaplains, but as human beings for another human being who happens to be touching your life at this time. This I believe is a responsibility we have toward each other. Perhaps this responsibility has been missing for too many years. We are simply their nurse and we shut off that fact at 3:30. Life isn't a turn on–turn off deal. Helen's physician never got to hear from her what a "ripoff" she thought he pulled. Fortunately, I told him; perhaps he will not do it to another patient.

When I go to see patients like Helen they frequently push me up against the wall with heavy questions—good questions—questions like: "I have an apartment that I am going to move into, but should I bother?" "I'm going to be discharged on Saturday. My husband and I used to go dancing a lot. Will we go dancing again?" These loaded questions are asking about life and death. If we develop good listening abilities we will hear what the patient is saying; we will be able to read between the lines and clarify these statements.

We are careful not to give a flippant, "Oh, sure, why don't you go ahead and move?" Rather we explore the reasons why the patient is asking these questions. Does she

have some feelings that perhaps she is not quite well enough to go home? What does she really mean?

"Do you mean to go home to die?"

"Yes."

And so for patients who keep asking and asking, I sometimes go back to the physician for clarification. "Doctor, Helen really wants to know what's going on. Did you tell her?" If the doctor answers, "I didn't think she could handle it," I will retort with, "Well, she's definitely asking questions now. When can I tell her you'll be in? How do you feel if I sort of talk with her some more and answer her questions truthfully?"

Sometimes physicians will go along with this and say, "That's okay." Yet you sometimes find physicians who say, "His wife doesn't want him to know, and I don't want you telling him either. There'll be hell raised around here."

You can try being patient with that physician for a few days. You can try to find the patient's wife during visiting hours or at her home or work, explain how you have talked with the patient, how he is very interested in knowing what is going on; and that is suspicious anyway. With what little health remains, the patient should perhaps do some things that he identifies as important for him during the remainder of his living. Then I think nothing can prevent our going in and listening to this patient—and answering his questions truthfully.

Again, it is our professional duty not to go bursting into the patient's room shouting, "Hey, you've got cancer. I know how to talk about that. Do you want to talk?" This is not at all appropriate. The important thing is to give this patient his choice of sharing his feelings if he wishes. If, after several requests of the physician to go to see this patient and to be totally honest with him, the physician does not comply and the patient is still asking questions, I have on several occasions given the patient the exact diagnosis he has asked for.

"Tell me the name of it."

"Is it important for you to know?"

"Yes, what is the name of the disease?"

"It is lymphosarcoma."

"Okay, thanks for telling me that."

Then I stay with the patient and we talk. I give him the opportunity to ask more questions. Many times the questions are not clinical or physiological but more in the context of "Does that mean I won't ever work again?"

"Yes. You are seriously ill with the disease. But maintain some aspect of hope in that your doctor has discussed with you chemotherapy or cobalt, and you have several options available. I will tell you the pros and cons of these options if you wish to have more information."

So I believe this patient will not jump out of the eleventh-story window. He is starting to "get a handle" on things. He has the name of the disease, the names of drugs, and some channels open for choices. The decision is now his to make. I find this a rather stable person who perhaps dies fairly well. By "well" I mean he dies "his way." Dying "his way," I think, means consistent with what he believes. He is the fellow who has probably been a fighter all his life and wants to fight death. This also is his right.

Please remember that we do not have the right to go into a patient's room and demand of him an easy death in order to make us more comfortable. We do not have the right to withhold pain medication; if the patient is in our hospital, there are some things we can do for him. Some persons might say "It might be well and good for you; you're a specialist and you have all the time you want." This is definitely an asset, but I have had some very good death and dying interviews that took place in a matter of 7 minutes. This is because both the patient and I talked very

openly and honestly with each other. We did not dance around and use all the "pretend" words. We got right down to the nitty gritty. I answered all of his questions truthfully, while I touched him and looked him in the eye, and remained for as long as he needed me, which was about 4 minutes.

I know nurses are busy passing out medication or doing preops, but we can have lunch with the patients and we can take coffee breaks with them. What is the matter with staying at the hospital half an hour after work? It is this involvement that I ask of you. It really is a gift, you know, and it is in the giving that we receive. Maybe it is legitimate, your trying to pass out medications to 35 patients. I have done it. It counts if you even take 1 minute to enter that patient's room, sit just for a moment—just a moment—and tell him that you want to be with him but you really can take no longer than you already have; that you do care about him and you want to listen; that now is not convenient, but that you will try to get back. This is what counts. It matters very much. All you are doing is being an honest human being.

We sometimes say, "I can't tell whether to believe him. His words tell me one thing but his actions tell me another." Our behavior as caring human beings should be consistent with our behavior as nurses. So my words are, "I really do like you, you know; I'll try to get back." Sometimes we even make promises. "Oh, I'll be back," and we never do get back. If it is a question of believing someone's words or his behavior, I think behavior is what we can justly believe.

For example, a person may say to you, "I really think I'm a good friend to you." But one day you ask "Will you give me a hand carrying these groceries up to my apartment?" The answer then becomes, "No, I can't do that right now." His behavior tells you that perhaps this is his true feeling for you. Words can be shallow and people can lie. But their behavior does not always lie.

Many times it takes only a few words, because your behavior can tell the patient that you really care and that you really want to be there. As you enter the patient's room go directly to him; stay close to him; physically touch him. Ask him what are some things you can help with?

I am sure you all have been taught about the little old lady who is lying in her bed, back to the hall, when you enter her room to answer the light: "What is it now, Mrs. Jones?"

"Well, I want the bedpan."

"You just had the bedpan."

"I know, but I need it again."

"Oh, all right."

And so you give her the bedpan, and she might urinate just a little. Then you abruptly rip the bedpan from under her, slam-banging into the bathroom. You wash your hands, but you do not bother to give Mrs. Jones a paper towel with soap on it to wash her hands. And then you hustle and bustle out of the room.

As you get to the door she says, "Nurse?"

"Yes, what is it now?"

"Could you please get me a drink of water?"

"Oh, all right."

You give her the water and plunk the pitcher down and do not hold the straw for her. She has had a stroke and cannot quite get the straw to her mouth. Meanwhile you stand there tapping your toe. "Can't you hurry up and slurp this down?" She does finally, and you rush to get to the door again.

"Nurse?"

"Now what is it?"

"Could you fix the window blind?"

What is she saying? She is saying, "Stay with me, please. I'm frightened."

Sometimes the dying are saying that too. But they are so wonderful about it. Unless they are desperate, they will not impose on

you because you have given all these cues that you cannot handle it, or that you do not care. Regardless of your words, if you are not comfortable and your words are true, both things click and then you are good. The dying check for cues; you get points if you sit on the patient's bed, if you look him in the eye, if you touch him, if you are honest, and if when you say you will be back you do come back. All of this is again that commitment of wanting to give and wanting to care. It is all very simple, you do not have to work at it. As you are learning from this textbook, I would want you all to ask yourselves repeatedly, "Who am I, and what am I good at?" "Do I want to be a nurse?" "What kind of nurse do I want to be?" "What kind of person do I want to be?" Write some of these things down and try to be consistent in your learning and your growing with who it is you want to be. In that quest, find out what you do well and then do it. It might not be working with death and dying. It might be a nursing in the gynecology clinic. But if you do it well and you feel good at it, continue to do it. Continue to feel good inside about your work.

I read a book called *I Ain't Much Baby but I'm All I've Got* by Jess Lair. In the book Jess talks about how we can tell when we are doing things well and how we can tell when we are pretty good with ourselves. He talks about that feeling of having a warm tummy. Other people call it a conscience. I want you all to get close to that warm tummy.

It is like giving nursing care to the patient who can tell no one how good it is—perhaps the comatose, dying person. It is very interesting. Studies have been done that show nurses usually try to isolate the patient who is terminally ill—the patient who is still alert and able to threaten them with the words, "I'm dying, aren't I? Please hold me, I'm awfully afraid." When the patient goes into a coma the nurses suddenly respond and work out their guilt for having isolated the patient by giving him excellent physical nursing care. It is safe now. He can no longer talk about it. We continue to give good mouth care, to administer back rubs, and to turn the patient every 2 hours because we know in our hearts that it should be done. There can be times when you are tired, when you have had a heavy assignment, and when you do not like death anymore. Perhaps you are tempted not to give the mouth care or not to turn the patient; who will know? He cannot tell. But you will know. And you will notice that you do not have that warm tummy feeling. That's a bad sign. Then what may happen is that we will forget what that warm tummy feels like and we will continue to do things like putting blue pads over messy sheets or not brushing the patient's mouth and teeth, or not turning him every 2 hours. We think we have gained some time or whatever; and all we have gained is a guilty conscience. What may happen then is that we know we are not doing it the way we should be doing it. We get to feeling a little guilty and perhaps do not look in the mirror as often as we should. We do not engage in as much introspection as we should, and we end up being a mean nurse.

Please stop and make sure that this does not happen to you. You have control of yourself. Find out what you do well and do it. Maintain your integrity and the patient's dignity. Sometimes you will get tired; however, and that is legitimate.

I was working with Mr. Snipes, a patient who had a carcinoma of the lung. He must have experienced several pulmonary emboli; he was bleeding badly, bringing much blood up from his mouth. We had changed the sheets three or four times that day. It was very hot and I was very tired; I had not had lunch, and I was not listening. Perhaps we can say that it is legitimate not to listen when you are hot and tired and you have been working hard on a patient. It was late; and I wanted to get home. I had blood all over me and everything else. Finally I got Mr. Snipes cleaned up for the last time. He took my hand, thanked me for the nursing care, and told me to take care of myself. I was very tired and was not listening. I said, "Okay, thank you, I will. Bye." I rushed to the door. When I got there, I suddenly realized what he was doing. Even though I was tired, I remembered to listen. I was slow in getting it, but I got it.

I went back to his bed again and took his hands and said, "You're saying good-bye aren't you?"

He said, "Yes."

"Then perhaps you won't be here tomorrow."

He answered, "No."

He knew that he was dying, that he could not make it through the night. I thanked him for what he had taught me and I told him something truthful, that I liked him. I thanked him for being my friend and for all I had learned. We said good-bye. The next morning it was not necessary for me to go to M-5 to find the empty bed, but curiosity took me there and the bed was empty.

Perhaps there is a lesson here, and that is, we should listen well, and we should tell people whenever they do nice things for us.

If Mr. Snipes had made it through the night, and if I had returned the next morning and found him alive as I have done with several patients, I would have rushed into his room and said, "You didn't die. You're still here."

And he would have answered, "Yes."

We would have sat and talked a little more. We would have had a little more time together; nothing would have been lost. We would not have lost anything by saying good-bye yesterday, even though he did not leave until tomorrow.

Sometimes when patients turn very bad, very quickly, someone—anyone—must get the patient's family there. You can tell the family, "The patient has drastically turned for the worse, and if you want to come in, I will be here when you get here." Some patients rally and that is wonderful; you still have lost nothing. The family was there in case the patient died. He did not die, not for a few days. We called the family back a second time and that time the patient did die. But we lost nothing. The family was very grateful.

There are times in our listening when we

have to make a judgment. Please have the courage to do that. I think now that in nursing our role models are changing to delightful instructors. They are not stiff-starched, stoic people who forbid us to cry, who force students to hide in the linen closet with their tears. Now, I think we have good role models. I am trying to be one myself. When I take little furry kittens into the pediatrics department I act as a role model; 3 weeks later one of the nurses on the floor brings in a puppy. I bring in a beer and a pizza to a 20-year old and 3 days later one of the staff nurses also goes out and gets him a beer and pizza, this is a good role model. I hope that it has been good for me because I have learned from it and I hope I can teach others. I am not being the death and dying nurse; I am simply being a patient's friend. This means I am helping him to help himself.

I think we should discuss one more area: giving patients permission to die. I had a lovely lady who was dying and doing quite a good job of it—rather painfully, but we were keeping that under control. She was close to death, had ovarian carcinoma with a terrible ascites, and her husband was having a problem with her dying. He did not want her to die, obviously. She was a good Christian woman, an active member of the church. Her husband, however, had not joined the church and was having a little problem dealing with that. He had some anger with God for taking his wife, who was a lovely person and never hurt anyone. Why should it be she? It was unfair. The patient, Mrs. Weller, sensed from her husband's words of encouragement that she did not have his permission to die.

He said, "Eat this pudding I brought you" and "Nurse, could you get her up in a chair?" when she was very close to death. While tapping her face he would say, "Come on, Mother, wake up, wake up."

Mrs. Weller was tired of being ill. We discussed this at great length. She believed in God and she believed in prayer. The congregation of the church had prayed for her to get well. After 2 or 3 days of this, she seemed to reach a plateau. She did not go on to death, but she definitely did not get better. She told me she thought perhaps the people's prayers should be changed, that when God was ready to take her He would, and that she was ready to go. Perhaps God's Spirit could touch her husband and let him know that she could not carry on any longer. Well, I relayed the message to Mr. Weller. Mr. and Mrs. Weller talked together about this, and within an hour Mrs. Weller died. I think she felt that she had my permission; the physicians had talked with her and had decided to give no more chemotherapy; but it was the husband who was the final person to give her his permission. She had not had it and it was important to her.

Please remember that in counseling families permission is an important thing. Sometimes it is hard to discern between giving a patient permission to die and asking the patient to give up prematurely. It is allowing the patient to know you are there to back him up in the fight for life as long as he wants it, but when he is finished fighting you can accept it in him, no matter when it is or why.

Do a few simple exercises to help you become more comfortable with death and dying. Take a piece of paper please, a rather large piece, and answer the following three questions quickly, the moment you have finished reading each one.

What color is death?
How big is it?
What does death sound like?

In the next exercise please complete each sentence beginning with 10 endings of your own.

Dying is like . . .
When I die . . .

This can be a difficult exercise. When you start getting into the fifth and sixth sentences and you have to do some brain racking for some good things, you are finally getting into the true nitty gritty of your thoughts. Please do this exercise and try to get all 10 or even 15 sentences completed.

Now turn your paper over, horizontally, and draw a straight line. On the left of the line write birth; on the right of the line write death. Somewhere along that line put an "X" where you are right now. Do not feel bad if you think you are young. Everyone puts the X close to birth. The point I am trying to make is that since none of us knows for sure where we are on that line, neither do we know for sure where the X is. It is important every day, too, to say "I love you."

Perspectives on the future of community health

☐ Part Four is made up of two chapters that are pertinent to current issues and concerns of community health care delivery—the issue of change processes in the delivery of primary health care and the concerns around the necessity for the evaluation of nursing care delivered in public health nursing agencies and home settings by the community health nurse.

Andrus and Mitchell describe and discuss changes needed in the system of primary health care delivery. They point out that primary care should be the center of patient management within the health care delivery system. Instead, primary care is relegated to a peripheral role without sufficient funding and manpower. To provide more effective primary health care, the nation's academic health institutions should concentrate more funding on educating a new generation of primary health care professionals.

The final chapter, contributed by Davidson, offers the community health nurse specific guidelines for action in evaluating the nursing care provided in public health agencies or in home settings. To provide more effective and more systematic care, nurses must learn to identify concurrent and retrospective review criteria; this will enable them to evaluate the outcome of their practice.

17

Change processes in primary care

Len Hughes Andrus and Ferd H. Mitchell, Jr.

The pressures for change in primary care are building today across a broad and contested front. Public demands for more responsive primary health care are creating tension and stress in the established delivery system. The growing importance of the self-care movement is strengthening the role of the individual in his or her own care and challenging the formal medical system. Legislators are moving to change existing programs and create new ones. Reimbursement agencies, planning organizations, private and public providers, and educational institutions are working to develop new plans and programs. However, despite these activities, the system has not been changing at a rate consistent with the pressures, which indicates large adjustments yet to come.

This article addresses some of the primary care change processes now taking place and discusses possible directions for the growth of primary care in the near future. Emphasis is on describing a possible transition route from the primary care model, which is predominant today, to an alternative one that utilizes team practice. We have concluded with a dis-

cussion of the problems and issues facing primary care and the American health care delivery system today.

THE PRIMARY CARE SYSTEM TODAY

Currently most primary care in the United States is provided through self-care,[1,2] as illustrated heuristically in Fig. 9. This is a testimonial to (1) the inherent strength of some individuals who have resisted a broad range of conditioning efforts to make them emotionally dependent on the present health care system and (2) the failures of this system to provide access for many others who have been conditioned to seek formal health care. The formal system is characterized more by inappropriate than by appropriate examples of primary care. For example, statistics of the American Medical Association[3] indicate that only 25% of the practicing physicians in office-based practices in this country are in the primary care fields of general practice, family practice, general internal medicine, and general pediatrics. The other 70% of physicians, who identify themselves as specialists and subspecialists, must derive their income from the handling of primary care cases or from secondary and tertiary care. In contrast to the physician distribution, it is estimated that over 75% of all patient care could be most

Portions of this material were presented at a 1976 Symposium on Health Planning and Primary Care sponsored by the American Association of Comprehensive Health Planners.

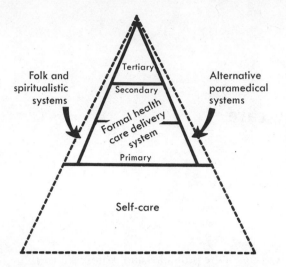

Fig. 9. Levels of health care. Folk and spiritualistic systems include shamans, medicine men, Faith healers, psychic surgery, Christian Science, and so on. Alternative paramedical systems include naturopaths, herbologists, chiropractors, meditation, behavior modification, hypnosis, homeopathy, encounter groups, and groups for smokers, alcoholics, weight control, and so on.

appropriately handled at the primary care level.[4] The distorted mix in the fields of practice has also promoted the inappropriate use of facilities; a prime example is the growth of nonurgent emergency room care because the patients have nowhere else to go.[5]

CHANGE PROCESSES TODAY

The processes of change in primary care are today advancing on several fronts—in the shift to self-care, in the trend toward new legislation, in examination of reimbursement policies, in planning activities, in the effort to try new provider practice patterns, and in pressures on educational institutions. The changes that have occurred are still limited compared with the mounting public forces, indicating that larger changes can be expected in the future.

Shift to self-care

Despite the fact that many people have abdicated their personal care to the formal medical systems, most care is still self-care. The return to and the growth of self-care is a current health trend that we believe will lead to better primary care. The public is examining alternatives to the present formalized health care system, and a movement is underway to take more responsibility for one's own health care as well as to participate in medical care decisions. Interest is increasing in metaphysics, parapsychology, organic food, natural childbirth, clean air, ecological factors, and behavioral programs. The media are full of health-related items. Self-care books, such as those by Senhart[1] and Samuels[2] are big sellers. Sociologists, economists, and philosophers are criticizing and questioning the present health care delivery system from broad perspectives.[6-9] Within and without the health care industry many questions arise as to whether the present physician-controlled medical care system has the commitment to deliver personalized comprehensive health care, for which primary care is the central focus.

Legislative trends

New legislation is needed to allow for innovation in the structure of our present delivery system. Legislators are concerned not only with the geographical and specialty maldistribution of providers but also with the increasing costs of secondary and tertiary care. They are starting to set priorities as to how much of the gross national product will be spent on the health care dollar. The increasing amount of legislative support for primary care is evidence not only of a financial concern but also of a new awareness by legislators that a more humanistic, consumer-oriented delivery system is possible and desirable.[10-13]

Reimbursement policies

Because of the present financial constraints on primary care,[14] reoriented reimbursement policies are needed. We must financially encourage preventive care, ambulatory care, continuity of care, and comprehensive care in opposition to in-patient, fragmented, subspecialty care. For the last few years, health maintenance organizations (HMOs) have been promoted as a new reimbursement philosophy that can change incentives through prepayment. However, in their present form HMOs have had only a limited impact on overall health care. History suggests that prepaid group practice with coverage for all will never grow without a supportive environment in terms of financial incentives, facilitating laws, and active community participation. HMOs now operate against the prevailing incentives provided for fee-for-service specialty medicine and against legislation that preempts community control of reimbursement. New incentives are needed to encourage the development of laws, regulations, benefits, and controls that will help bring about needed reimbursement reforms. Unfortunately the changes in this area have been slow.

Planning

As the Health System Agencies and other planning groups address the issues discussed in this article, they are faced with programs that interrelate political, social, and economic issues in a personal way for every individual. The unique features of health care planning require a broad definition of the planning process and require planners to become interacting participants in the developmental activities of their communities; otherwise, plans become library materials rather than blueprints for change. A new planning emphasis on primary care can be effective only if individual planners will get intimately involved in the new primary care programs. Whether planning for new clinics, new private practices, new educational programs, new financial incentives, or new organizational approaches to primary care; planners who do not implement are impotent.

Provider practice patterns

In meeting the nation's primary health care deficit, the original emphasis was on defining needs in terms of physician shortages and seeking solutions through increased physician production. Dissatisfaction with the physician production rate led to the development of nurse practitioner (NP) and physician's assistant (PA) programs that were originally designed as another mechanism to extend the productivity of the physician. The training of nurse practitioners and physician assistants grew dramatically between 1970 and 1978; the number of programs in the United States has increased from less than 20 of each program to 198 nurse practitioners and 57 physician's assistants programs; and the number of graduates has increased from a few hundred to 12,000 nurse practitioners and 8600 physician assistants.[15] A major evolution of the nurse practitioner/physician's assistant concept has accompanied this growth. Although nurse practitioner and physician's assistant graduates were originally conceived of as physician extenders, they have outgrown this concept to challenge some of the most sacred tenets of medical practice. They are stimulating intense role examinations among physicians, nurse practitioners, physician assistants, nurses, aides, and other general team members.

Educational institutions

Coupled with the above, there are strong pressures being brought to bear to create change processes in physician education. Here in the bastion of the existing delivery system, the pace of change is at its slowest. But even here change is taking place, and at an ever-accelerating rate. One major action in medical education has been the establishment of the family practice movement. The Millis[16] and Willard[17] reports of 1966 were important points in the family practice movement. During its first decade of existence the number of family practice residencies has grown from 30 to almost 350, and the number of residents in training or trained has grown from zero to over 5400.[18]

The parallel growths of family practice residencies and NP/PA practitioner programs have not automatically led to structural changes in the delivery system or to the development of the team concept of care. However, these programs have provided the nurturing ground for new perspectives of existing problems and have stimulated innovative efforts in creating new models of care. This is all a part of the change process.

Who should provide primary care?

Primary care must include access and availability as well as the opportunity for first contact with the patient. It consists of the following components: (1) diagnosis and treatment of common ailments; (2) psychological evaluation; (3) socioeconomic appraisal; (4) preventive medicine; (5) patient education; and (6) total patient management. It is generally accepted that the physician, who has had the most extensive training in pathophysiology, is the person best equipped to diagnose and treat disease processes. The question as to what kind of physicians are needed (family physicians versus internists for adults and pediatricians for children versus a combination of these specialties and others) is a current burning academic and political issue. But they are only a part of a larger issue. A serious basic question is Does a physician always have to make the diagnosis and prescribe the treatment? What about nonphysi-

cian, primary care practitioners such as nurse practitioners or physician's assistants? And if these new health care professionals can participate in the diagnosis and treatment of common ailments, then what kind of practitioners should deliver primary care? Should they be physician's assistants and nurse practitioners who are generalists; Medex;[19] primary care associates;[20] or family nurse practitioners[21]? Or should they be specializing midlevel practitioners such as pediatric associates or pediatric nurse practitioners; adult nurse practitioners; geriatric nurse practitioners; or OB/GYN nurse practitioners? The same question must be asked at a different level: If these midlevel practitioners can participate in the diagnosis and treatment of disease, could not some of the more basic first-level health care professionals such as licensed vocational nurses or community and family

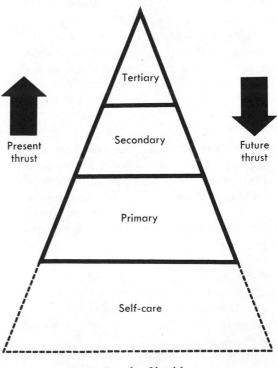

Fig. 10. Levels of health care.

health aides participate in physical assessment and therapeutic skills? Again, consideration must be given to generalists versus specialists such as emergency room technicians, family planning aides, health educators, psychiatric aides, and so forth. And finally, one is faced with the question How many of the functions that constitute the diagnosis and treatment of disease could be done just as well by the patient?

The emphasis, we believe, should be on more self-care; we believe in reversing the trend that has made people more attitudinally dependent on increasingly specialized health care providers and on the concommittant technology. The present thrust of the formal health care delivery system it toward pulling people into and through primary care toward secondary and tertiary care. We think that the thrust of the future should be toward self-responsibility (Fig. 10).

DELIVERY SYSTEM OPTIONS

It is obvious that there are many approaches to health care. The question is Which of these are the most effective, efficient ways of providing comprehensive health care, of which primary health care is a major component? In the past the approaches have been dictated mainly by economic factors and by the special interests of the professional providers.

Supermarket approach

Supermarket approaches are based on the premise that the patient, through an organized triage and referral system will find his or her way to the appropriate care counter. The client enters the system either personally or by reference or through a telephone call, and any complaint is referred to the group involved in such management (that is, one has a sore throat and may be referred directly to the ear, nose, and throat department). Modifications of this approach are present today in large medical centers and large multispecialty groups. The problem with the supermarket approach is that it is based on the following premises: (a) patients' ailments can be categorized; (b) they can always be sent to a specific and appropriate department, specialty, or subspecialty clinic; and (c) this departmentalization will provide high-quality care.

The limitation to this system is that it is difficult to categorize illnesses (for example, a backache). Most people have multiple complaints and ailments rather than a simple presenting illness, and some present with a complaint unrelated to the real reason for their consulting the health care system. It is a provider-oriented approach, which is based on the "pigeonholes" or "diagnosis-decision trees" of the medical model; it is not a holistic approach to the patient. The approach of the worried well and the worried sick[22] implies clear-cut differences in conceptualization, which uses the medical model to separate the mind and the body. It is a fragmented, time-consuming, and expensive approach, and in its present form it underutilizes many of the special skills and talents of primary care providers, while at the same time it overutilizes subspecialists for the tasks that do not require their expertise as consultants.

Primary physician model

Considerable controversy exists over the selection of the most desirable primary physician model for team care. Some groups, especially in academic centers,[23] recommend internists and pediatricians (with or without obstetricians) as the primary care physicians. Petersdorf[24] has recommended internist and pediatrician teams in urban areas and family practice physicians in rural areas. Parker[25] advocates the family physician as the preferred selection for all teams. We are advocates of the family practitioner as the key provider on all primary health care teams. In addition to having the general practitioner's broad knowledge of diseases and episodic treatment, the physician who specializes in family practice has training in the behavioral sciences and is dedicated to the concept of total comprehensive health care. As a generalist, he or she can treat both sexes and all ages; moreover, his experience with the family as a social group permits him to recognize the influence of family dynamics on individual illnesses. This is simply not possible if each family member were to go to a separate specialist. We believe, for reasons stated below, that the family physician working in a team setting is the most effective and efficient model provider of primary care.

Multispecialty approach

Group practice includes fewer than 20% of the nonfederal physicians engaged in patient care, excluding interns and residents.[3] These data are clouded by the fact that not all of the multispecialty groups are involved in primary health care. A majority of the groups have three to four physicians, which limits the spectrum of care that can be given by such a multispecialty approach. The prevailing complaints by patients are that they lack continuity and a personalized relationship with providers. Large multispecialty groups such as Kaiser-Permanente are now turning toward the course of the Health Plan of Puget Sound;[26] they are shifting toward an emphasis on primary care. Many multispecialty groups are faced for the first time with taking care of the entire population and thus are developing departments of family practice.[27]

The problem in the multispecialty models is a dual one: there are not enough people trained and committed to primary health care, and there is a lack of institutional commitment to the facilities, support functions, and numbers and kinds of providers needed to deliver high-quality primary health care.

Team approach

Primary health care teams are made up of providers who have close, continuing interpersonal relationships and who work toward the goal of providing comprehensive care to a common group of patients. The composition of the team may include persons from three levels of training—the physicians, midlevel practitioners (physician's assistants or nurse practitioners), and health workers or aides. This group makes up the so-called nuclear primary health care team. As discussed above, pediatricians and internists with or without obstetricians are sometimes proposed as the physician team members; however, it is hard even getting internists to work with internists or pediatricians to work with pediatricians. Parker[25] advocates the family physician as a key provider in the primary health care team; being a generalist, the family physician can act as a backup for treatment of both sexes and all ages. The goal of most family practice programs is to turn out a generalist physician who recognizes that the maintenance of health and the prevention of disease or illness requires cooperation not only with other physicians but also with nonphysician team members.

The roles of nonphysician primary care practitioners in a team practice should remain as flexible as possible so that the team can adapt to the patients it serves, the community, and the interests of its provider members. The key to good team operation is a specific definition of responsibilities for all members and a close spirit of cooperation shared among team members. Much national effort is presently going into learning about team dynamics and team building and into the development of written protocols that define how all midlevel providers will relate to the team physicians.[28]

The nuclear health care team, consisting of a physician, nurse practitioner or physician's assistant, and family health worker aides, may not by itself represent a stable model that its perpetuity rests precariously on the presence of one physician. An ideal minimum-sized primary group practice team may be composed of several teams, each consisting of one family physician, two midlevel practitioners, and four aides. With three nuclear teams the group can work as a unit and also cover each other on nights and weekends. Such a practice could handle 60 to 80% of the health care needs of a community of 8000 to 10,000.

PROBLEMS AND ISSUES
Competing forces

It has been popular during the past decade to describe the health care industry in the United States as a "nonsystem." But this point of view is an illusion. The present form and function of health care are a resultant solution to competing social and individual pressures in our society where action is rationally related to pressures. We have a system, then, that follows prescribed political and economic rules and relationships; what we do not have is a system that is rationally designed to deliver health care!

Planners are faced with the challenge of conceptualizing rational system changes that can be implemented in the general environment set by the political and economic factors. Through a process of planned change, the system can evolve in new directions. Within the present system there are many competing factors generated by public expectations and demands, provider expectations and demands, goals of the educational institutions, profit-oriented drives by groups in the private sector, self-enhancement drives by nonprofit organizations, and political determinations by legislators and government agencies. The individual patient can easily be lost and alone among the collisions of so many strong groups. In contrast to these forces, there is an increased emphasis on the growth

of new systems of care based on self-healing and self-understanding and the concept of the individual being a key member of his or her own health care team.

Issues in team practice

The major issues in team practice pivot around the concepts of independence, dependence, and interdependence. In a strict legal interpretation, the physician is responsible for all activities of the team, and all team members act under his specific direction. However, the team concept requires that the members of the team move from strict relationships of independence and dependence and be able to function in relationships of interdependence. The legal status of nonphysician primary care practitioners has undergone a great change during the past decade. Most states now have laws that facilitate the use of midlevel practitioners in a setting that is adequately supervised by a physician. Requiring the geographical presence of the physician with the physician's assistant, as in California, was an earlier blow to the potential for remote rural coverage by physician's assistants. Legislation has just been passed reversing this requirement.[29] Fortunately this geographic restriction has not applied to family nurse practitioners, and we have many examples of rural sites being served by nurse practitioners, with telephone backup by a physician in another location.[30] Practice has preceded law by many years, although much of what we and others have done may not have been sanctioned according to the technical definitions of the law.

Another major legal issue today is the one of malpractice. The physician's malpractice fees have been either not affected or raised only $200 to $300 per year as a result of adding a midlevel practitioner. In addition, many physician's assistants and family nurse practitioners carry their own malpractice insurance through their various professional organizations at relatively low fees. However, the present malpractice costs do seriously limit the services that are provided by primary care practitioners, especially in a high-risk state like California. More and more rural physicians have stopped delivering babies because of the high malpractice rates,[30] since obstetrical care may increase the family physician's insurance from $4,500 to $21,700.* Better solutions to the malpractice problem must be found in order not to penalize primary care teams or inhibit their functioning.

Reimbursement issues

Our current delivery system maximizes reimbursement to the traditional hospital-based specialities and subspecialties. There is broad third-party coverage for inpatient care and for ambulatory care provided through the emergency room setting but very limited coverage for ambulatory office visits or preventive care that can reduce hospital admissions. The primary physician and the primary care team are often the only ones whom the public must pay directly, and office calls are usually either not covered by insurance or are reimbursed by the insurance company at a disproportionately low rate. Patients may complain about office costs since they do not perceive the higher costs that they are paying through third-party payors for emergency and inpatient care. Expansion of specialty care and instrumentation account for much of the high costs of medical care in the United States.[32]

Experience has shown that nurse and physician's assistants are financially viable if reimbursement rates are the same for all providers of a given service, and the very existence of the team concept is dependent on this approach to reimbursement.

---

*Rates for the northern California area, the Travelers Insurance Co.

Architectural issues

Much of the past architectural design of the private office has been based on the solo practice model, and as such these facilities are also based on the physician model with little provision for skilled team awareness by the designers. Design can limit patient flow and minimize the opportunity for patient education in group meetings. As attitudinal obstacles toward team care have been reduced, architectural limitations have become a major deterrent to team effort. Private and government architects are now redesigning primary care facilities since form can indeed determine function.[10,33]

Quality of care issues

The general attitude of physicians in the past, whether private practitioners or professors, has been that nonphysician care means second-rate care. Although this attitude persists, it is waning. Many studies have indicated that the quality of care actually increases with team effort.[34] The primary health care team is distinguished by its focus on comprehensive health care as a goal. Included in this care are an understanding of patient management, patient education, and the ability to link with secondary and tertiary care to provide the best in total patient care.

CONCLUSIONS

We have developed a distorted health care system without a coordinated port of entry. Instead of making primary care the center of the patient's management and of the system, we have relegated primary care to a peripheral role; it is inadequately housed, inefficiently funded, and understaffed. Our efforts at health education should be directed toward educating the patient rather than toward deifying technologies or mystifying the health care industry. Our educational institutions must assume a greater responsibility for the numbers, kinds, and distribution of its products.

We cannot provide primary health care without the commitment of this nation's academic health care institutions. We must train a new generation of primary care physicians, nurse practitioners, and physician's assistants (for whom we believe the family practice model to be the best) who are committed to the wholistic, humanistic approach to primary health care, which means providing education for physicians and allied health care professionals in a team setting, facilitating team utilization, and providing continuing education for group professional satisfaction.

Changes in primary care and the health care delivery system are occurring at a slow pace as decades of resistance are being overcome by intense public pressure. Because of the long period of time during which the system has been unresponsive to public need, we can expect an escalation of the change process in the future. With active participation by the public and planners, our present system can evolve into one that can more adequately serve the people.

REFERENCES

1. Senhart, K. W.: How to be your own doctor, New York, 1975, Grosset & Dunlap, Inc.
2. Samuels, M., and Bennett, H.: The well body book, New York, 1973, Random House, Inc.
3. American Medical Association: Profile of medical practice, 1977 ed., Chicago, 1977, The Association.
4. Rabin, D. L., and Spector, K. K.: Ambulatory care in the community: implications for medical education, paper presented at convention of the Association of American Medical Colleges, San Francisco, 1976.
5. Andrus, L. H.: The emergency room ripoff, J. Fam. Pract. 2:147-148, 1975.
6. Fuchs, V. R.: Who shall live? Health, economics and social choice, New York, 1974, Basic Books, Inc., Publishers.
7. Lee, P. R., and Silverman, M. R.: Pills, profits and politics, Berkeley, 1974, University of California Press.
8. Illich, I. P.: Medical nemesis: the expropriation of health, London, 1975, Calder & Boyars, Ltd.
9. Ginzberg, E., and Oston, M.: Men, money and medicine, New York, 1970, Columbia University Press.
10. Health Professions Education Act of 1976, PL 94-484.
11. Health Maintenance Organization Act of 1973, PL 93-222.
12. Health Planning and Resources Development Act of 1974, PL 93-641.
13. Experimental Health Manpower Pilot Projects, AB 1503, Ch. 1350, California Statutes.
14. Blendon, R. J.: The reform of ambulatory care: a financial paradox, Med. Care 14:526-534, 1976.
15. Data from American Nursing Association and Association of Physician's Assistant Programs.
16. Millis, J. S.: The graduate education of physicians, 1966, Council on Medical Education, Chicago, American Medical Association.
17. Willard, W. R.: Meeting the challenge of family medicine, report of the Ad Hoc Committee on Education for Family Practice, Council on Medical Education, Chicago, 1966, American Medical Association.
18. Data from Academy of Family Physicians.
19. Smith, R. A.: Towards solving the great training robbery, Pharos 33(2):44-52, 1974.
20. Primary care associate program syllabus, Palo Alto, Calif., 1976, Stanford University.
21. Andrus, L. H., and Fenley, M.: Assistants to primary physicians in California, Western J. Med. 122:80-86, 1975.
22. Garfield, S. R.: Evaluation of an ambulatory medical-care delivery system, N. Engl. J. Med. 294:426-431, 1976.
23. Alpert, J. J.: Graduate education for primary care: problems and issues, J. Med. Educ. 50:123-128, 1975.
24. Petersdorf, R. G.: Highlights of the April 1976 Board of Regents Meeting, Bull. Am. Coll. Physicians 17:6-7, 1976.
25. Parker, A.: The diversions of primary care: blueprints for change, Sun Valley, Idaho, April 1973, Sun Valley Forum on National Health.
26. Schwartz, M. E.: Maintaining health on Puget Sound, Fam. Plann. Perspect. 6:72-73, 1974.
27. Primary care: who'll do it in a multi-specialty group? Group Pract. 22:26-29, 1973.
28. Runyan, J. W.: Primary care guide, New York, 1975, Harper & Row, Publishers, Inc.

29. State of California Administrative Code, Section 1379.22.

30. Andrus, L. H., and Fenley, M.: Educational evolution of a family nurse practitioner program to improve primary care distribution, J. Med. Educ. **51**:317-324, 1976.

31. Health manpower study of selected health professions in California, Sacramento, 1976, Secondary Post Graduate Education Commission.

32. Perlman, L. V., Maham, T., and Wallace, C.: Primary care, Intern. Med. Residencies **136**:111-113, 1976.

33. Wagner, C.: Ambulatory care facilities required for academic programs in primary health care and family medicine and dentistry, Washington, D.C., 1977, Bureau of Health Manpower, U.S. Department of Health, Education, and Welfare.

34. Spitzer, W. O., et al.: The Burlington randomized trial of the nurse practitioner, N. Engl. J. Med. **290**:251-256, 1974.

18

Evaluating home health care

Sharon V. Davidson

Methods employed for the evaluation of professional nursing services in a home health care agency setting are fluid and in an evolutionary state. There is no right or wrong method of evaluating quality care; the important factor is that some type of methodology is being effectively used for improving care.

Evolutionary state? Yes, especially when you consider that among the first efforts to assess the adequacy of medical and nursing care and its impact on recipients can be found in *Notes on Matters Affecting the Health, Efficiency and Hospital Administration of the British Army* by Florence Nightingale in 1858.[1] Since 1858, professionals have seen many different approaches to assessing quality assurance mechanisms in nursing.

The profession developed a check list to assess the quantity and licensure of personnel, based on the philosophy that an adequate staffing pattern of registered nurses assured quality patient care. A check list also evaluated whether or not simple tasks were completed.

Patient care conferences were introduced as an informal method for evaluating nursing services with revisions of written nursing care plans. This conference method requires that each group of nurses rediscover deficiencies,

and it lacks identification of patterns of care.

Criteria evaluations approached the evaluation of nursing services by establishing criteria statements to assess rendered care; for example, A new diabetic patient self-administers insulin correctly three times before discharge. With these types of statements medical records can be evaluated for compliance or deficiencies.

Phenuff developed extensive criteria evaluation through a check list system that could be used to evaluate completion of nursing services and is available with a specific form for home health agencies.

Retrospective audits were developed by the Joint Commission on Accreditation of Hospitals to review medical care and then were adapted to review nursing care. A retrospective audit is a closed chart review that evaluates the health, activity, and knowledge of a discharged patient and is useful in determining patterns of nursing care of both a correct and a deficient nature. Retrospective audits can reflect structure (the buildings, organizations), process (the procedure for care), or outcome (the desired effects of care).

Program evaluation and clinical record review were introduced into the evaluative activities of a home health agency as a requirement of the Medicare Law. Program evaluation is concerned with policy, administration, and clinical record review. It is also known as the 60-day continuous review, which assures that established policies are followed in providing services.[2]

Standards for practice in the major clinical areas of nursing were developed and released by the American Nurses Association. The standards have attempted to identify the nurse's responsibility for monitoring the quality of care and services.

The major force for quality care has been the formalization of quality assurance programs in health care, mandated in Public Law 92-603—the 1972 amendment to the Social Security Act—which provided for the creation of professional standards review organizations (PSROs).[1]

This law mandates that all care covered for payment under federal programs, independent of the delivery system, is subject to review by the PSRO. Therefore, the skilled nursing services provided by a home health agency and paid for by Medicare are subject to review. The question is what type of review?

The PSRO Program Manual emphasizes that the Professional Standards Review Organizations are expected, over a period of time, to provide evidence that non-physician health care practitioners are involved in the following activities: (1) development and ongoing modification of names, criteria, and standards for their area of practice; (2) development of review mechanisms to be used for peer assessment of the performance of non-physician health care practitioners; (3) conduct of health care review of non-physician health care practitioners by their peers; (4) working with established continuing education programs to assure utilization of results of review in educational efforts and (5) where appropriate, participation by both physicians and non-physicians health care practitioners in utilization service committee activities.[1]

Even though the PSRO has begun its enforcement of the law through the acute care facilities, its planning includes phasing into long-term care, ambulatory care, and home health care. The professional nurse in the home health care agency is involved in combination with a physician advisory group in review for utilization purposes. In addition, nurses will be required to develop standards, criteria, and norms; to undergo peer assessment and evaluation; to couple the results of the health care review with continuing education activities within their own profession of nursing; and to develop area-wide profile analyses.[2]

A new dimension generated by the PSRO in the evolutionary process of nursing audit activities has resulted in a logical, systematic approach to the assessment of nursing quality assurance known as nursing care evaluation (NCE). This comprehensive system incorporates the following components:

Nursing Care Evaluation (NCE)—the combined analysis of concurrent and retrospective nursing review.

Concurrent nursing care review or concurrent nursing audit—the evaluation of nursing care of a patient while that care is being rendered.

Retrospective nursing care review or retrospective nursing audit—the evaluation, after discharge of the patient, of the quality of nursing care that was rendered.[6]

Continuing education—an educational program for members of the nursing staff, presented to improve the quality of patient care, based on the problems or deficiencies identified during the review process.

Profile Analysis—the evaluation of the effectiveness of nursing review components, the identification of review priorities, and comparison with other local nursing groups.[1]

A comprehensive NCE system in a home health agency is not to be confused with program evaluation that is currently being performed.

METHOD OF NURSING AUDIT IN HOME HEALTH AGENCY

Professional nursing staffs of home health care agencies must work cooperatively to determine the scope and type of evaluation or review activities that will be involved in assessing the quality of rendered nursing care. The development of a plan with realistic time frames is imperative in initiating a comprehensive NCE program, which should include the following components.

Concurrent nursing care review

This is an evaluation concerned with the identification of nursing care priorities and the provision of optimal nursing services while the patient is still receiving care from the home health care agency. A concurrent nursing audit is an "open chart" review for evaluating the quality of nursing care that patients are receiving. It is a vehicle by which variations from standard criteria for individual and group practice can be identified in time to realize a qualitative improvement in the ongoing care of the audited patient.

The concurrent nursing audit has existed formally and informally for some time. Making rounds to a group of patients receiving skilled home services is an audit, although a potentially ineffective one when not done for a specific purpose. The concurrent nursing care review component of NCE offers an objective means to evaluate care and implement immediate corrective nursing action that will benefit patients for the time period during which they receive services from the home health agency.

Supervisors have conducted concurrent nursing evaluation through daily reviews of nursing documentation or with patient-centered conferences. Subjectively the supervi-

sor compares the patient's progress with the goal of the care. Nursing actions and interventions are reexamined, and modifications in the nursing care plan are implemented. This type of nursing audit has a narrow focus of one patient and unique individual patient criteria; also identification of variations or deficiencies in nursing care approaches are completed in isolation.

Failure to communicate with the whole staff the outcome of conference audits prevents the result from benefiting more patients and precludes identification of patterns of care. Consequently the same deficiency may occur in the care of several other patients and the deficiency must be rediscovered in each case. The application of concurrent review criteria within each nursing unit of a home health agency can provide objective evaluation to identify deficiencies and motivate immediate corrective action and continuing education programs. Failure to return to the standard should be recorded. Failure of the nurses to conduct concurrent audits and to take corrective action is in itself a process defect that will be discovered when the undesirable outcome is audited retrospectively.[2]

Retrospective nursing care review

This method is for identification of deficiencies in the organization and administration of nursing care, for correction of deficiencies through education and administrative change, and for periodic reassessment of performance to assure that improvements or changes have been maintained. Retrospective review provides a means of determining the effectiveness of the concurrent review component as well as of identifying patterns of nursing care that require comprehensive evaluation. This process is also used in validating and revising criteria, norms, and standards.

A "closed chart" review of predetermined outcomes for the purpose of identifying variations in care, patterns of nursing care, or nursing care under a set of specific conditions is accomplished through retrospective review. A well-developed evaluation system generates valid statistics on norms or trends and becomes the basis for future criteria development. This method depends on the documentation of care. If the medical record does not reveal a nursing care component, then it must be assumed that the component was missing. Immediately the need for more diligent documentation is recognized as well as the need for an efficient data retrieval system. The mere existence of a retrospective audit system can improve the documentation of nursing care that is being rendered in a home health care agency.

VALUE OF EVALUATION

Professional nurses in a home health agency may feel that NCE, with concurrent and retrospective review, presents problems since patients may actively receive skilled home services for many years, and the desired outcome for the patient may be a peaceful death. Even though large numbers of patients are served by the home health agency for long periods of time—even years—concurrent review can be used to improve care by developing subacute concurrent criteria and maintenance criteria.

Retrospective evaluation of nursing care may be accomplished even though the patients are still actively receiving services by determining to review the charts of patients who receive care during a specific period of time such as January 1980 back through January 1979. All patient charts that fall within the problem area identified for review would be evaluated whether services were concurrent or retrospective.

Implementation of an NCE program requires the nursing staff to develop and ratify criteria to be used in evaluating the nursing care on a concurrent and retrospective basis before the NCE studies can be completed. Criteria can be developed along the lines of medical diagnosis or nursing problems.

The results or deficiencies identified during the evaluation system should be linked to the home health agency's educational program. Cooperation between agencies, professional organizations, and educational institutions will enhance the availability of continuing education programs based on audit results. After staff participation in educational programs, a reaudit at a predetermined future date is indicated to assess changes in the professional's behavior. The emphasis of review activities is not intended to be punitive but rather to improve the quality of nursing care through the education of the practicing nurse.[1]

A profile analysis is the last component of nursing care evaluation, a component just beginning to evolve. Ideally, with the cooperation of the PSROs, results of nursing audits will be compared and analyzed on a regional basis. Profiles allow for identification of local, state, and national patterns of nursing care and relate through a feedback system to continuing education programs and topic selection for evaluation.

NCE FORMAT

A format for writing concurrent and retrospective review criteria is a critical element. Consistency and understanding of criteria format from the acute care facility to the home health agency represents the movement of patients along a health continuum. Also, a criterion that is not met on one level of care affects the initiation of nursing care by another agency. The patient moves from acute to subacute to maintenance care, and nursing criteria should be developed to allow for this type of progression.

Table 12 illustrates the criteria format for

Table 12. Nursing care evaluation in a home health agency*

Topic _____   Code: _____

Subacute home care	Maintenance home care
Concurrent review criteria	*Concurrent review criteria*
I. Identification of patient's physical and psychological needs and/or concerns.	I. Identification of patient's physical and psychological needs and/or concerns.
II. Recommended nursing action consistent with diagnosis.	II. Recommended nursing action consistent with diagnosis.
A. Nursing services in the home (must include some skilled nursing services).	A. Nursing services in the home (must include some skilled nursing services if Medicare is to cover payment).
B. Health education.	B. Health education.
III. Indicators for change of status.	III. Indicators for discharge.
A. Adaptation of health status to complete subacute care.	A. Adaptation of health status.
B. Examples of nonprofessional personnel that may be utilized when status changes.	B. Final report to primary physicians' office.
Retrospective review criteria	*Retrospective review criteria*
I. Health	I. Health
II. Activity	II. Activity
III. Knowledge	III. Knowledge
Complications	*Complications*

*From Davidson, S. V.: Community nursing care evaluation, Fam. Community Health 1(1):37-35, April 1978.

home health care criteria. The categories of criteria are the same for each level of care; only the criteria elements change from level to level.

One of the most efficient methods for criteria development is through an intra-agency criteria committee. Nursing representatives from an acute care, ambulatory care (or physician's office), and long-term care facility and a home health agency should cooperatively develop progressive criteria. This is also an excellent means of improving communication and sharing responsibility for patient improvement.

Table 13 is a completed format for the NCE in a home health agency for the subacute care criteria of diabetes mellitus juvenile. The development of criteria should begin following the identification of the most frequently

occurring diagnosis or nursing problems that are to be evaluated. Criteria for 80% of the admissions should be determined, realizing that frequently home health patients will have more than one chronic illness, in which case more than one set of criteria may be appropriately applied.

As the acceptance of nursing care criteria becomes more prevalent, when a patient is accepted by a home health agency for care a notation should be made on his transfer records of which criteria have been successfully completed during the acute phase of illness. This will allow the nurses in the home health agency to recognize acute care criteria that must be met before subacute criteria can be applied.

Table 14 illustrates a criterion element compatible with progressive nursing criteria.

Table 13. Nursing care evaluation in a home health agency: completed format*

Topic: *Diabetes mellitus, juvenile*   Codes: *250, 250.3, 250.4*   Date: *November 30, 1979*

Subacute criteria	Standard			Exceptions	Special instructions for data retrieval
	100%	Expected %	Actual %		
Concurrent					
Identification of patient's physical and psychosocial needs and/or concerns					
Control of disease condition after release from hospital.	X	90	92	Presence of secondary disease	See nursing history and physical exam.
Development of a high level of physical and emotional health.	X	95	95	None	See nurse's notes, diabetic flow sheet.
Continuation of normal growth with freedom from hypoglycemic reactions.	X	95	95	None	See nurse's notes, growth charts.
Increased ability for self-care.	X	95	96	Child age/development	See diabetic flow sheet, nurse's notes.
Ability to deal with feelings related to chronic disease condition including guilt, rejection, decreased independance, changes in body image, daily injections, or unsuspected insulin reactions.	X	95	90	None	See nurse's assessment and nurse's notes, look for refer to social services or counselor if indicated.
Recommended nursing action consistent with diagnosis					
NURSING SERVICE					
Perform nursing assessment to evaluate level of physical and emotional health, growth, presence of hypoglycemic reactions, acetone in urine, presence of glycosuria that exceeds 1000 mg/100 ml four times daily.	X	95	89	None	See nursing history, assessment and nursing notes.
Survey patient's response to medical management including insulin dosage regulated with diet, sleep, exercise, and fluids.	X	95	90	None	See nurse's notes, diabetic flow sheet.
Evaluate patients ability to administer insulin according to orders with close observation by family for reactions.	X	95	99	None	See nurse's notes, diabetic flow sheet.
Monitor activity requirements and prevent infection.	X	95	94	None	See nurse's notes.

Assess coping ability and discuss methods to deal with feelings.	X	95	96	None	See nurse's notes.
Encourage independence and assist parents in not being overprotective.	X	95	97	None	See nurse's notes.

HEALTH EDUCATION

Review signs and symptoms of insulin shock, diabetic acidosis, and appropriate actions to take should either occur.	X	95	95	None	See nurse's notes.
Assess transfer of diet instructions and dietary restrictions to home environment with repeated instructions as necessary.	X	95	95	None	See nurse's notes.
Coach on methods of preventing skin irritations and infections, skin hygiene, immunizations and dental care.	X	95	97	None	See nurse's notes.
Reenforce instruction on sterilization of insulin injection equipment, techniques for drawing up proper dosage, proper techniques for administering insulin, name of insulin, dosage, frequency, importance of rotating sites of injection, and relationship of activity to diet to insulin in diabetic control.	X	95	99	Sterilization of equipment may not be taught if disposable needles and syringes are used.	See nurse's notes, diabetic flow sheet.
Teach methods of maintaining records of urine testing, blood sugars, insulin administration, and presence of hypoglycemic reactions for presentation to physician during continued medical followup visits.	X	95	81	If patient too young to maintain records, teach a parent.	See nurse's notes, diabetic flow sheet.

Indicators for change of status

ADAPTATION TO HEALTH STATUS TO COMPLETE SUBACUTE CARE

Administer own insulin for 30 days.	X	95	92	None	See nurse's notes.
Appearance of glycosuria and acetone not more than five times in 30 days.	X	95	92	None	See nurse's notes.
Demonstrates an understanding of health teaching and successfully transferred learning from acute care hospital to home environment.	X	95	96	None	See nurse's notes.

*From Davidson, S. V.: Community nursing care evaluation, Fam. Community Health 1:37-55, April 1978.

Continued.

Table 13. Nursing care evaluation in a home health agency: completed format—cont'd

Topic: *Diabetes mellitus, juvenile* Codes: *250, 250.3, 250.4* Date: *November 30, 1979*

Subacute criteria	Standard 100%	Standard Expected %	Actual %	Exceptions	Special instructions for data retrieval
Returned to normal activities for age including school, sports, parties, games, and so forth.	X	95	97	None	See nurse's notes.
Increasing independence under parental supervision.	X	95	96	None	See nurse's notes.
Selects lunch from school cafeteria according to diet plan.	X	95	95	Absence of school lunch program in which case can select lunch box meal.	See nurse's notes.
School health nurse reconfirms student's adherence to diet, activity, absence of insulin reactions, and coping with diabetes.	X	95	95	Absence of school health nurse.	See nurse's notes for communication with school health nurse
Retrospective					
Health					
Urine free of glycosuria and acetone.	X	95	96	None	See nurse's notes.
Blood sugars less than 120 mg/100 ml of blood.	X	95	97	None	See nurse's notes.
Growth appropriate for age.	X	95	95	None	See nurse's notes.
Weight loss regained.	X	95	95	None	See nurse's notes.
Activity					
Administers own insulin correctly, including proper dosage and technique.	X	95	97	None	See nurse's notes.
Selects correct diet from school lunch program on a daily basis, also can select after school snacks according to meal plan.	X	95	97	None	See nurse's notes.
Participates in school activities, sports, youth activities and so forth.	X	95	95	None	See nurse's notes.
Maintains own insulin injection equipment.	X	95	90	None	See nurse's notes.
Tests urine for glycosuria and acetone before breakfast, prelunch, presupper, and before bedtime.	X	95	89	None	See nurse's notes.

Wears medi-alert identification.	X	95	81	None	See nurse's notes.
Knowledge					
Can state type of insulin, action, frequency of administration and side effects.	X	95	95	None	See nurse's notes.
Family members understand signs and symptoms of insulin shock and diabetic coma and know appropriate action to take.	X	95	92	None	See nurse's notes.
Can discuss the interrelationship of diet, activity, control of infections, sleep and insulin to control of diabetes.	X	95	93	None	See nurse's notes.
Demonstrates understanding of importance of continuous medical followup care by having maintained diabetic record and completed at least one medical visit in last month.	X	95	94	None	See nurse's notes.
Complications					
Dehydration	Criteria same as for acute care.				

Table 14. Criterion element from acute, subacute, and maintenance categories.

Acute

Correctly selects menu for two days before discharge

Subacute

Selects lunch from school cafeteria according to diet plan

Maintenance

Understands diet exchanges and modifies diet selection without presence of glycosuria

---

It is obvious that if the acute criterion of menu selection has not been accomplished during hospitalization, it will be difficult for the patient to succeed in selecting his school lunch or in modifying his diet without developing glycosuria.

The home health agency nurse will need to be familiar with each level of criteria because the patient being visited in the home may be in an acute phase instead of a subacute phase. Also, the nurse should utilize the criteria to assess the patient's progress. Remember that all of the acute care criteria must be met before the subacute criteria become appropriate.

Criteria sets are not easy to write. The first criteria set is the most difficult to complete, but the more criteria sets that are developed, the easier the task becomes for the nursing personnel. There is no right or wrong way to develop criteria sets. The criteria sets should reflect the level of care being rendered by a given facility. It is possible during criteria development to have lengthy discussions of peculiarities that various nursing personnel wish to include in the criteria. Since the criteria must be ratified by the professional whose performance is being evaluated, the addition of idiosyncrasies is not a problem and will be eliminated during the ratification period.

Text continued on p. 240.

Table 15. Audit criteria—prenatal and postpartum*

Criterion	Standard (%)	Exception	Instructions and definitions for data retrieval
Concurrent			
Identification of patient's physical and psychosocial needs and/or concerns			
1. Understanding of physiological changes of pregnancy	100	None	Check prenatal visit form or nurse's notes for documentation of patient's concerns, for example, weight gain, gastrointestinal distress, increased urination.
2. Understanding of danger signs of pregnancy	100	None	Check prenatal visit form or nurse's notes for evidence of discussion of danger signs, for example, bleeding, edema, headache.
3. Understanding changes in relationship with significant others	100	Disinterest	Check nurse's notes for documentation of discussion regarding sibling rivalry, relationship with significant others, parenting role.
4. Awareness of emotional changes of pregnancy	100	None	Check nurse's notes for evidence of documentation of ambivalent feelings toward pregnancy, introversion, passivity, change in body image, changes in sexual desire, increased sensitivity.
5. Awareness of changes in nutritional needs	100	None	Check nurse's notes or prenatal visit form for discussion of needs: 1 quart milk, 6-8 ounces meat, 2 tablespoons fat, 2 slices enriched or whole grain bread plus ½ cup cereal, 1 cup yellow vegetable, 1 cup another vegetable, 1 citris and another fruit, minimum 4 glasses of water.
Recommend nursing action consistent with diagnosis			
NURSING SERVICES			
6. Provide counseling for	100	None	Check nurse's notes and prenatal visit form for discussion of nursing services and health education.
a. Physiological changes of pregnancy			
b. Danger signs of pregnancy			
7. Provide support in regard to changes in emotional status and relationships with significant others	100	None	Check nurse's notes for discussion of indicators for discharge to management by physician.

Criterion	Standard	Exceptions	Source of validation
8. Secure diet history	100	Diet history done by women, infants, and children clinic	Check prenatal visit form, nurse's notes, or women, infants, and children clinic questionnaire for evidence of diet history.
9. Referrals as needed			
a. Women, infants, and children clinic	100	Patient disinterest in women, infants, and children clinic	Check nurse's notes for referral to women, infants, and children clinic when weight gain is inappropriate (increase 2 pounds per week or decrease 1/2 pound per week after first trimester), less than 12 months interconceptional period, more than 5 deliveries.
b. Physician or prenatal clinic	100	None	Check nurse's notes for presence of danger signs of pregnancy, for example, bleeding, persistent headaches, blurred vision, dizziness, edema, fainting.
c. Mental health	100	None	Check nurse's notes for documentation of persistent problems with emotional lability or changes with significant others.
HEALTH EDUCATION			
10. Explain via use of visual aid or pamphlets	100	Unable to read or blind	Check nurse's notes or prenatal visit form for documentation of instruction in reference to normal changes in pregnancy (see No. 1) and danger signs (see No. 2).
a. Normal physiological changes of pregnancy			
b. Danger signs			
11. Discuss possible changes in emotional status and relationship with significant others; encourage to read pamphlets on these areas	100	Unable to read or blind	Check nurse's notes or prenatal visit form for documentation (see No. 3).
12. Instruct on adequate diet for pregnancy by use of nutritional pamphlets and discussion	100	None	Check nurse's notes and prenatal visit form for documentation of instructions (see No. 3).
13. Review patient's plan for transportation to hospital, care of home and siblings, infant care, and supplies	100	None	Check nurse's notes or prenatal visit form for evidence of documentation.

*These criteria were developed at the Nursing Division of the El Paso County Health Department, Colorado Springs, Colorado, by S. Barton, D. Malone, R. Falsetto, and D. Nadler, all public health nurses.

Continued.

Table 15. Audit criteria—prenatal and postpartum—cont'd

Criterion	Standard (%)	Exception	Instructions and definitions for data retrieval
Indicators for discharge to health supervision; private physician, record closure			
14. Referral to other services as needed after postpartum check by private physician	100	Referral not required	Check nurse's notes for evidence of documentation.
15. Client becomes eligible for Medicaid or over income for prenatal clinic	75	Record open for other reason	Check nurse's notes for evidence of documentation.
16. Client moves	100	None	Check nurse's notes for evidence of documentation.
17. Client fails to comply with clinic protocol	100	None	Check nurse's notes for evidence of documentation.
Retrospective			
Health			
1. Decreased lochia	100	None	Check newborn postpartum assess sheet or nurse's notes for evidence of documentation.
2. Episiotomy healed	100	C-section, infection	Check newborn postpartum assess sheet or nurse's notes for evidence of documentation.
3. Cesarean section wound healing	100	Vaginal delivery, infection	Check newborn postpartum assess sheet or nurse's notes for evidence of documentation.
4. Elimination patterns within normal limits	100	Constipation, urinary tract infection, diarrhea	Check newborn postpartum assess sheet or nurse's notes for evidence of documentation.
5. Absence of edema of extremities	100	None	Check newborn postpartum assess sheet or nurse's notes for evidence of documentation.
6. Resolution of problems identified during prenatal period	100	Complications referred for appropriate treatment	Check newborn postpartum assess sheet or nurse's notes for evidence of documentation.
Activity			
7. Resumption of normal sexual activity	100	Discord in relationship with significant others, complications	Check nurse's notes for evidence of documentation.

	Standard (%)	Exception	Instructions and definitions for data retrieval
8. Reintegration into relationship with significant others	100	Postpartum depression, absence of significant others	Check newborn postpartum assess sheet or nurse's notes for evidence of documentation.
Knowledge			
9. Knows birth control options are available	100	Tubal ligation at time of delivery	Check postpartum assess sheet or nurse's notes for evidence of documentation of discussion.
10. Knows activity limitations and needs	100	None	Check postpartum assess sheet or nurse's notes for evidence of documentation of discussion.
11. Understands community resources available for assistance	100	Needs being met	Check postpartum assess sheet or nurse's notes for evidence of documentation of discussion.
12. Understands signs and symptoms of complications and when to report to physician, that is, heavy bleeding, fever, toxemia, failure of family interaction, mastitis, urinary tract infection	100	None	Check postpartum assess sheet or nurse's notes for evidence of documentation of discussion. Go to appropriate complication card for critical nursing management.

Table 16. Audit criteria: newborn, postpartum assessment*

Criterion	Standard (%)	Exception	Instructions and definitions for data retrieval
Concurrent			
Identification of patient's physical and psychosocial needs and/or concerns			
1. Development of bonding	100	None	Check postpartum assessment and/or nurse's notes for documentation of eye contact, cuddling, talking to child, using name and/or appropriate sex (at least two of these), and discussion of father's involvement.
2. Understanding of proper infant feeding			
a. Bottle feeding	100	None	Check postpartum assessment and/or nurse's notes for "adequate" feeding pattern (2–3 ounces every 3–4 hours), "tolerated well," formula preparation, and proper bottle technique discussed.

*These criteria were developed at the Nursing Division of the El Paso County Health Department, Colorado Springs, Colorado, by S. Barton, P. McAtter, J. Rosenthal, and Diana Nakai, all public health nurses.

Continued.

Table 16. Audit criteria: newborn, postpartum assessment—cont'd

Criterion	Standard (%)	Exception	Instructions and definitions for data retrieval
b. Breast feeding			Check postpartum assessment and/or nurse's notes for documentation of discussion of baby activity at breast and time on each, fluid intake and diet of mother, and feeding environment.
3. Understanding proper infant skin care	100	None	Check postpartum and/or nurse's notes for documentation of discussion of cord care, scalp and genital care, and bathing.
4. Healthful environment	100	None	Check postpartum assessment and/or nurse's notes for documentation on sanitation in home, stimulation (change of position or environment for child), and safety; check for "documentation" of recognition of rest of family (siblings, father).
Recommended nursing action consistent with diagnosis NURSING SERVICES			
5. Physical assessment of newborn	100	None	Check postpartum assessment for completed newborn assessment sheet, documentation in postpartum assessment or nurse's note of quality of cry, muscle tone, reflexes including Babinski, rooting, sucking, Moro grasp and support.
6. Referrals as needed a. Physician	100	None	Check postpartum assessment or nurse's notes for referral to physician for 6-week check if normal; check for documentation of immediate physician referral when any abnormalities are noted in postpartum assessment or nurse's notes.
b. Women, infants, and children clinic	100	None	Check for referral to women, infants, and children clinic if nutritional need is documented in nurse's notes or postpartum assessment.
c. Mental health	100	None	Check for documentation of referral to psychiatric care if emotional problems or needs are documented in postpartum assessment or nurse's notes.
7. Encouraging parental roles and feelings	100	None	Check postpartum assessment or nurse's notes for documentation of public health nurse's reinforcing and/or supporting the parent's roles.

HEALTH EDUCATION

8. Demonstrate and have parents return demonstration for feeding, diaper changing, cord care and circumcision care, and taking axillary temperatures.	100	No circumcision done; cord gone	Check nurse's notes or postpartum assessment for documentation of feeding, diaper changing, cord care, circulation care and auxiliary temperatures, and of physician that parents returned demonstration on each.
9. Write instructions or leave booklet for infant feeding and formula preparation.	100	Breast feeding	Check postpartum assessment or nurse's notes for documentation that public health nurse wrote instructions for parents on infant feeding (time pattern, amount) and formula, or left infant care booklet.
10. Instruction on infant care and dressing	100	None	Check postpartum assessment or nurse's notes for documentation that public health nurse instructed parents on general care (handling) and dressing.
11. Instruction on infant safety in the home	100	None	Check postpartum assessment or nurse's notes for documentation that public health nurse instructed parents on home safety for infant.
12. Instruction on signs and symptoms of illness	100	None	Check postpartum assessment or nurse's notes for documentation that public health nurse explained to parents signs and symptoms of vomiting, diarrhea, fever, loss of appetite, irritability, rash.
13. Discuss parental roles and needs	100	None	Check postpartum assessment or nurse's notes for documentation of discussion between public health nurse and parents of their parental role and needs.
14. Instruct on growth and development for first 3 months of life	100	None	Check postpartum assessment or nurse's notes for documentation of growth and development teaching done with parents.

Indicators for discharge to well child clinic or pediatrician

15. Mother correctly demonstrates proper infant care methods	100	None	Check postpartum assessment or nurse's notes for documentation that parent correctly demonstrated infant handling, feeding (including formula preparation if bottle fed, breast care if breast fed), dressing, bathing, and skin care.
16. Family has assumed parenting role	100	Single parent	Check postpartum assessment or nurse's notes for documentation that both family intact and mother caring adequately for infant.
17. Any medical problems being monitored by a physician	100	None	Check postpartum assessment or nurse's notes for documentation that, for any medical problems noted on chart, child is being seen by physician.

Continued.

Table 16. Audit criteria: newborn, postpartum assessment—cont'd

Criterion	Standard (%)	Exception	Instructions and definitions for data retrieval
18. Parents know growth and development	100	None	Check postpartum assessment or nurse's notes for documentation of instruction of growth and development to parents and documentation of their knowledge of process.
19. Family meeting its other needs appropriately	100	None	Check postpartum assessment or nurse's notes for documentation that family is meeting its other needs, for example, recreation, social, spiritual.
Retrospective			
Health			
1. Assessment done; no gross abnormalities	100	Medical problems being followed by physician	Check postpartum assessment for completed newborn assessment; no gross abnormalities.
2. Diet tolerated	100	None	Check postpartum assessment and/or nurse's notes for documentation of "good" feeding tolerance.
3. Weight and height increasing proportionately	100	None	Check growth chart in record.
4. Safe, healthful environment	100	None	Check postpartum assessment and/or nurse's notes for documentation of safe, clean, stimulating home.
Activity			
5. Alert and responsive	100	None	Check postpartum assessment and/or nurse's notes for documentation of alert and responsive newborn.
6. Mother demonstrates proper handling and infant care comfortably	100	None	Check postpartum assessment and/or nurse's notes for documentation of mother's ability to correctly and comfortably handle newborn, bathing, feeding, and dressing.
7. Family meeting its other needs appropriately	100	None	Check postpartum assessment and/or nurse's notes for documentation that family is meeting its other needs, for example, recreation, social, and sexual.
8. Family has followed through with any referrals and medical care as needed	100	None	Check postpartum assessment and/or nurse's notes for documentation that if a referral has been made the family has followed through with appointment.

Table 17. Audit criteria: complications

Critical nursing management	Health education	Instruction for data retrieval
Congenital anomalies		
Observe, report, and record the presence of anomaly (hip click, abnormal heart sounds, hearing loss, visual problems, hydrocephalus, asymetrical gluteal folds).	Explanation to parents: reinforce and evaluate teaching already done to parents regarding anomaly.	Check nursing notes for description of anomaly and parent teaching, for example, cause and treatment.
Report pertinent information to physician.	Provide parents with information about pertinent signs and symbols.	Notify physician of pertinent information, for example, hip click, lack of response to noise, extra heart sound, inability to follow object.
Report effect of anomaly on family.		Describe attitudes and responses of parents and significant others.
Provide necessary supportive measures and services to patient and family.		Check nursing notes for supportive services in referral to crippled children's service or other appropriate agency, emotional support, for example, ventilation of feelings.
Cyanosis		
Observe, report, and record symptoms of cyanosis, for example, circumoral pallor, degree of mottling, location of cyanosis (extremities, trunk, nailbeds).	Instruct parents in identifying cyanotic signs.	Check nursing notes for observation of signs of cyanosis and parent education.
Monitor patient for causative factors of cyanosis.	Instruct parents in identifying causative factors.	Check nursing notes for causative factors of cyanosis, for example, feeding, crying, defecation, general activity, rest.
Notify physician of condition.	Instruct parents to schedule visit with physician.	Check nursing notes for documentation of physician notification and parent instruction and follow through.
Observe, report, and record administration of appropriate medication.	Instruct parents in administration of medication, dosage, side effects.	Check nursing notes for administration of medications, documentation of parents' description of side effects of drugs.

Continued.

Table 17. Audit criteria: complications—cont'd

Critical nursing management	Health education	Instruction for data retrieval
Diarrhea		
Excessive bowel movements (more than 6/day); report color, consistency, odor, presence of blood or mucus; axillary fever above 100.5°; distension of stomach; excessive water passage (diaper will be soaked); signs of dehydration (sunken eyes and mouth, skin and tongue looking dry).	Contact physician if any of these symptoms noted; stop all solid foods and milk; offer clear liquids (tea, water, sugar water), Kool-Aid for 12-18 hours; begin with 2-3 ounces every 2-3 hours; gradually increase 4-5 ounces every 4-6 hours; if condition improves after 12-18 hours begin to use half-strength formula or skim milk for next 12-18 hours; increase volume slowly; resume normal diet the following day.	Check nursing notes for observation of diarrhea and parent education.
Feeding intolerance		
Observe, report, and record:		
1. Projectile vomiting	Teach mother/family; notify physician of projectile vomiting and bloody stools if symptoms persist.	Check nursing notes for documentation of above.
2. Frequent vomiting during and after feeding	Teach mother to add foods gradually one at a time, beginning with vegetables.	
3. Diarrhea	Teach mother to keep discharge journal.	
4. Eczema		

5. Abdominal distension-flatus
6. Colic (painful cry)
7. Pale, semisolid, foul-smelling, greasy stool
8. Failure to gain weight
9. Bloody stool or vomitus
10. Constipation

Fever (persistent, above 100.5° F axillary)

Observe, report, and record level of dehydration and presence of other symptoms, infection, increased respiration and heart rates, decreased urinary output; report to physician if axillary temperature is over 100.4° F; force fluids as ordered; implement fever-reducing measures: fever sponges, antipyretic therapy as ordered.

Teach mother to take axillary temperature and monitor pulse and respiration every 4 hours for 24 hours; document and observe urinary intake and output measurements and record; alert family to possibility of convulsions; teach mother/family to follow regimen ordered by physician.

Check nurse's notes for description of underlying causes of elevated temperature; description of fever-reducing measures; teaching techniques employed to monitor temperature and reduce fever; record vital signs on follow-up visit; document follow through by mother/family.

Vomiting

Note amount, frequency, force, coughing with vomiting; relationship to feeding; dietary changes; scant urine; increased irritability; twitchiness; signs of abdominal pain (knee-chest position); blood in vomit; enlarged abdominal lymph nodes.

Stop all feeding 2-4 hours; Coca-Cola syrup, antiemetic (as prescribed by physician).

Check record for:
1. Symptoms of vomiting and diarrhea
   a. Number, color, consistency of stool
   b. Blood in stool or vomit
   c. Fever
   d. Development of hydration
   e. Evidence of abdominal pain
2. Evidence of teaching:
   a. Symptoms of vomiting and diarrhea
   b. Dietary regimen

Two additional sets of concurrent and retrospective audit criteria are presented in Tables 15 and 16. Table 15 presents concurrent and retrospective audit criteria for prenatal and postpartum visits that are designed specifically for the community health nurse in the public health or community health nursing agency. These criteria can be used in the prenatal clinic setting and are specific for ages 19 to 35. Excluded from the study should be patients with known histories of pathology or chronic disease, for example, diabetes, hypertension, heart disease, miscarriage, stillbirths, prematurity, and drug use (methadone clinic patients).

Table 16 presents concurrent and retrospective criteria for newborn and postpartum assessment. The audit study specifications are as follows:

Describe: Newborn postpartum assessment.
Include: Male and female, all races, no socioeconomic bounds, up to first 3 visits, initial age at first visit under 14 days.
Exclude: Over 14 days, initial home visit, congenital abnormalities: cleft lip, cleft palate, hydrocephalus, or microcephalus, clubfoot, cardiac problems, etc.
Study objectives: Revise postpartum assessment; add support, Babinski, and Moro reflexes.
Study to go back as far as 12 months if necessary to obtain 20 records.

Table 17 shows audit criteria for the following complications found in the audits in Tables 15 and 16: congenital abnormalities, cyanosis, diarrhea, feeding intolerance, fever (axillary temperature above 100.5° F), and vomiting.

Nurses in the home health nursing agency now have an opportunity to evaluate their performance and determine the items that should be available in criteria sets. The development of criteria, standards, and norms will provide professionals in home health agencies with a voice about the acceptable levels of practice when the PSRO begins review activities. Ratification of criteria, measurement of care, correction of deficiencies, and implementation of continuing education programs are necessary before home health agencies will be ready to be part of PSRO profile analysis within a region or state. The professional concerned about elevating the quality of care in home health agencies should not wait for the PSRO to become operational. Instead, work should begin now, and professionals should be ready to say to the PSRO, "These are our standards, criteria, and norms for utilization—as opposed to those developed by the PSRO."

SUMMARY

Completion of the evolutionary process for nursing care evaluation is several years in the future. Professional nurses in all fields of employment must become interested, invest time, and provide action for the systematic improvement of patient care. It is hoped that the information provided in this chapter will serve as a catalyst to thought and action for nursing evaluation in home health and community nursing agencies.

REFERENCES

1. Davidson, S. V., ed.: Nursing care evaluation, St. Louis, 1977, The C. V. Mosby Co.
2. Davidson, S. V.: Community nursing care evaluation, Fam. Community Health 1(1):37-55, 1978.

SUGGESTED READING

Davidson, S. V., ed.: Nursing care evaluation, St. Louis, 1977, The C. V. Mosby Co.

Index

A

Abuse, child; *see* Child abuse
Abuse, sexual, of children, 90
Abusive behavior, susceptibility of families to, 91-92
Accountability in occupational health nursing, 174-175
Accreditation and quality of care, 164
Active listening, 83-84
Acute care, occupational health nursing and, 167
Acute care teams, 6, 7
Acute stage of rape response, 142-143, 146
Administrative skill in occupational health program, 171
Administrators of health facility, 8
Adolescence, definition of, 124-127
Adolescent(s)
    nurse and, in changing social structure, 124-134
    using alcohol and tobacco, 129
    using marijuana and other drugs, 129
Adult rape victim, response of, 142-143
Advocates, consumer, 8
Age of rape victim, developmental, emotional style and, 151
Age of rape victim, postrape reactions and, 141
Agent in child abuse, 90-91
Aide, school health, concept of, 181
Alcohol, adolescents using, 129
Alternate life-styles and family, 60-69
Anger, resolving of, in divorce process, 74
Architecture of private office, health care issues in, 218
Assault, sexual; *see* Rape
Assimilation and biculturism, 42
Audit, nursing, method of, in home health agency, 223-224
Audit criteria
    complications, 237-239
    newborn, postpartum assessment, 233-236
    prenatal and postpartum, 230-233
Auxiliary personnel in school health program, 184-191; *see also* School health aide concept

Aversive racism, 50

B

Barrier methods of contraception, 101
"Battered child" syndrome, 89
Bicultural experiences, health care implications and, 39-59
Bicultural group versus minorities, 41-42
Bicultural health care, interactions in, 54-57
Bicultural health care, nurse's role in, 55-56
Bicultural identification, degrees of, 44-54
Bicultural people, identification of, 39-40
Biculturism
    concepts related to, 40
    differentiating terms related to, 41
    theoretical evolution in, 42-44
Biological variables of adolescence, 124-126
Blitz rape, 148-149
Budgeting process in occupational health program, 171

C

Care
    home health, evaluation of, 221-240
    nursing, 222-224
    patient, conferences, 221
    plan(s) of, 158-160
    primary, change processes in, 211-220
Categories of those educated, change in, 11
Causes of divorce, 73
Certification for pediatric nurse practitioner, 19-20
Certification, quality of care and, 164
Challenges for family planning, 107-109
Change
    capacity for, of health system, 4
    in categories of those educated, 11
    in content of education 11-12
    in education for new health system, 9-15
    in educational process, 12-14
    in educators, 9-11

Change—cont'd
generators of, 8-9
process of, 80
change in, 14-15
in primary care, 211-220
today, 212-215
in relationship, status of, in divorce, 79-82
in views of individual's responsibility for personal health, 29-36
where health workers are educated, 14
Characteristics of rural areas compared to urban areas, 113
Check list system, evaluation with, 221
Child abuse
community health nursing intervention to minimize effects of, 92-95
occurrence of, 89-90
patterns of, in family unit, 89-95
role of nurse in intervention in, 92-95
Child rape victim, response of, 142
Childbearing, social factors influencing decisions about, 103-104
Children in divorce process, 73-76
Children, goal of marriage and, 70-71
Chronic disease conditions, management of, occupational health nursing, and, 167
Client-nurse trust in child abuse intervention, 92
Clinical record review, 221-222
"Closed chart" review, 224
Cohabitation, 65, 67
Collectives, college, 67
Comfort with death and dying, 198
exercises to increase, 206
Communes, 62-63
Communicable diseases, control of, school health service and, 178-181
Community
models of adolescent health care in, 127-133
organization in, action through, 121-122
relationships in, in rural health care systems, 120
Community health, perspectives on future of, 209-240
Community health care systems in rural areas, 113-123
Community nursing, family-centered, in the 1980s, 1-36
Community nursing, intervention of, to minimize effects of child abuse, 92-95
Company policy and occupational health program, 171
Concreteness in child abuse intervention, 93
Concurrent nursing care review, 223
Condescending, 53
Conferences, patient care, 221
Confidence rape, 149-150
Congenital defects, risk of, and age of mother, 102
Consent, inability to, rape, 150
Consumer advocates, 8

Consumers of health care, role of, in health system, 5
Content of education for health workers, changes in, 11-12
Continuing education for health system members, 5
Continuum as tool in decision making, 85
Contraceptives
failure of, 99-100
need for better, 108
revolution in use of, 97-101
technology of, 100-101
Contract, mutually defined, in child abuse intervention, 92-93
Contract divorce, 76
Control of communicable diseases, school health service and, 178-181
Control practices, fertility; see Contraceptives
Coping problems of single-parent families subsequent to separation and divorce, 70-88
Cost
confrontation of reality of, 30-32
health care
effect of health professionals on, 30-31
health maintenance organizations and, 32
private sector and, 31-32
public sector and, 31
Cost effectiveness, change in health system and, 4
Counseling, mental health, occupational health nursing and, 167
Counseling services and family planning programs, 106-107
Crisis
child abuse and, 91-92
intervention in, 82
life, divorce as, 71-72
life, theory of, 83
Criteria
audit
complications, 237-239
newborn, postpartum assessment, 233-236
prenatal and postpartum, 230-233
development of, 229
elements of, from acute, subacute, and maintenance categories, 229
sets of, 229
Cultural continua with variables affecting bicultural identities, 46-47
Cultural enlightenment, 55
Cultural enrichment, 48-50
Cultural identities and biculturism, 43-44
Cultural racism, 50
Current issues in pediatric nurse practitioner role, 26-27
Custody, problems of, in divorce, 76
Cycle, race relation, Parks' theory of, 42
Cytogenetics in occupational health care, 175

D

Damage to child in divorce process, 75
Death, 194-207
  with dignity, 163
  leading causes of, 128
Decision making, continuum as tool in, 85
Decisions, family planning, influences on, 103-104
Decline of fertility, causes of, 97
Defence of family planning, need for, 108
Degrading, 51
Delivery systems, options in, 215-217
Dependence in team practice, 217
Depersonalizing, 52
Despising, 52
Developmental age and emotional style of rape victim, 151
Developmental stage of rape victims, 151-153
Deviance, social, biculturism and, 42-43
Diagnostic framework for victims of sexual assault, 145-155
Die, permission to, 206
Discounting in health care, 54-55
Discounting, phenomenon of, 51-54
Disease(s)
  communicable, control of, school health service and, 178-181
  management of chronic, occupational health nursing and, 167
  prevention of, emphasis of health system on, 4
Disease prevention teams, 6-7
Disguising, 52
Divorce, 70-88; *see also* Divorce process
  causes of, 73
  children and, 73-76
  grief process as part of, 72-73
  kind of, 76-78
  life after, 78
  as a life crisis, 71-72
  reasons for, 73
Divorce process; *see also* Divorce
  child as victim of, 74
  damage to child in, 75
  Kübler-Ross's stages of grief applied to, 72
  organization of, 71, 72
  resolving of anger in, 74
Domestic colonialism, 43
Dominative racism, 50
"Door, the," 126, 131-132
Drugs, adolescents using, 129
Dyads, nuclear, 66
Dying patient, 194-207

E

Economic benefits of family planning, 101-103
Education

Education—cont'd
  additional, for school nurse, 182
  changes in content of, 11-12
  changing, for new health system, 9-15
  consumer health, in rural health care systems, 123
  continuing, for health system members, 5
  family planning programs and, 106-107
  health
    future of, 32-34
    for 1980s and beyond, 3-16
    occupational health nursing and, 167
    in school health services, 180
  of health workers, changes in location of, 14
  patient, effect of design of, 218
Educational background, diverse, role confusion among school nurses and, 187
Educational institutions, primary care, 213-214
Educational preparation of school nurse, 189
Educational process, changes in, 12-14
Educational programs for pediatric nurse practitioners, 18-19
Educational programs for school nurse practitioners, 131
Educators
  changes in, 9-11
  within health system, 9
  inservice, school nurses as, 181
Effectiveness of school nurse role, improving, 190
Elements of rural health care system, 119-120
Elimination of school nursing positions, 185-186
Emergency medical services in rural areas, 118-119
Emotional involvement of nurse with dying patient, 198
Emotional style of rape victim, 151-152
Enlightenment, cultural, 55
Enrichment, cultural, 48-50
Environmental teams, 5-7
Equipment for home care, 160-161
Ethnicity, 41
Ethnocentrism, 50
Evaluation
  of home for feasibility of home care, 158
  of home health care, 221-240
  nursing care, 222-223
    format of, 224-240
    value of, 224
Evaluators, 8-9
Evolution
  and change in education, 14-15
  of new life-style, 81
  theoretical, in biculturism, 42-44
Examination
  medical, in school health nursing, 179-180
  physical, occupational health nursing and, 167
  of rape victim, 137-138

Exercises to increase comfort with death and dying, 206
Expansion of scope of family planning, 107-108
Expectations, inappropriate, in child abuse, 90
Extended care teams, 6, 7
Extended family, 66

F
Failure of contraceptives, 99-100
Family(ies)
    alternate life-styles and, 60-69
    definition of, 61
    with elderly parent, home health care services for, 156-165
    feelings of, toward rape victim, effect of, 150
    life-styles of, today, 37-110
    rape victim and, 153
    single-parent, coping problems of, subsequent to separation and divorce, 70-88
    size of, health and, 102
    susceptibility of, to abusive behavior, 91-92
Family planning
    decisions about, influences on, 103-104
    definition of, 101
    future of, 107-109
    network of, 105-106
    process of, 101-104
    programs for, 104-107
        as primary health care provider, 106
        services provided by, 106-107
    services of, direct providers of, 106
    in United States, 96-110
Family system, diagram of, 86
Family unit, child abuse patterns, in, 89-95
Family-centered community nursing in the 1980s, 1-36
Fearing, 54
Feasibility of home care, 157-158
Federal assistance and support of school nursing programs, 189
Federal government involvement in family planning programs, 105
Female battered divorce, 77
Fertility in United States, 96-110
Financial aspects of home health care, 164-165
Financial justification for family planning, 105
Financial sources for home health care, 164
"Floating team" concept of rape treatment, 136
Form, referral information, 161
Form, sexual battery, 138-139
Format of nursing care evaluation, 224-240
Funding, increased, for family planning, need for, 109
Funding of rural health care systems, 120
Future
    of adolescent health care, 133
    of communes, 62-63

Future—cont'd
    of community health, perspectives on, 209-240
    of family planning, 107-109
    growth of primary care in, 211
    of health promotion and education, 32-34

G
Games in divorce, 77
Gay parents, 63-64
Goal of marriage, children and, 70-71
Golden age families, 66
Grief
    child's, over divorce, 75
    Kübler-Ross's stages of, applied to divorce process, 72
    process of, as part of divorce, 72-73
Group marriage, 65
Group process in child abuse intervention, 94
"Growing pains" of pediatric nurse practitioner role, 24-26
Growth of primary care in future, 211
"Guidelines on Short-Term Continuing Education Programs for Pediatric Nurse Associates," 18
Guilt
    child's feelings of, in divorce, 73-74
    in confidence rape, 149
    as defense against vulnerability in rape, 150

H
Hamilton, Alice, 174
Handicapped child, needs of, emphasis of school health program on, 183
Healing process, recycling as part of, 83
Health
    benefits to, of family planning, 101-103
    family size and, 102
    optimum, components of, 182
    personal, changing views of individual's responsibility for, 29-36
    World Health Organization's definition of, 124
Health agency, home, method of nursing audit in, 223-224
Health agency, home, nursing care evaluation in, 225
Health board and rural health care system, 114-116
Health care
    adolescent, 124-134
    approaches to, 215
    bicultural interactions in, 54-57
    in community, adolescent, models of, 127-133
    comprehensive, 3
    cost of, 30-32
    discounting in, 54-55
    home, evaluation of, 221-240
    home, services of, for family with elderly parent, 156-165

Health care—cont'd
  implications of bicultural experiences and social inter-
    actions on, 39-59
  systems of, community, in rural areas, 113-123
  team approach to, 216-217
  volunteer workers in, 5
Health data specialists, 8
Health education
  consumer, in rural health care systems, 123
  for 1980s and beyond, 3-16
  occupational health nursing and, 167
  in school health services, 180
Health facility, administrators of, 8
Health insurance, national systems of, health system
    and, 4
Health maintenance, emphasis of health system on, 4
Health maintenance organizations, 213
  cost of health care and, 32
  pediatric nurse practitioner in, 20
Health maintenance teams, 6-7
Health manpower, 3-16
Health ombudsmen, 8
Health Plan of Puget Sound, 216
Health professionals, effect of, on cost of health care,
    30-31
Health professionals, roles and tasks of, 4-5
Health professions, ethnic minorities in, 6
Health program in Harlem, school, 130-131
Health service, 111-207
Health services, school, 178-193
Health system
  educators within, 9
  managers of, 7-8
  new, changing education for, 9-15
  new, staffing in, 5-9
  in 1980s and beyond, 3-5
Health teams, 5-6
Health training for 1980s and beyond, 3-16
Health workers, need for operationalized concepts for,
    40-41
Health-related enterprises, managers of, 8
Helping people, intervention process in, 82-87
High school, nurse practitioners in, 131
History
  of development of school nurse role, 178-186
  of emerging role of pediatric nurse practitioner, 17
  of family planning programs, 104-105
HMOs; see Health maintenance organizations
Home, evaluation of, for feasibility of home care, 158
Home, family, transfer of hospitalized parent to, 160-
    162
Home care
  evaluation of, 221-240
  feasibility of, 157-158
  services of, for family with elderly parent, 156-165

Home health agency, method of nursing audit in, 223-
    224
Home health agency, nursing care evaluation in, 225
Home health care, evaluation of, 221-240
Home health care, services of, for family with elderly
    parent, 156-165
Homosexual family, 63-64
Honesty about feelings about death, 195, 199-200
Host in child abuse, 91

I

Identification, bicultural, degrees of, 44-54
Identification of bicultural people, 39-40
Identities, bicultural, cultural continua with variables
    affecting, 46-47
Identities, cultural, biculturism and, 43-44
Illness, prevention of, 4
Implementation of program of nursing care evaluation,
    224
Implementation of rape program, protocol for, 147-148
Inability to consent rape, 150
Incest, 90
Independence in team practice, 217
Information form, referral, 161
Inservice educator, school nurse as, 181
Inspection, medical, in school health services, 179
Insurance
  health, national systems of, health system and, 4
  malpractice, occupational health program and, 172
  malpractice, for physician's assistants and nurse prac-
    titioners, 217-218
Insurance companies and home health care, 164
Insurance contracts and home care visits, 163
Integration stage of rape response, 143, 147
Intensive care teams, 6, 7
Interdependence in team practice, 217
Intervention
  community health nursing, to minimize effects of child
    abuse, 92-95
  crisis, 82
  nursing, in divorce, 84-87
  process of, in people helping, 82-87
Involvement, emotional, of nurse with dying patient,
    198
Issues, health care
  in architecture of private office, 218
  in primary health care, 217-218
  in quality of care, 218
  in reimbursement, 218
  in team practice, 217-218

K

Kaiser-Permanente, 216
Kübler-Ross's stages of grief applied to divorce process,
    72

L

Law enforcement agencies and rape victim, 153-154
"Laying on of hands," 163
Legal agencies and rape victim, 153-154
Legal barriers to family planning, need to remove, 108
Legislative trends in primary care, 212
Life after divorce, 78
Life, quality of, concern about, effect on childbearing, 103-104
Life crisis, divorce as, 71-72
Life crisis, theory of, 83
Life-styles
    alternate, family and, 60-69
    family, today, 37-110
    new, evolution of, 81
Listening, active, 83-84
"Living together," 67
Loss in divorce, 73
Love, 70-71

M

"Mainstreaming" of handicapped children, 185
Maintenance of health, 29-36
Male battered divorce, 77
Malpractice, 217-218
Malpractice insurance and occupational health program, 172
Management, better, for family planning programs, need for, 109
Management of health system, 5
Management specialists, 8
Managers of health system, 5, 7-8
Managers of health-related enterprises, 8
Manpower, health, 3-16
Marijuana, adolescents using, 129
Marriage, 70-71
    group, 65
Maslow's hierarchy of needs, 80
Maturation, rate of, and nutritional status, 124-125
Media and rape, 145
Medicaid, home health care and, 164-165
Medical agencies, rape victim and, 153-154
Medical care of rape victim, 135-144
Medical examination in school health services, 179-180
Medicare, home health care and, 164-165
Mental health counseling and occupational health nursing, 167
Method of nursing audit in home health agency, 223-224
Minorities, ethnic, in health professions, 6
Minorities versus bicultural groups, 41-42
Monogamy, 61-62
Morbidity, age of mother and, 102
Mortality, maternal and infant, age of mother and, 102
Mortality, patient, 194-204

Mother, age of, maternal and infant morbidity and mortality and, 102
Motivations for childbearing, 103
Multispecialty approach to health care, 216

N

National Institute of Occupational Safety and Health, 172
NCE; *see* Nursing care evaluation
Needs
    for family planning, 107
    future, for school nurse, 189-192
    Maslow's hierarchy of, 80
Neglect, occurrence of, 89-90
"Neogamy," 66
Network of family planning, 105-106
    expansion of, 107
NIOSH; *see* National Institute of Occupational Safety and Health
"Nonparenthood" couples, 66
Nonprofessional assistants in school health program, 181, 184, 191
Nontraditional family, 65-67
NP; *see* Nurse practitioner(s)
Nuclear dyads, 66
Nuclear primary health care team, 216
Nurse
    adolescent and, in changing social structure, 124-134
    role of
        alternate life-styles and, 67-68
        in child abuse intervention, 92-95
    school
        historical development of role of, 178-186
        problems confronting, 186-188
Nurse practitioner(s), 213
    in high school, 131
    pediatric, role of, 17-28
    physician conflicts with, 25
    school, educational programs for, 131
    school, role of, 185, 192
Nurse practitioner research, 22-24
Nursing
    community, family-centered, in 1980s, 1-36
    occupational health, 166-177
    quality assurance mechanisms in, 221
    school, problems in and prospects of, 178-193
Nursing audit, method of, in home health agency, 223-224
Nursing care, primary, 163-164
Nursing care evaluation, 222-223
    format of, 224-240
    in home health agency, 225
        completed format, 226-229
    program of, implementation of, 224
Nursing care review, concurrent, 223

Nursing services for worker, 166-167
Nutrition in home care, 162
Nutritional status and rate of maturation, 124-125

O

Occasional family, 67
Occupational health nursing, 166-177
Occupational Safety and Health Act of 1970, 171, 172
Ombudsmen, health, 8
"Open chart" review, 223
Openness about feelings about death, 195, 199-200
Operationalized concepts, need for, for health workers, 40-41
Options in delivery systems, 215-217
Organization of divorce process, 71, 72
OSHA; *see* Occupational Safety and Health Act of 1970
Outreach programs in family planning, need for, 103
Outward adjustment stage of rape response, 143, 146-147

P

PA; *see* Physician's assistant
Parent, elderly, home health care services for family with, 156-165
Parental rejection as child abuse, 89
Parenting, single, rules for, 75-76
Parentless families, 66
Parents Anonymous, 94
Parks' theory of race relation cycle, 42
Paternalism and biculturism, 43
Pathological orientation and biculturism, 42-43
Patient, dying, desires of, 195, 196
Patient care conferences, 221
Patient flow, effect of design of private office on, 218
Patterns of fertility, changes in, 96-97
Patterns, provider practice, in primary care, 213
Pediatric nurse associate; *see* Pediatric nurse practitioner
Pediatric nurse practitioner, 17-28
Peer group, support of, and nurse practitioner, 25
People helping, intervention process in, 82-87
Permission to die, 206
Personality adjustment, premorbid, 154-155
Personnel in rural health care systems, 119
Personnel, trained family planning, need for, 108
Phenomenon of discounting, 51-54
Physical examinations and occupational health nursing, 167
Physician conflicts with nurse practitioner, 25
Physician's assistant, 213
Plan(s) of care, 158-160
Planning in primary care, 213
Planning specialists, 8
PNA; *see* Pediatric nurse practitioner
PNP; *see* Pediatric nurse practitioner

POMR; *see* Problem-oriented medical record system
Population, concern about size of, and effect on childbearing, 103-104
Population, study, for rape crisis demonstration project, 148
Postrape reactions, age of rape victim, 141
Practice, scope of, for pediatric nurse practitioner, 20-22
Practitioner, nurse; *see* Nurse practitioner
Premorbid personality adjustment, 154-155
Prevention of disease, 29-36
Primary care
    change processes in, 211-220
    growth of, in future, 211
    improved, and self-care, 212
    organized, in rural health care system, 120-121
    in schools, 127
    who should provide, 214-215
Primary care system today, 211-212
Primary health care, family planning programs as provider of, 106
Primary nursing care, 163-164
Primary physician model approach to health care, 215
Privacy in home care, 158-160
Private sector, cost of health care and, 31-32
Problem(s)
    confronting school nurse, 186-188
    of custody in divorce, 76
    in primary health care, 217-218
Problem solving, process of, 83
Problem-oriented medical record system, 34
    in home care, 160
Process of change, 80
    in primary care, 211-220
    today, 212-215
Process of family planning, 101-104
Process of healing, recycling as part of, 83
Process of problem solving, 83
Professional standards review organizations, 222
Program(s)
    for family planning, 104-107
    health care, evaluation of, 221-222
    rape, implementation of, protocol for, 147-148
Promotion, health, 29-36
Prophylaxis against venereal disease, 140
Prospects, future, for school nurse, 189-192
Protection, game of, and dying patient, 199
Protocol for rape program implementation, 147-148
Provider practice patterns in primary care, 213
Providers, direct, of family planning services, 106
Pseudoadjustment stage of rape response, 146-147
PSROs; *see* Professional standards review organizations
Psychological variables of adolescence, 126-127
Psychology of Birth Planning, 103
Pubertal stages, Tanner, 125

Public information on family planning, need for, 108
Public sector, cost of health care and, 31

Q

Quality of care, issues in, 218
Quality assurance in home health care, 164
Quality assurance, mechanisms of, in nursing, 221

R

Race, 41
Race relation cycle, Parks' theory of, 42
Racism, problems with, 50-51
Rape, types of, 148-150
Rape crisis demonstration project, 147-155
Rape crisis syndrome, 146-147
  fear in, 149
Rape experience, meaning of, 152
Rape victim
  age of, postrape reactions and, 141
  child, response of, 142
  developmental stage of, 151-153
  diagnostic framework for, 145-155
  effect of family feelings toward, 150
  emotional style of, 151-152
  family and, 153
  law enforcement agencies and, 153-154
  legal agencies and, 153-154
  medical agencies and, 153-154
  medical care of, 135-144
  significant others and, 153
  social network and, 153-154
Reasons for divorce, 73
Record keeping in occupational health program, 171
Record keeping as problem in school nursing, 183
Recycling as part of healing process, 83
Referral information form, 161
Reimbursement issues, 218
Reimbursement policies in primary care, 212
Relationship change, status of, in divorce, 79-82
Research and change in education, 15
Research, nurse practitioner, 22-23
Research findings for rape crisis demonstration project, 148-155
Research process, evaluative, stages within, 23
Researchers, 8-9
Responsibility of individuals for personal health, changing views of, 29-36
Restorative care teams, 6, 7
Retrospective nursing care review, 223-224
Review, concurrent nursing care, 223
Review, retrospective nursing care, 223-224
Revolution, contraceptive, 97-101
Role(s)
  of consumers of health care in health system, 5
  of health professionals, 4-5

Role(s)—cont'd
  multiple, of occupational health nurse, 168-169
  nurse
    and alternate life-styles, 67-68
    in bicultural health care, 55-56
    in child abuse intervention, 92-95
  of pediatric nurse practitioner, 17-28
  of school nurse
    historical development of, 178-186
    improving effectiveness of, 190
    limiting of, 188
  of school nurse practitioner, 185, 192
  of women, effect of, on childbearing, 103
Role confusion among school nurses, 187
"Rooming-together" families, 66
Rules for single parenting, 75-76
Rural areas, community health care systems, 113-123

S

Same-sex unrelated families, 66
Sanger, Margaret, and family planning, 104
Scheduling of home care visits, 162-163
School health aide concept, 181
"School health council" concept, 183
School health programs, 128-131, 178-193
School Health Project Bill, 130
School health services, 178-193
School nurse, historical development of role of, 178-186
School nurse, problems confronting, 186-188
School nurse practitioner role, 185, 192
School nursing, problems in and prospects of, 178-193
Scope of family planning, expansion of, 107-108
Scope of practice for pediatric nurse practitioner, 20-22
Self-blame in confidence rape, 149
Self-care
  emphasis on, 215
  improved primary care and, 212
  shift to, 212
  in United States, 211
  versus other types of care, 212
Self-concept, inadequate, in child abuse, 90
Separation, 70-88
Services
  delivery of, in rural health care system, 117-118
  nursing, for worker, 166-167
  provided by family planning programs, 106-107
  in rural health care system, 119-120
  utilization of, 122-123
Sexual abuse of children, 90
Sexual assault; *see* Rape
Sexual battery form, 138-139
Sexual experience and meaning of rape to victim, 152
Shocker-shockee divorce, 76

Significant others, involvement with, rape victim and, 152-153

Single parenting, rules for, 75-76

Single-parent family(ies), 64-65

coping problems of, subsequent to separation and divorce, 70-88

Size of family and health, 102

SNP; *see* School nurse practitioner role

Social deviance and biculturism, 42-43

Social factors influencing decisions about childbearing, 103

Social interactions and health care implications, 39-59

Social isolation in child abuse, 91

Social network and rape victim, 153-154

Social Readjustment Rating Scale, 84

Sociological variables of adolescence, 127

Southwest Minnesota Health Care Enterprises, 121-122

Staffing in the new health system, 5-9

Status of women, effect of, on childbearing, 103

Stereotyping, 52

Sterilization, surgical, as contraceptive, 98, 100-101

Stress, 84

Struthers, Lina Rogers, 179

Study population of rape crisis demonstration project, 148

Style, emotional, of rape victim, 151-152

Subculture, 41

Supermarket approach to health care, 215

Support by peer group and nurse practitioner, 25

System(s), delivery, options in, 215-217

System(s) of primary care today, 211-212

T

Tanner pubertal stages, 125

Tasks of health professionals, 4-5

Team approach to health care, 216-217

Team practice, issues in, 217-218

Team teaching, 12-13

"Teamwork" philosophy of school health program, 183

Technology of contraceptives, 100-101

Temporary family, 67

Terms, differentiation of, related to biculturism, 41

"The Door," 126, 131-132

Theory, life crisis, 83

Tobacco, adolescents using, 129

Traditional medical center models for adolescent health care, 132-133

Training, health, for 1980s and beyond, 3-16

Transfer of hospitalized parent to family home, 160-162

Trends, legislative, in primary care, 212

Types of rape, 148-150

U

Underutilization of school nurses, 188

Unions, occupational health and, 170-171

University of Colorado Medical Center School Nurse Practitioner Program, 131

Utilization of services in rural health care systems, 122-123

V

Value of evaluation, 224

Venereal disease, prophylaxis against, 140

Verbal battery as child abuse, 89

Victim of divorce process, child as, 74

Victim, rape; *see* Rape victim

Victimization and biculturism, 43

Visits, home care, scheduling of, 162-163

Volunteer workers in health care, 5

Vulnerability, guilt as defense against, in rape, 150

W

Wald, Lillian, 179

Willing and unwilling partner divorce, 77

Women, status and roles of, effect on childbearing, 103

Worker, nursing services for, 166-167

World Health Organization, definition of health, 124